Image-Guided Radiation Therapy

IMAGING IN MEDICAL DIAGNOSIS AND THERAPY

William R. Hendee, Series Editor

Quality and Safety in Radiotherapy
Todd Pawlicki, Peter B. Dunscombe, Arno J. Mundt, and
Pierre Scalliet, Editors
ISBN: 978-1-4398-0436-0

Adaptive Radiation Therapy
X. Allen Li, Editor
ISBN: 978-1-4398-1634-9

Quantitative MRI in Cancer
Thomas E. Yankeelov, David R. Pickens, and
Ronald R. Price, Editors
ISBN: 978-1-4398-2057-5

Informatics in Medical Imaging
George C. Kagadis and Steve G. Langer, Editors
ISBN: 978-1-4398-3124-3

Adaptive Motion Compensation in Radiotherapy
Martin J. Murphy, Editor
ISBN: 978-1-4398-2193-0

Image-Guided Radiation Therapy
Daniel J. Bourland, Editor
ISBN: 978-1-4398-0273-1

Forthcoming titles in the series

Informatics in Radiation Oncology
Bruce H. Curran and George Starkschall, Editors
ISBN: 978-1-4398-2582-2

Image Processing in Radiation Therapy
Kristy Kay Brock, Editor
ISBN: 978-1-4398-3017-8

Proton and Carbon Ion Therapy
Charlie C.-M. Ma and Tony Lomax, Editors
ISBN: 978-1-4398-1607-3

Monte Carlo Techniques in Radiation Therapy
Joao Seco and Frank Verhaegen, Editors
ISBN: 978-1-4398-1875-6

Stereotactic Radiosurgery and Radiotherapy
Stanley H. Benedict, Brian D. Kavanagh, and
David J. Schlesinger, Editors
ISBN: 978-1-4398-4197-6

Cone Beam Computed Tomography
Chris C. Shaw, Editor
ISBN: 978-1-4398-4626-1

Handbook of Brachytherapy
Jack Venselaar, Dimos Baltas, Peter J. Hoskin, and
Ali Soleimani-Meigooni, Editors
ISBN: 978-1-4398-4498-4

Targeted Molecular Imaging
Michael J. Welch and William C. Eckelman, Editors
ISBN: 978-1-4398-4195-0

IMAGING IN MEDICAL DIAGNOSIS AND THERAPY

William R. Hendee, Series Editor

Image-Guided Radiation Therapy

Edited by

J. Daniel Bourland

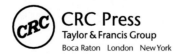 CRC Press
Taylor & Francis Group
Boca Raton London New York

CRC Press is an imprint of the
Taylor & Francis Group, an **informa** business

A TAYLOR & FRANCIS BOOK

CRC Press
Taylor & Francis Group
6000 Broken Sound Parkway NW, Suite 300
Boca Raton, FL 33487-2742

First issued in paperback 2020

© 2012 by Taylor & Francis Group, LLC
CRC Press is an imprint of Taylor & Francis Group, an Informa business

No claim to original U.S. Government works

Version Date: 20111208

ISBN-13: 978-0-367-57678-3 (pbk)
ISBN-13: 978-1-4398-0273-1 (hbk)

Library of Congress Cataloging-in-Publication Data

Image-guided radiation therapy / editor, J. Daniel Bourland.
       p. ; cm. -- (Imaging in medical diagnosis and therapy)
    Includes bibliographical references and index.
    ISBN 978-1-4398-0273-1 (hardback : alk. paper)
    I. Bourland, J. Daniel. II. Series: Imaging in medical diagnosis and therapy.
    [DNLM: 1. Radiotherapy, Computer-Assisted--methods. 2. Image Processing, Computer-Assisted--methods. 3. Radiation Oncology--methods. WN 250.5.R2]

616.07'57--dc23   2011049464

**Visit the Taylor & Francis Web site at
http://www.taylorandfrancis.com**

**and the CRC Press Web site at
http://www.crcpress.com**

To my family—my wife, Beth, my daughter,
Rebekah, and my sons, John and Peter.

Contents

Series Preface

Advances in the science and technology of medical imaging and radiation therapy are more profound and rapid than ever before, since their inception over a century ago. Further, the disciplines are increasingly cross-linked as imaging methods become more widely used to plan, guide, monitor, and assess treatments in radiation therapy. Today, the technologies of medical imaging and radiation therapy are so complex and so computer driven that it is difficult for the persons (physicians and technologists) responsible for their clinical use to know exactly what is happening at the point of care, when a patient is being examined or treated. The person best equipped to understand the technologies and their applications are medical physicists, and these individuals are assuming greater responsibilities in the clinical arena to ensure that what is intended for the patient is actually delivered in a safe and effective manner.

The growing responsibilities of medical physicists in the clinical arenas of medical imaging and radiation therapy are not without their challenges, however. Most medical physicists are knowledgeable in either radiation therapy or medical imaging, and expert in one or a small number of areas within their discipline. They sustain their expertise in these areas by reading scientific articles and attending scientific talks at meetings. In contrast, their responsibilities increasingly extend beyond their specific areas of expertise. To meet these responsibilities, medical physicists periodically must refresh their knowledge of advances in medical imaging or radiation therapy, and they must be prepared to function at the intersection of these two fields. How to accomplish these objectives is a challenge.

At the 2007 annual meeting of the American Association of Physicists in Medicine in Minneapolis, this challenge was the topic of conversation during a lunch hosted by Taylor & Francis Publishers and involving a group of senior medical physicists (Arthur L. Boyer, Joseph O. Deasy, C.-M. Charlie Ma, Todd A. Pawlicki, Ervin B. Podgorsak, Elke Reitzel, Anthony B. Wolbarst, and Ellen D. Yorke). The conclusion of this discussion was that a book series should be launched under the Taylor & Francis banner, with each volume in the series addressing a rapidly advancing area of medical imaging or radiation therapy of importance to medical physicists. The aim would be for each volume to provide medical physicists with the information needed to understand technologies driving a rapid advance and their applications to safe and effective delivery of patient care.

Each volume in the series is edited by one or more individuals with recognized expertise in the technological area encompassed by the book. The editors were responsible for selecting the authors of individual chapters and ensuring that the chapters were comprehensive and intelligible to someone without such expertise. The enthusiasm of volume editors and chapter authors has been gratifying and reinforces the conclusion of the Minneapolis luncheon that this series of books addresses a major need of medical physicists.

Imaging in Medical Diagnosis and Therapy would not have been possible without the encouragement and support of the series manager, Luna Han of Taylor & Francis Publishers. The editors and authors, and most of all I, are indebted to her steady guidance of the entire project.

William Hendee
Series Editor
Rochester, MN

Preface

This book presents key image-guided radiation treatment (IGRT) technologies for external beam radiotherapy and caps a multidecade phase of technology development in the realm of conformal, customized radiation treatment. This development phase has been somewhat brief and vigorous, with new IGRT innovations such as increased image fidelity and adaptive radiotherapy continuing through the present day. IGRT had been in development in earnest since the early 1990s as a desired companion to intensity-modulated radiation treatment (IMRT). It was known at the time that beam-intensity modulation would be proven to enable beamlets of radiation dose to be formed and delivered to give highly conformal treatment to target volumes, while at the same time providing avoidance of even nearby normal structures. IMRT was being developed with pathways that were based on particular technological features of each vendor's designs for their multileaf collimators (MLCs) and linear accelerators, e.g., leaf design (width, height, focus, speed, etc.), dose rate control, error checking, and gantry motion control. In a previous decade, the 1980s into the mid-1990s, three-dimensional conformal radiation treatment (3D-CRT) had been developed such that for the first time, using static pretreatment 3D images from computed tomography (CT), anatomical volumes could be identified and segmented for the target, normal structures, and the external contour. As 3D-CRT and IMRT technologies developed, it was recognized that confirming "correct" treatment geometry for every individual fraction might be important, since daily variations in treatment position and the locations of internal structures would lead to blurring (degradation) of the cumulative dose distribution. Thus, IGRT was born from the important requirement for verifying the correct target and normal tissue positions before "beam-ON."

While IGRT technologies are new, the importance of correct patient positioning was recognized very early on and proven with clinical studies. Early important IGRT-related activities of relevance include the following: (1) the development of patient immobilization devices and weekly port field imaging in the 1960s–1970s that paved the way for today's more precise and accurate daily radiation treatments, and (2) in the 1950s–1960s, the addition of a kilovoltage x-ray tube to cobalt teletherapy devices, side-mounted on the gantry head, to provide quality portal images with reasonable contrast and much better sharpness than those obtained with megavoltage gamma rays from a nominal 2-cm diameter cobalt-60 source.

Similar to differing designs and implementations for 3D-CRT and IMRT, IGRT technologies show a richness and creativity that were driven by particular linear accelerator designs, each with existing unique advantages and limitations, as well as the visions of the medical physicists, clinicians, and engineers who conceived of "in-room imaging" immediately before or during treatment. In some cases, image-guidance was an "add-on" to existing linear accelerator designs, either free-standing additions or coupled to the gantry, or took advantage of the megavoltage treatment beam to use it for imaging. In other approaches, new basic designs for both treatment and imaging were conceived and implemented that used either kilovoltage or megavoltage imaging and abandoned the conventional C-arm linear accelerator gantry designs. Additional radiological, ultrasound, and optical technologies have provided alternative means to determine or assist with target and/or patient position, including near real-time monitoring for fast feedback of treatment position. In particular, anatomical and biological imaging using CT and positron emission tomography have contributed to the understanding of target volume boundaries and biological behavior, including the effects and accommodation of physiological motion (e.g., respiratory, cardiac, and other) on radiation treatment accuracy, precision, and clinical outcome. Similarly important, computing and imaging science software algorithms and tools serve as the infrastructure to integrate the various IMRT processes into a procedure that can be readily implemented in the clinic. The results of these modalities, software tools, and imaging treatment geometries are a wealth of hybrid IGRT technologies and devices for coupled imaging + treatment inside the radiation treatment room—these IGRT technology classes are reviewed herein.

This book benefits from having nationally and internationally known authors who actively participated in the development of IGRT, imaging, and ancillary technologies. Their expertise is evident in the descriptions of IGRT technologies and their clinical uses and impact. The editor expresses his great appreciation for their important and excellent contributions to make this publication possible such that medical physicists, clinicians, and trainees will profit from their intellect, insight, and scientific curiosity for the benefit of patient care.

J. Daniel Bourland

Acknowledgment

The expert editorial and logistical assistance of Luna Han, Taylor & Francis Group, is hereby acknowledged. This work would have not been possible without her patient and persistent reminders and her invaluable oversight and advice.

Editor

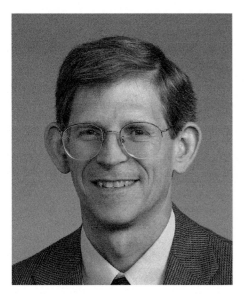

J. Daniel Bourland, PhD, received his PhD in medical and health physics from the University of North Carolina (UNC) at Chapel Hill. He was on the radiation oncology faculty at UNC-Chapel Hill and the Mayo Clinic, and is now professor, Department of Radiation Oncology, Wake Forest University (WFU). He teaches medical physics graduate students in the WFU Departments of Biomedical Engineering and Physics and is co-director for physics for his department's NIH-funded T-32 fellowship program. He is a Fellow of the American Association of Physicists in Medicine (AAPM), and past/current board member for the AAPM, the American Institute of Physics, and the Society of Directors of Academic Medical Physics Programs. He has served as associate editor for the journal *Medical Physics*. Dr. Bourland is a diplomate of the American Board of Radiology (ABR) in therapeutic radiological physics and serves on the ABR written and oral examination boards. He is known for his educational activities and has published in the areas of convolution-based radiation dose calculations, where his dose computation algorithm was used in the first commercial IMRT planning system, and automated shape-based treatment planning for stereotactic radiosurgery. He is fortunate to have "grown-up" during the eras of development for 3D-CRT, IMRT, and IGRT. His current research interests include imaging in radiation treatment, bioeffects from radiological terrorism, and small animal irradiations.

Contributors

Hidefumi Aoyama
Department of Radiology Oncology
Hokkaido University
Sapporo, Japan

Gerard Bengua
Department of Medical Physics
Hokkaido University
Sapporo, Japan

J. Daniel Bourland
Department of Radiation Oncology
Wake Forest School of Medicine
Winston-Salem, North Carolina

Kristy K. Brock
Radiation Medicine Program
Princess Margaret Hospital
University Health Network
and
Department of Radiation Oncology
University of Toronto
Ontario, Toronto, Canada

Yusuf E. Erdi
Department of Medical Physics
Memorial Sloan-Kettering Cancer
   Center
New York, New York

Zhanrong Gao
Morristown Medical Center
Morristown, New Jersey

Devon Godfrey
Department of Radiation Oncology
Duke University
Durham, North Carolina

Carnell J. Hampton
Department of Radiation Oncology
Wake Forest School of Medicine
Winston-Salem, North Carolina

Masayori Ishikawa
Department of Medical Physics
Hokkaido University
Sapporo, Japan

Patrick A. Kupelian
Department of Radiation Oncology
M.D. Anderson Cancer Center Orlando
Orlando, Florida

Katja M. Langen
Department of Radiation Oncology
M.D. Anderson Cancer Center Orlando
Orlando, Florida

Thomas Rockwell Mackie
Department of Medical Physics
University of Wisconsin
Madison, Wisconsin

Sanford L. Meeks
Department of Radiation Oncology
M.D. Anderson Cancer Center Orlando
Orlando, Florida

Janelle A. Molloy
Department of Radiation Medicine
University of Kentucky
Lexington, Kentucky

Olivier Morin
Department of Radiation Oncology
Helen Diller Family Comprehensive
   Cancer Center
University of California San Francisco
San Francisco, California

Martin J. Murphy
Department of Radiation Oncology
Massey Cancer Center
VCU Health System
and
School of Medicine
Virginia Commonwealth University
Richmond, Virginia

Sadek A. Nehmeh
Department of Medical Physics
Memorial Sloan-Kettering Cancer
   Center
New York, New York

Gustavo Hugo Olivera
21st Century Oncology, Inc
Madison, Wisconsin

Rikiya Onimaru
Department of Radiology Oncology
Hokkaido University
Sapporo, Japan

Jean Pouliot
Department of Radiation Oncology
Helen Diller Family Comprehensive
   Cancer Center
University of California San Francisco
San Francisco, California

Lei Ren
Department of Radiation Oncology
Duke University
Durham, North Carolina

Michael B. Sharpe
Radiation Medicine Program
Princess Margaret Hospital
University Health Network
and
Department of Radiation Oncology
University of Toronto
Ontario, Toronto, Canada

Shinichi Shimizu
Department of Radiology Oncology
Hokkaido University
Sapporo, Japan

Hiroki Shirato
Department of Radiology Oncology
Hokkaido University
Sapporo, Japan

Jeffrey H. Siewerdsen
Department of Biomedical Engineering
Johns Hopkins University
Baltimore, Maryland

Jan-Jakob Sonke
Department of Radiation Oncology
Netherlands Cancer Institute
Antoni van Leeuwenhoek Hospital
Amsterdam, the Netherlands

Ken Sutherland
Department of Medical Physics
Hokkaido University
Sapporo, Japan

Minoru Uematsu
Radiation Oncology
UAS Oncology Center
Kagoshima, Japan

Michael Velec
Radiation Medicine Program
Princess Margaret Hospital
University Health Network
Ontario, Toronto, Canada

Twyla R. Willoughby
Department of Radiation Oncology
M.D. Anderson Cancer Center Orlando
Orlando, Florida

James R. Wong
Morristown Medical Center
Morristown, New Jersey

Q. Jackie Wu
Department of Radiation Oncology
Duke University
Durham, North Carolina

Fang-Fang Yin
Department of Radiation Oncology
Duke University
Durham, North Carolina

Sua Yoo
Department of Radiation Oncology
Duke University
Durham, North Carolina

1

Optical and Remote Monitoring IGRT

Sanford L. Meeks
Department of Radiation Oncology

Twyla R. Willoughby
Department of Radiation Oncology

Katja M. Langen
Department of Radiation Oncology

Patrick A. Kupelian
Department of Radiation Oncology

1.1 Introduction

Radiation therapy dose distributions have become more focused, often utilizing sharp dose gradients to deliver high doses to target volumes while sparing nearby normal structures. Hence, knowledge of the tumor's location is critical during treatment to optimize therapy and minimize complications. Multiple factors affect the location of a target volume, including daily set-up variations that occur between treatment days (interfraction errors) and changes that occur while the patient is undergoing daily treatment (intrafraction motion). These uncertainties can be large enough to potentially compromise the ability to deliver a curative dose of radiation. Optical and image-guided radiation therapy systems have played a significant role in improving the precision of patient treatment. Optical and remote monitoring systems are attractive for image-guided radiation treatment because they can make fast, accurate 3D measurements to verify patient's position in real time without coming into contact with the patient. Furthermore, these systems require no ionizing radiation to make these measurements. This chapter reviews the concepts, technology, and clinical applications of optical tracing and remote monitoring systems currently in use for image-guided radiation therapy.

1.2 Optical Tracking Using Markers

Tracking is the process of measuring the location of instruments, anatomical structures, and/or landmarks in 3D space and in relationship to each other in real time. Systems for tracking and motion capture for interactive computer graphics have been explored for more than 30 years. Various technologies have been tested for determining an object's location, including mechanical [1–3], electromagnetic [4–7], acoustic [8–10], inertial [11,12], and optical [13–16] position sensors. These technologies have all been used in either image-guided surgery or image-guided tracking in radiation therapy, but the most common tracking technology used in radiation therapy has been optical tracking.

Optical tracking determines an object's position by measuring light either emitted or reflected from an object. The hallmark of optical-tracking systems is their high spatial resolution and measurement in real time; such systems can resolve the position of a point source within a fraction of a millimeter and report at a rate of 10 Hz or faster. Several marker-based optical systems have been developed for radiation therapy, all of which track infrared markers attached to the patient's external surface [17–25]. These markers may either be active or passive (see Figure 1.1). Active markers are infrared light-emitting diodes (IRLED) that require an electrical power source for operation, whereas passive markers are spheres or disks coated with a surface that reflects the infrared light emitted from an external source. Most often, this reflective surface is either a paint or film that has highly reflective glass beads imbedded in it. Charged couple device (CCD) cameras are most often used to detect the emitted or reflected IR light. CCD cameras are a collection of light-sensitive cells that can be arranged in either a 1D or 2D matrix. When light passes through a lens and strikes a CCD cell, electrons are produced in proportion to the amount of light incident on the cell. The charge collected per cell provides a pixel luminance value; a 2D CCD array thus provides a 2D digital image of the target, with brighter pixels corresponding to a higher light intensity incident on the cell and darker pixels corresponding to lower light

(a)   (b)

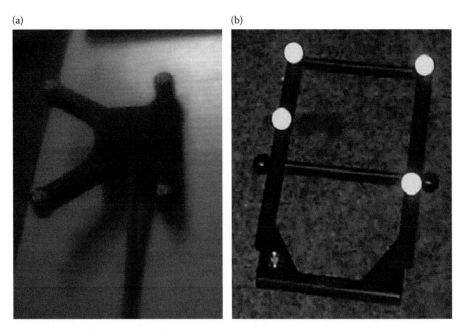

FIGURE 1.1 Examples of (a) active and (b) passive rigid-body arrays used in medicine. Active systems require a source of power and are therefore wired. Passive systems are wireless but require an external source of infrared light.

intensity incident on the cell. This digital image can be analyzed to determine the pixel with the highest intensity. In the simplest example of optical measurement, called photogrammetry, the distance between two points, which lie on a plane parallel to the image plane, can be determined by determining their distances on the image. If the scale of the image is known, the actual distance between the points can be calculated by dividing the measured distance by the scale of the image.

Stereophotogrammetry makes it possible to determine the 3D coordinates of an object using multiple cameras. Each camera in a 2D CCD array determines a ray in 3D. When an optical system uses two 2D CCDs, the intersection of the 3D rays from the cameras determines a point in space and hence the 3D marker location through triangulation. An individual point object can be tracked using stereophotogrammetry. However, the ability to track the location of a single marker by itself is not sufficient to track the location of a target (point) inside the patient. An optical-tracking system can track a collection of markers on the patient's external surface. Assuming a rigid-body relationship exists between the markers and the internal target point, the location of the target point can be found by determining the location of the collection of markers. The translation between the planned positions of a set of optical markers and the actual, detected marker positions is relatively simple to determine by finding the vector difference between the center of the fiducial array in the treatment plan and as detected on the actual patient. However, determining the rotations (around three axes), which when performed would best align one set of optical marker positions to the other, is a slightly more complicated mathematical problem. The positions of the optical markers relative to the target volume, together with the desired marker positions relative to treatment

isocenter, are determined during CT simulation. In the treatment room, the real marker positions are measured relative to the linear accelerator isocenter using the CCD camera systems described previously; rigid-body mathematics then determine marker displacements. The mathematics required for optical guidance are simply those required to determine the relationship between the markers' locations in CT simulation relative to their location in the treatment room. Exhaustive details of the mathematics used in optical guidance can be found in the literature [21,26–29], and a brief description is given here. We can denote the desired marker coordinates from the CT images as a 3×1 column matrix $\vec{p}_I = \begin{pmatrix} x_I \\ y_I \\ z_I \end{pmatrix}$, while the optically measured room coordinates of the markers are $\vec{p}_R = \begin{pmatrix} x_R \\ y_R \\ z_R \end{pmatrix}$. One must determine the relationship between these two vectors and, hence, determine the misalignment of the patient at the time of treatment relative to the time of virtual simulation. The geometric transformation between $\vec{p}_I$ and $\vec{p}_R$ can be represented by a 3×3 transformation matrix $Q_{I \to R}$ as

$$\vec{p}_R = Q_{I \to R} \vec{p}_I \qquad (1.1)$$

An arbitrary finite motion of a rigid body can be considered as the sum of two independent motions: a linear translation of some point in the rigid body plus a rotation about that point. Therefore, we may rewrite Equation 1.1 in terms of a 3×3 rotation matrix, $\hat{R}$, and a 3×1 translation matrix, $\hat{T}$:

$$\vec{p}_R = \hat{R} \vec{p}_I + \hat{T} \qquad (1.2)$$

Only three noncoplanar points with known positions in both room and image coordinates are required to solve this equation. However, using more points reduces the statistical noise and increases the accuracy in determining the transformation matrices [26]. Hence, most optical-tracking systems require a minimum of four markers for patient localization, and some use up to six markers. Assuming that N points are used, $\hat{R}$ and $\hat{T}$ are the solution of the following least-square fit equation:

$$\varepsilon^2 = \sum_{k=1}^{N} \left\| \vec{p}_{R,k} - \left(\hat{R} \vec{p}_{I,k} + \hat{T} \right) \right\|^2 \qquad (1.3)$$

It is useful to change Equation 1.3 by referring all points to the centroids $\vec{p}_{R,C}$ and $\vec{p}_{I,C}$ of the sets of points in room and image space using the centroid coincidence theorem (13). The centroids are determined using the geometric averages of the points in both coordinate systems:

$$\vec{p}_{R,C} = \frac{1}{N} \sum_{k=1}^{N} \vec{p}_{R,k}, \text{ and} \qquad (1.4)$$

$$\vec{p}_{I,C} = \frac{1}{N} \sum_{k=1}^{N} \vec{p}_{I,k} \qquad (1.5)$$

Equation 1.3 can therefore be written in terms of $\vec{p}_{R,k}'' = \vec{p}_{R,k} - \vec{p}_{R,C}$ and $\vec{p}_{I,k}'' = \vec{p}_{I,k} - \vec{p}_{I,C}$:

$$\varepsilon^2 = \sum_{k=1}^{N} \left\| \left(\vec{p}_{R,k}'' - \hat{R} \vec{p}_{I,k}'' \right) + \left(\vec{p}_{R,C} - \hat{R} \vec{p}_{I,C} - \hat{T} \right) \right\|^2, \text{ or} \qquad (1.6)$$

$$\varepsilon^2 = \sum_{k=1}^{N} \left\| \left(\vec{p}_{R,k}'' - \hat{R} \vec{p}_{I,k}'' \right) \right\|^2 - 2 \left(\vec{p}_{R,C} - \hat{R} \vec{p}_{I,C} - \hat{T} \right)$$

$$\sum_{k=1}^{N} \left(\vec{p}_{R,k}'' - \hat{R} \vec{p}_{I,k}'' \right) + N \left\| \vec{p}_{R,C} - \hat{R} \vec{p}_{I,C} - \hat{T} \right\|^2 \qquad (1.7)$$

Since sums $\sum_{k=1}^{N} \left(\vec{p}_{R,k}'' \right)$ and $\sum_{k=1}^{N} \left(\hat{R} \vec{p}_{I,k}'' \right)$ are equal to zero, Equation 1.7 can be simplified as

$$\varepsilon^2 = \sum_{k=1}^{N} \left\| \left(\vec{p}_{R,k}'' - \hat{R} \vec{p}_{I,k}'' \right) \right\|^2 + N \left\| \vec{p}_{R,C} - \hat{R} \vec{p}_{I,C} - \hat{T} \right\|^2 \qquad (1.8)$$

The translation minimizing Equation 1.8 is the difference between vector of the image centroid and the rotated room centroid:

$$\hat{T} = \vec{p}_{I,C} - \hat{R} \vec{p}_{R,C} \qquad (1.9)$$

Consequently, to determine the rotation, we have to minimize

$$\varepsilon_R^2 = \sum_{k=1}^{N} \left\| \left(\vec{p}_{R,k}'' - \hat{R} \vec{p}_{I,k}'' \right) \right\|^2 \qquad (1.10)$$

Several different algorithms can be used to determine the best-fit rotation $\hat{R}$ from Equation 1.10. Since this is a minimization problem, iterative optimization algorithms can be used. Several different optimization algorithms have proven effective, including simulated annealing and various downhill algorithms such as the downhill simplex and the Hooke and Jeeves pattern search algorithm [29].

While downhill optimization algorithms are sufficient solution of the absolute orientation as applied to stereotactic radiotherapy using rigid sets of optical fiducials, nonrigid-body tracking and/or other image systems used in conjunction with optical tracking increase the statistical noise in the optimization and decrease the reliability of these simple algorithms [26]. Closed-form solutions to the absolute orientation problem work equally well for well-behaved solution spaces and for noisy data sets and are most often used in commercial systems. The minimum of Equation 1.10 is achieved when for all $k \in N_N$ we have $\vec{p}_{R,k} = \hat{R} \vec{p}_{I,k}$. This can be rewritten in terms of a simple matrix equation:

$$\begin{bmatrix} X_{R,1} & X_{R,2} & \cdots & X_{R,N} \\ Y_{R,1} & Y_{R,2} & \cdots & Y_{R,N} \\ Z_{R,1} & Z_{R,2} & \cdots & Z_{R,N} \end{bmatrix} = \hat{R} \begin{bmatrix} X_{I,1} & X_{I,2} & \cdots & X_{I,N} \\ Y_{I,1} & Y_{I,2} & \cdots & Y_{I,N} \\ Z_{I,1} & Z_{I,2} & \cdots & Z_{I,N} \end{bmatrix} \qquad (1.11)$$

where (X, Y, Z) represent the Cartesian coordinates of the points p. Equation 1.11 represents an overdetermined linear set of equations that can be solved by using the singular value decomposition theorem. This theorem uses a decomposition of the $(N \times 3)$ matrix into the product of two orthogonal matrices. After decomposition, the solution of Equation 1.11 can be determined by inverting the corresponding orthogonal matrices. This closed-form solution gives the rotation that minimizes the least-square problem stated in Equation 1.10.

Another closed-form algorithm that can be used to solve Equation 1.10 is the solution presented by Horn using quaternion theory [26,30]. Quaternions can be thought of as a complex number with three different imaginary parts:

$$\dot{q} = q_0 + i q_x + j q_y + k q_z \qquad (1.12)$$

where q_0 is the real part and q_x, q_y, and q_z are the imaginary parts associated with the three imaginary numbers i, j, and k, respectively. In what follows, we will work with unit quaternions, that is, quaternions for which $\|\dot{q}\| = 1$, since they can be used to express rotations using the isomorphism:

$$\vec{r}_1 = R \vec{r}_0 \rightarrow \dot{r}_1 = \dot{q} * \dot{r}_0 * \dot{q}' \qquad (1.13)$$

where the rotation transform R from a point r_0 to a point r_1 is written in terms of the quaternion $\dot{q}$ and its conjugate $\dot{q}^t$. Expanding Equation 1.10 and using the fact that rotations are orthogonal linear transformations, one finds

$$\varepsilon_R^2 = \sum_{k=1}^{N} \|\vec{p}_{R,k}'\|^2 + \sum_{k=1}^{N} \|\vec{p}_{I,k}'\|^2 - 2 \sum_{k=1}^{N} \vec{p}_{R,k}' \cdot \hat{R}\vec{p}_{I,k}' \qquad (1.14)$$

Therefore, minimizing Equation 1.14 corresponds to maximizing the last term in

$$\xi = \sum_{k=1}^{N} \vec{p}_{R,k}' \cdot \hat{R}\vec{p}_{I,k}' = \sum_{k=1}^{N} \hat{R}\vec{p}_{I,k}' \cdot \vec{p}_{R,k}' \qquad (1.15)$$

which can be written in terms of quaternions using Equation 1.13:

$$\xi = \sum_{k=1}^{N} \dot{q} * \dot{p}_{I,k} * \dot{q}^t * \dot{p}_{R,k} \qquad (1.16)$$

Using the matrix representation of quaternion multiplication [30], one can rewrite Equation 1.16 as

$$\xi = \dot{q}^T \left(\sum_{k=1}^{N} N_k \right) \dot{q} = \dot{q}^T N \dot{q} \qquad (1.17)$$

where the N_k are 4×4 matrices formed of the coefficients of the points $\vec{p}_{I,k}$ and $\vec{p}_{R,k}$. Horn showed that the unit quaternion maximizing Equation 1.17 is the eigenvector corresponding to the largest positive eigenvalue of N. Since N is a 4×4 matrix, this corresponds to finding the roots of the fourth-degree characteristic polynomial of N. This quaternion corresponds to a closed-form solution of the rotation minimizing the least-square problem stated in Equation 1.10.

The first commercially available optical-tracking system for radiation therapy was originally developed at the University of Florida [18,21,31–34] and is commercially available as part of Varian's optical guidance platform (Varian Medical Systems, Inc., Palo Alto, CA). This system uses the Polaris position sensor unit (Northern Digital, Inc., Waterloo, Ontario), which is an array of two 2D CCD cameras, to optically track the position of 4–6 either active or passive infrared markers arranged in a planar array to form a rigid body (see Figure 1.2). The Polaris CCD camera unit is mounted in the ceiling above the linear accelerator. A stable mounting point is important, as the camera location will serve as the frame of reference for patient positioning. As in all tracking systems, a calibration procedure is required to transform the coordinate system from the camera system's native coordinate system to the linear accelerator's coordinate system. This procedure uses a calibration apparatus that places passive markers at known coordinates relative to the machine isocenter (see Figure 1.3). An optical measurement of the apparatus is obtained, thereby establishing a transformation matrix from camera coordinates to room coordinates. After this calibration, the position of any infrared marker in the room may be determined relative to the isocenter.

Patient localization is accomplished through the detection of an optical reference array containing four passive markers. This reference array is attached to a custom bite plate that links to the maxillary dentition of the patient to form a rigid system. The biteplate and reference array are placed and imaged during the virtual simulation CT scan, and the image coordinates of the reflective markers are determined as part of the virtual simulation. During treatment planning, the desired target, or

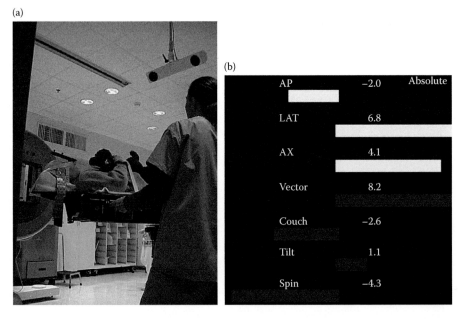

FIGURE 1.2 Example optical guidance platform. (a) The physical setup, where a rigid-body passive array is attached to a patient through a biteplate mechanism. The position of the passive array is optically measured using the infrared illuminators and CCD cameras of a Polaris system, which is rigidly mounted in the ceiling. The therapist positions the patient using real-time feedback from (b) a display that shows the patient's displacement from isocenter (in mm) along the three principal axes, plus the rotational misalignments (in degree) about each of these axes.

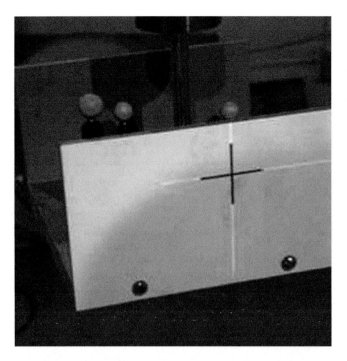

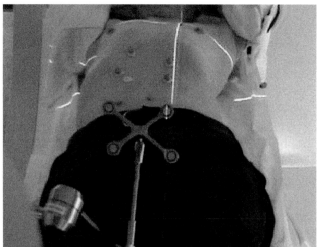

FIGURE 1.4 Body markers used for Novalis ExacTrac system. Reflective markers with an adhesive backing can be placed directly on the patient's skin for tracking the patient's position.

FIGURE 1.3 Example of an array for establishing a calibration between the camera coordinate system and the machine isocenter. The array is positioned relative to isocenter by either aligning scribe marks with the room lasers or by using a rigid front pointer that attaches to the head of the machine. In this example, the positions of passive markers with known geometry relative to isocenter are optically measured and a calibration matrix is established.

isocenter, coordinates are determined in CT space. The centers of the spherical fiducial markers in the optical reference array are also localized in CT space, thus determining their positions relative to the treatment isocenter and defining a stereotactic coordinate system. During patient setup, optical tracking determines the patient's position and reports the displacement from isocenter in real time. The system reports the translational misalignments along three orthogonal axes and the rotational misalignment about each of these axes. The patient is monitored in real time (at a rate of approximately 10 Hz) during treatment delivery, with deviations in position displayed in bar-graph form at the treatment console for easy interpretation by the operator (or similar statement). This system has been shown to have an accuracy of 1.1 mm in patient studies [21] and has been used for fractionated stereotactic radiotherapy of intracranial and skull base tumors [31,33–36] and for frameless radiosurgery of intracranial metastases [32,37,38].

The ExacTrac system (BrainLab, Munich, Germany) is operationally similar to Varian's optical-tracking system described previously, except it allows tracking of nonrigid sets of optical markers [25,39,40]. ExacTrac employs two 2D infrared cameras, which are rigidly mounted in the ceiling of the linear accelerator vault, to track passive optical markers ("body markers") that are attached to the patient (see Figure 1.4). A calibration procedure similar to the one described for the Varian system is used to transform the coordinate system from the camera's native

coordinate system to the linear accelerator's coordinate system. An optical measurement of a calibration apparatus is obtained, thereby establishing a transformation matrix from camera coordinates to room coordinates. After this calibration, the position of any infrared marker in the room may be determined relative to the isocenter.

The body markers are attached to the patient using an adhesive backing prior to CT scanning. The marker position is referenced with a tattoo or ink marking to aid reapplication for each treatment fraction. Standard CT images are acquired and then sent to the treatment planning workstation, where the target volume and isocenter are defined and the plan is completed. The isocenter is established relative to the coordinate system defined by the body markers, which are later used for positioning. At the time of treatment, the internal target is positioned at the linac isocenter based on optical tracking of the external fiducials. This method assumes that a rigid-body relationship exists between the external markers and the internal target. This rigid-body relationship is more easily maintained for intracranial treatments than for stereotactic body radiotherapy, in which both inter- and intrafraction 3D localization is affected by the accuracy of refixation of skin markers (i.e., *remarking error*), respiratory motion, and skin or other soft tissue deformation [17,25,41].

1.3 Optically Guided Imaging Systems

One of the weaknesses of optical tracking is that it relies on tracking the patient's surface, and the external surface may not always be an accurate surrogate for tumor motion. Hence, optical tracking has been integrated with x-ray and ultrasound imaging to determine the position of internal anatomy targets relative to isocenter. Systems have been developed for optical and ultrasound guidance, including the SonArray system (Varian Medical Systems, Palo Alto, CA), the BATCAM (BestNomos,

Pittsburgh, PA), and the Clarity System (Resonant Medical, Quebec, Canada). In the SonArray system, which is a part of Varian's optical guidance platform, the 3D ultrasound data sets are generated through optical tracking of free-hand acquired 2D ultrasound data [26,28]. The operator holds the ultrasound probe and manipulates it over the anatomical region of interest. The raw 2D data are transferred to a computer workstation using a standard video link. The position and angulation of the ultrasound probe in any arbitrary orientation is determined using an array of four IRLEDs attached to the probe. Similar to the system for intracranial optical tracking, the Polaris camera system is used to determine the positions of the IRLEDs, and this information is input to the computer workstation. The position of each ultrasound pixel can therefore be determined using the IRLEDs, and an ultrasound volume can be reconstructed by coupling the position information with the raw ultrasound data.

In addition to building the 3D image volume, optical guidance is used to determine the absolute position of the ultrasound volume in the treatment room coordinate system. Because the relative positions of the ultrasound volume and the ultrasound probe are fixed, the knowledge of the probe position in the treatment room coordinate system at the time of data acquisition is sufficient to determine the position of the image volume relative to the linear accelerator isocenter. The determination of the relative position of the image and probe corresponds to a calibration step that is performed at the time of system installation.

Ultrasound localization has been used for conformal and intensity-modulated radiotherapy of prostate radiotherapy [42] and for patient localization for patients undergoing extracranial radiosurgery for a variety of abdominal, paraspinal, and pelvic lesions [27,43]. The CT is acquired with the patient immobilized in the same position as that will be used during the radiotherapy treatment in order to maintain a generally consistent position of mobile anatomy. The CT images are transferred to a 3D treatment planning system where the tumor volume and normal structures of interest are delineated. On the day of the treatment, the patient is placed in the same immobilization cushion that was used during CT scanning. The patient is initially set up relative to isocenter using conventional laser alignment. A 3D ultrasound volume is then acquired and reconstructed in the computer workstation. The target volume and critical structure outlines, as delineated on the planning CT scans, are overlaid on the acquired ultrasound volume in relation to isocenter. The contours determined from the CT scans are then manipulated until they align with the anatomic structures on the ultrasound images. The amount of movement required to align the contours with the ultrasound images determines the magnitude of the target misregistration with isocenter based on conventional set-up techniques. The target is then placed at the isocenter by tracking an infrared array attached to the treatment couch, which allows precise translation from the initial position to the 3D ultrasound determined position. Once all of the setup information has been verified using repeat ultrasound acquisition and coregistration, treatment proceeds as planned. Ultrasound-IGRT is covered more completely in a separate chapter.

Similar to combined ultrasound-optical tracking, BrainLab's Novalis Body system integrates two kilovoltage x-ray tubes and amorphous silicon flat panel imagers with the Exactrac optical-tracking system [25,39,40,44]. The patient is prepositioned on the treatment couch based on the ExacTrac Body Markers. Typically, these markers are not placed as a rigid body, but rather are placed individually on the patient's skin, forming a nonrigid body for tracking purposes. Two digital stereoscopic x-ray images are acquired immediately prior to treatment. The ExacTrac software uses the initial CT scan, which was used during planning, to automatically calculate a set of stereoscopic digitally reconstructed radiographs (DRRs) that serve as a reference image set for patient positioning. The software then uses a mutual information algorithm to automatically register the digital x-ray images with the DRRs and hence determine any misalignment of the patient's bony anatomy [24,45].

X-ray imaging is particularly well suited for alignment of tumor volumes that maintain a rigid relationship to bony anatomy, such as intracranial tumors or paraspinal tumors. In these situations, aligning the bony anatomy as seen on the x-ray images with the bony anatomy from the treatment planning CT scan will adequately place the tumor at isocenter. For soft-tissue targets that are not fixed relative to bony anatomy, high Z (e.g., gold) implanted fiducials can be used as a surrogate for tumor visualization on x-ray projection images. For prostate cancer treatments, patients typically have three gold markers placed in the prostate transrectally under ultrasound guidance prior to CT simulation and treatment planning. These implanted markers are then used to indicate the prostate position on planar x-ray images. Compared with techniques such as transabdominal ultrasound or even pelvic CT scans, the interpretation of the actual location of the prostate gland is easier and more objective using implanted markers [46–48]. However, this technique requires the implanted markers to be reliable surrogates of prostate position. A review of 56 cases treated at M.D. Anderson Cancer Center Orlando (MDACCO) demonstrated that no true "migration" of the seeds occurs, and patients can be reliably positioned using intraprostatic markers [49].

Other mobile soft-tissue targets, such as lung or liver tumors, can be implanted with marker seeds to allow visualization on x-ray imaging. Patients undergoing radiation therapy at MDACCO for small early stage lung cancer are implanted with small metallic markers using the superDimension®/Bronchus system, which is a radio-frequency signal-based bronchoscopy guidance system referenced to an initial set of CT images. A review of 23 lung cancer patients implanted with gold markers indicated that implanted lung marker seeds are stable within tumors throughout the treatment duration [50].

1.4 Optical Tracking for Gated Imaging and Radiotherapy

Varian's Respiratory Gating system (Varian Inc., Palo Alto, CA) uses optical tracking of a reflective marker box detected by a

1D video camera system [20]. The patient's respiratory cycle is obtained by optically tracking the motion of the box placed on the patient's chest or abdomen. This system can be interfaced with many different vendors' multislice CT-scanners to form a 4D image acquisition system. After a CT study has been obtained in 4D mode, the chest-wall motion trace recorded using Varian's Respiratory Gating system is used to bin CT images that have been acquired in Cine mode into a number of breathing phases. These binned CT studies can then be used to determine a motion envelope of the tumor using virtual simulation. This motion envelope can then be used in treatment planning as a 4D-GTV, or one can use this technique to decide in which breathing phases to gate the radiation therapy treatment (usually around the expiration phase) and create a radiation treatment plan using only those CT image sets for treatment planning that correspond to the selected treatment gating phase. Clearly, this system has the inherent assumption that the external marker box is an acceptable surrogate for internal tumor motion. It has been shown that this is not always a reliable assumption [51].

BrainLab has developed a similar system for gated x-ray acquisition and treatment delivery based on the optically guided stereoscopic x-ray system described previously [39,52]. In this system, body markers placed on the patient's chest and/or abdomen are used with a 2D stereo CCD camera system to determine the patient's breathing pattern. The breathing pattern is used to select a trigger point for x-rays and treatment delivery (see Figure 1.5). With the linear accelerator turned on, a gridded electron gun is used to restrict the treatment beam until the breathing pattern coincides with this trigger point. The trigger point is generally selected to coincide with end expiration where there is a longer duty cycle in which the x-ray beam is on. Once a trigger point is selected the user obtains x-ray images of an implanted fiducial for localization and treatment verification. The system is designed to take x-ray images when the

patient's breathing cycle matches a trigger level as determined by body markers. A single x-ray image from one of the stereoscopic imagers is obtained at a time, followed by acquisition of the complementary view from the second imaging system. With the triggering of the system set to a single line on the breathing curve, the patient should be in the same location for each of the two stereoscopic x-rays; thus, an acceptable pair of stereoscopic x-ray images is obtained. Only one identifiable point is necessary to correlate the x-ray images with the planning CT. More points clearly give better geometry, and at least three points are required to calculate the rotational differences in the patient position relative to the CT scan. Based on the localization images, the patient is repositioned such that the target is at the isocenter of the beam for the phase of breathing cycle corresponding to the trigger level. The radiation treatment beam is then gated based on this breathing cycle. The user can determine what percentage of the breathing cycle around the x-ray trigger level is to be used to deliver radiation. The default level is 20%, but this window should be determined for an individual patient based on the overall motion of the target and the amount of motion that is to be allowed during treatment. After the beam ON is pressed, the gridded gun is synchronized with the trigger point to automatically turn the radiation beam on when the body markers fall within the treatment window and off when they are outside of the treatment window.

1.5 Markerless Optical Tracking of Patient's External Surface

All of the techniques discussed so far rely on detection of markers attached to the patient's surface. The AlignRT system (Vision RT Ltd., London, UK) uses close-range photogrammetry with speckle projection to track the patient's surface in real time, without the use of markers [53,54]. The system hardware consists

(a) (b)

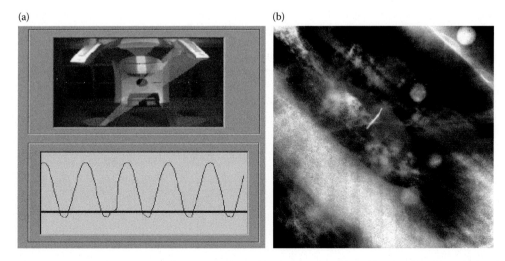

FIGURE 1.5   In the Novalis ExacTrac gating system, (a) a sinusoidal breathing pattern is established by optical tracking of fiducial markers placed on the patient's abdomen as illustrated in Figure 1.4. A trigger point is established near end expiration; this trigger point is represented by the horizontal line on the sinusoidal breathing pattern. Stereoscopic x-rays can be obtained when the patient's position matches this trigger point. (b) Implanted markers are clearly visible on the x-ray image and can be used to verify the patient's location relative to the linac isocenter.

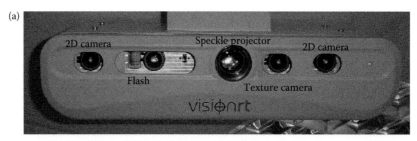

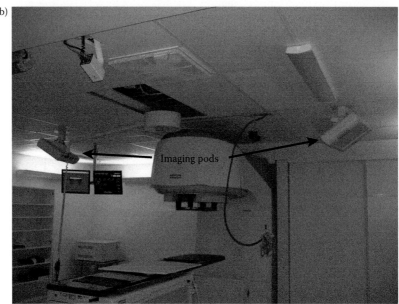

FIGURE 1.6 Set-up for VisionRT system. (a) A close-up of a VisionRT imaging pod, including the speckle projector and CCD cameras. (b) The mounting of the imaging pods in the ceiling of the treatment room.

of two ceiling-mounted imaging pods that are interfaced to software running on a standard PC (see Figure 1.6). Each imaging pod contains two CCD cameras for stereophotogrammetry, an additional CCD camera for texture image acquisition, one clear flash unit, one flash unit projecting a speckle pattern, and a slide projector that produces a continuous speckle projection for dynamic imaging. Speckle refers to an optically projected pseudorandom gray-scale pattern. The speckle provides sufficient unique information to allow reconstruction of the surface and stereo matching of the acquired surface to a reference surface. Each pod covers only a portion of the body surface, and data from both pods are merged to form an integrated surface model. The six cameras are calibrated relative to the linac coordinate system using a calibration plate with a printed grid. The software identifies points in the calibration grid and correlates the system's camera coordinate system to the linac coordinates. This calibration process merges each pod's surface data to form a smooth transition at the match line.

To date, the system has been used primarily for aligning patients undergoing breast irradiation [54]. Clinical use of the system requires acquisition of a reference surface model. This acquisition can be done during the first treatment session or during simulation using a second imaging system. At subsequent treatment sessions, the system can be used as an alignment tool

by comparison of the reference surface with a surface model acquired in the treatment room. During the alignment process, the software calculates the optimal rigid-body transformation that best aligns the patient's surface at the daily treatment with the reference surface. Phantom studies have shown that alignment accuracy is better than 0.8 mm and 0.1° [53]. The system also has a continuous acquisition mode in which the speckle pattern is projected continuously and image data are acquired at a frequency of 7 Hz. This continuous data acquisition mode can be used for real-time monitoring, studying surface motion due to breathing, and for respiratory-gated capture, which minimizes breathing motion artifacts. These latter techniques are currently under development for clinical use.

1.6 Laser Tracking of Patient's Position

Similar to the markerless infrared optical-tracking systems, 3D scanning lasers can be used to scan a surface of the patient and to compare this surface to a reference surface of the patient for alignment purposes. Examples of such laser positioning systems are the Galaxy (LAP America, Boca Raton, FL) and Sentinel (C-RAD, Uppsala, Sweden). Laser tracking with the Galaxy system uses a narrow-line laser and mirror mounted on a galvanometer to sweep the fan-shaped laser beam [55]. The laser line is swept along the patient at a rate of 2500 Hz with a step time of less than 300 μs in order to determine contour lines along the patient. A complementary metal-oxide semiconductor (CMOS) camera captures the laser line on the patient at a frame rate of up to 50 frames per second, thereby capturing the patient profile frame by frame. Knowing the absolute positions of the camera and laser, the system can back project each illuminated pixel along the light rays. This computer-calculated back projection produces one 3D contour per camera image. Multiple contours are combined to form a surface. The surface scanned during treatment can be directly compared to a reference surface, such as the skin detected by the CT scanner used for treatment planning. Using a surface registration algorithm, set-up errors can be detected. The time resolution for capturing patient surfaces within a normal detection volume and with a resolution of approximately two contours/cm is about 1 image/s. For respiratory motion monitoring, the scan rate is increased in frequency over a truncated region specified by the user, and the temporal resolution may reach 20 images/s.

To ensure that all coordinate systems are aligned, a special calibration process is used. System calibration is performed by imaging and scanning a reference object of known size and shape, adjusting the geometrical parameters until the back projected dataset matches the known reference dataset. This calibration corrects for the absolute position of the reference object, the true focal length, and lens distortions. The detected translational and rotational deviations between the reference and the scanned image are compensated for to ensure that the patient surface generated by the LC system is really given in the equipment coordinate system. In a rigid phantom, the positioning accuracy of the system is better than 1.6 mm (1.1 ± 0.5), and the reproducibility is better than 0.1 mm [55].

1.7 Radiofrequency Tracking of Patient's Position

Numerous investigators have demonstrated that targets such as the prostate, focal liver tumors, and lung tumors move with respect to traditional positioning references of the skin and skeleton. A comprehensive review of these studies is given in the literature [56]. Pretreatment localization using ultrasonography and x-ray imaging have been demonstrated, as discussed previously, but the current systems are unsuited for continuous monitoring of internal anatomy during treatment. Predictive systems that combine external references with periodic radiographic verification have also been described, but it is not clear that the external surface motion always correlates directly with the motion of the internal target [51].

The Calypso 4D Localization System (Calypso Medical Technologies, Seattle) is designed to provide accurate, precise, objective, and continuous target localization during external beam radiotherapy (see Figure 1.7). One or more wireless transponders (Beacons™) are implanted in the patient before acquisition of a treatment planning CT scan. Each Beacon consists of an AC electromagnetic resonance circuit encapsulated in glass. The Beacons can be implanted using a 14-gauge needle in the same manner that gold markers are implanted for x-ray localization [49,57]. The coordinates of the Beacons and the corresponding isocenter from the treatment plan are entered into the Calypso

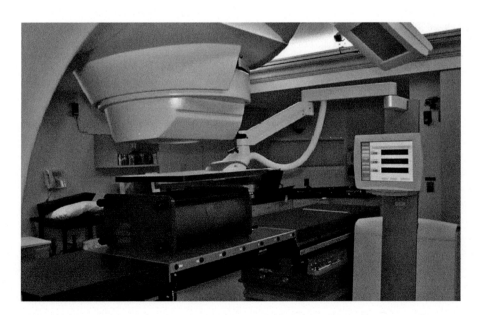

FIGURE 1.7 The Calypso system requires a magnetic source and receiver coil array placed over the patient to determine the transponder positions. The array is tracked in real time relative to the isocenter through the use of an infrared optical-tracking system. The system calculates the table translations that are necessary to move the beacons to positions that best match the locations determined from the treatment planning CT scan. These translations are shown in an easy to read user interface that allows the therapist to shift the table to the desired location.

system. When the patient is to be positioned for radiotherapy, a magnetic source and receiver coil array is used to determine the transponder positions. The electromagnetic array is tracked in real time relative to the isocenter through the use of an infrared optical-tracking system registered with the isocenter. With the position and orientation of the antenna array known, detected locations of the RF beacons inside the patient can be converted to room or treatment machine coordinates, in similar fashion to the optically tracked ultrasound system discussed earlier. The system determines the best geometric fit of these transponders to the planned coordinates that were entered into the system. From this fit, the system calculates the table translations that are necessary to move the beacons to positions that best match the locations determined from the treatment planning CT scan. These translations are displayed in an interface that guides the therapist to shift the table to the desired location. The position data are updated at a rate of 10 Hz, providing continuous feedback for initial positioning of the target and subsequent monitoring of the target position during treatment.

A comparison between the measured and known positions has established a submillimeter accuracy of the system for well-known, in-phantom locations [58]. The *in-vivo* accuracy for prostate localization has been tested by Willoughby et al. [59]. The system localizations were compared with radiographic localization of the transponders, and an average 3D difference of 1.5 ± 0.9 mm was seen between the two localization techniques. However, the two localization techniques were not used simultaneously, and a required time delay of 3–5 minutes between the two localizations could have had contributed to the observed differences between the two localization techniques [59].

1.8 Tracking Radioactive Sources

The RealTrack (Navotek Medical Ltd., Israel) system is designed to localize and track radioactive sources within the body. A novel radioactive implantable soft tissue marker (approximately 50 μCi of ^{192}Ir) has been developed for radiographic and/or radioactive target localization [60]. The marker has been designed to be visible on x-ray, CT, and MR images while producing minimal artifact on CT and MRI. The source emits photons that are detected by an array of detectors that is attached to the head of the linear accelerator. These detectors are designed to localize the source in 3D space and to track its location in real time. In phantom, the accuracy of tracking a static target has been shown to be approximately 0.6 mm while the accuracy of tracking a dynamic target is approximately 1 mm [61]. The first version of the system is designed for use in prostate radiotherapy and is an investigational device at the time of this writing.

1.9 Summary

Optical and remote monitoring IGRT systems enable accurate patient set-up, respiratory correlated radiotherapy, collision avoidance, and adaptive radiation therapy. The systems provide cost-effective methods for enabling high-precision radiotherapy and have minimal effect on treatment efficiency. Furthermore, these creative systems are minimally invasive and deliver minimal or no additional ionizing radiation to the patient. Because of these advantages, optical and remote monitoring systems can be expected to play a continued role in improving the precision of radiation delivery. Currently, methods are under development to allow 4D dose calculations using motion traces from real-time tracking systems as input [62–67]. Future uses of these systems can be expected to include real-time adaptive therapy methods that take the dosimetric effects of inter- and intrafraction motion into account and allow real-time treatment corrections based on this feedback [66–68].

References

1. Reinhardt, H.F. and H. Landolt, CT-guided "real time" stereotaxy. *Acta Neurochir Suppl (Wien),* 1989. **46**: pp. 107–8.
2. Watanabe, E., et al., Three-dimensional digitizer (neuronavigator): new equipment for computed tomography-guided stereotaxic surgery. *Surg Neurol,* 1987. **27**(6): pp. 543–7.
3. Zamorano, L., Z. Jiang, and A.M. Kadi, Computer-assisted neurosurgery system: Wayne State University hardware and software configuration. *Comput Med Imaging Graph,* 1994. **18**(4): pp. 257–71.
4. Kuipers, J.B., *SPASYN*—an electromagnetic relative position and orientation tracking system. *IEEE Trans Instrum Meas,* 1980. **29**: pp. 462–6.
5. Meskers, C.G., et al., Calibration of the "Flock of Birds" electromagnetic tracking device and its application in shoulder motion studies. *J Biomech,* 1999. **32**(6): pp. 629–33.
6. Milne, A.D., et al., Accuracy of an electromagnetic tracking device: A study of the optimal range and metal interference. *J Biomech,* 1996. **29**(6): pp. 791–3.
7. Wagner, A., et al., Virtual image guided navigation in tumor surgery – technical innovation. *J Craniomaxillofac Surg,* 1995. **23**(5): pp. 271–3.
8. Hata, N., et al., Development of a frameless and armless stereotactic neuronavigation system with ultrasonographic registration. *Neurosurgery,* 1997. **41**(3): pp. 608–13; discussion 613–4.
9. Reinhardt, H.F. and H.J. Zweifel, Interactive sonar-operated device for stereotactic and open surgery. *Stereotact Funct Neurosurg,* 1990. **54–55**: pp. 393–7.
10. Roberts, D.W., et al., A frameless stereotaxic integration of computerized tomographic imaging and the operating microscope. *J Neurosurg,* 1986. **65**(4): pp. 545–9.
11. Zhou, H., H. Hu, and Y. Tao, Inertial measurements of upper limb motion. *Med Biol Eng Comput,* 2006. **44**(6): pp. 479–87.
12. Zhu, R. and Z. Zhouh, A real-time articulated human motion tracking using triaxis inertial/magnetic sensors package. *IEEE Trans Neural Syst Rehabil Eng,* 2004. **12**(2): pp. 295–302.
13. Colchester, A.C., et al., Development and preliminary evaluation of VISLAN, a surgical planning and guidance system using intra-operative video imaging. *Med Image Anal,* 1996. **1**(1): pp. 73–90.

14. Nolte, L.P., et al., Clinical evaluation of a system for precision enhancement in spine surgery. *Clin Biomech (Bristol, Avon),* 1995. **10**(6): pp. 293–303.

15. Rohling, R., et al., Comparison of relative accuracy between a mechanical and an optical position tracker for image-guided neurosurgery. *J Image Guid Surg,* 1995. **1**(1): pp. 30–4.

16. Smith, K.R., K.J. Frank, and R.D. Bucholz, The NeuroStation – a highly accurate, minimally invasive solution to frameless stereotactic neurosurgery. *Comput Med Imaging Graph,* 1994. **18**(4): pp. 247–56.

17. Baroni, G., G. Ferrigno, and A. Pedotti, Implementation and application of real-time motion analysis based on passive markers. *Med Biol Eng Comput,* 1998. **36**(6): pp. 693–703.

18. Bova, F.J., et al., The University of Florida frameless high-precision stereotactic radiotherapy system. *Int J Radiat Oncol Biol Phys,* 1997. **38**(4): pp. 875–82.

19. Kai, J., et al., Optical high-precision three-dimensional position measurement system suitable for head motion tracking in frameless stereotactic radiosurgery. *Comput Aided Surg,* 1998. **3**(5): pp. 257–63.

20. Kubo, H.D., et al., Breathing-synchronized radiotherapy program at the University of California Davis Cancer Center. *Med Phys,* 2000. **27**(2): pp. 346–53.

21. Meeks, S.L., et al., Image localization for frameless stereotactic radiotherapy. *Int J Radiat Oncol Biol Phys,* 2000. **46**(5): pp. 1291–9.

22. Menke, M., et al., Photogrammetric accuracy measurements of head holder systems used for fractionated radiotherapy. *Int J Radiat Oncol Biol Phys,* 1994. **29**(5): pp. 1147–55.

23. Rogus, R.D., R.L. Stern, and H.D. Kubo, Accuracy of a photogrammetry-based patient positioning and monitoring system for radiation therapy. *Med Phys,* 1999. **26**(5): pp. 721–8.

24. Soete, G., et al., Clinical use of stereoscopic X-ray positioning of patients treated with conformal radiotherapy for prostate cancer. *Int J Radiat Oncol Biol Phys,* 2002. **54**(3): pp. 948–52.

25. Wang, L.T., et al., Infrared patient positioning for stereotactic radiosurgery of extracranial tumors. *Comput Biol Med,* 2001. **31**(2): pp. 101–11.

26. Bouchet, L.G., et al., Calibration of three-dimensional ultrasound images for image-guided radiation therapy. *Phys Med Biol,* 2001. **46**(2): pp. 559–77.

27. Meeks, S.L., et al., Ultrasound-guided extracranial radiosurgery: technique and application. *Int J Radiat Oncol Biol Phys,* 2003. **55**(4): pp. 1092–101.

28. Tome, W.A., et al., Commissioning and quality assurance of an optically guided three-dimensional ultrasound target localization system for radiotherapy. *Med Phys,* 2002. **29**(8): pp. 1781–8.

29. Yang, C.C., et al., A comparison of 3-D data correlation methods for fractionated stereotactic radiotherapy. *Int J Radiat Oncol Biol Phys,* 1999. **43**(3): pp. 663–70.

30. Horn, B.K., Closed-form solution of absolute orientation using unit quaternions. *J Opt Soc Am,* 1987. **4**(4): pp. 629–42.

31. Buatti, J.M., et al., Preliminary experience with frameless stereotactic radiotherapy. *Int J Radiat Oncol Biol Phys,* 1998. **42**(3): pp. 591–9.

32. Ryken, T.C., et al., Initial clinical experience with frameless stereotactic radiosurgery: analysis of accuracy and feasibility. *Int J Radiat Oncol Biol Phys,* 2001. **51**(4): pp. 1152–8.

33. Tome, W.A., et al., A high-precision system for conformal intracranial radiotherapy. *Int J Radiat Oncol Biol Phys,* 2000. **47**(4): pp. 1137–43.

34. Tome, W.A., et al., Optically guided intensity modulated radiotherapy. *Radiother Oncol,* 2001. **61**(1): pp. 33–44.

35. Keshavarzi, S., et al., Initial clinical experience with frameless optically guided stereotactic radiosurgery/radiotherapy in pediatric patients. *Childs Nerv Syst,* 2009. **25**(7): pp. 37–44.

36. Lu, H., et al., Optically guided stereotactic radiotherapy for lacrimal sac tumors: a report on two cases. *Technol Cancer Res Treat,* 2008. **7**(1): pp. 35–40.

37. Kamath, R., et al., Initial clinical experience with frameless radiosurgery for patients with intracranial metastases. *Int J Radiat Oncol Biol Phys,* 2005. **61**(5): pp. 1467–72.

38. Furuse, M., et al., Frameless stereotactic radiosurgery with a bite-plate: our experience with brain metastases. *Minim Invasive Neurosurg,* 2008. **51**(6): pp. 333–5.

39. Tenn, S.E., T.D. Solberg, and P.M. Medin, Targeting accuracy of an image guided gating system for stereotactic body radiotherapy. *Phys Med Biol,* 2005. **50**(23): pp. 5443–62.

40. Yan, H., F.F. Yin, and J.H. Kim, A phantom study on the positioning accuracy of the Novalis Body system. *Med Phys,* 2003. **30**(12): pp. 3052–60.

41. Weiss, E., et al., Interfractional and intrafractional accuracy during radiotherapy of gynecologic carcinomas: a comprehensive evaluation using the ExacTrac system. *Int J Radiat Oncol Biol Phys,* 2003. **56**(1): pp. 69–79.

42. Patel, R.R., et al., Rectal dose sparing with a balloon catheter and ultrasound localization in conformal radiation therapy for prostate cancer. *Radiother Oncol,* 2003. **67**(3): pp. 285–94.

43. Ryken, T.C., et al., Ultrasonographic guidance for spinal extracranial radiosurgery: technique and application for metastatic spinal lesions. *Neurosurg Focus,* 2001. **11**(6): pp. e8.

44. Verellen, D., et al., Quality assurance of a system for improved target localization and patient set-up that combines real-time infrared tracking and stereoscopic X-ray imaging. *Radiother Oncol,* 2003. **67**(1): pp. 129–41.

45. Soete, G., et al., Setup accuracy of stereoscopic X-ray positioning with automated correction for rotational errors in patients treated with conformal arc radiotherapy for prostate cancer. *Radiother Oncol,* 2006. **80**(3): pp. 371–3.

46. Langen, K.M., et al., Evaluation of ultrasound-based prostate localization for image-guided radiotherapy. *Int J Radiat Oncol Biol Phys,* 2003. **57**(3): pp. 635–44.

47. Scarbrough, T.J., et al., Comparison of ultrasound and implanted seed marker prostate localization methods: implications for image-guided radiotherapy. *Int J Radiat Oncol Biol Phys,* 2006. **65**(2): pp. 378–87.

48. Serago, C.F., et al., Comparison of daily megavoltage electronic portal imaging or kilovoltage imaging with marker

seeds to ultrasound imaging or skin marks for prostate local-ization and treatment positioning in patients with prostate cancer. *Int J Radiat Oncol Biol Phys,* 2006. **65**(5): pp. 1585–92.

49. Kupelian, P.A., et al., Intraprostatic fiducials for localization of the prostate gland: monitoring intermarker distances during radiation therapy to test for marker stability. *Int J Radiat Oncol Biol Phys,* 2005. **62**(5): pp. 1291–6.

50. Kupelian, P.A., et al., Implantation and stability of metallic fiducials within pulmonary lesions. *Int J Radiat Oncol Biol Phys,* 2007. **69**(3): pp. 777–85.

51. Ionascu, D., et al., Internal-external correlation investiga-tions of respiratory induced motion of lung tumors. *Med Phys,* 2007. **34**(10): pp. 3893–903.

52. Willoughby, T.R., et al., Evaluation of an infrared camera and X-ray system using implanted fiducials in patients with lung tumors for gated radiation therapy. *Int J Radiat Oncol Biol Phys,* 2006. **66**(2): pp. 568–75.

53. Bert, C., et al., A phantom evaluation of a stereo-vision sur-face imaging system for radiotherapy patient setup. *Med Phys,* 2005. **32**(9): pp. 2753–62.

54. Bert, C., et al., Clinical experience with a 3D surface patient setup system for alignment of partial-breast irradiation patients. *Int J Radiat Oncol Biol Phys,* 2006. **64**(4): pp. 1265–74.

55. Brahme, A., P. Nyman, and B. Skatt, 4D laser camera for accurate patient positioning, collision avoidance, image fusion and adaptive approaches during diagnostic and ther-apeutic procedures. *Med Phys,* 2008. **35**(5): pp. 1670–81.

56. Langen, K.M. and D.T. Jones, Organ motion and its manage-ment. *Int J Radiat Oncol Biol Phys,* 2001. **50**(1): pp. 265–78.

57. Kupelian, P., et al., Multi-institutional clinical experience with the Calypso System in localization and continuous, real-time monitoring of the prostate gland during external radiother-apy. *Int J Radiat Oncol Biol Phys,* 2007. **67**(4): pp. 1088–98.

58. Balter, J.M., et al., Accuracy of a wireless localization system for radiotherapy. *Int J Radiat Oncol Biol Phys,* 2005. **61**(3): pp. 933–7.

59. Willoughby, T.R., et al., Target localization and real-time tracking using the Calypso 4D localization system in patients with localized prostate cancer. *Int J Radiat Oncol Biol Phys,* 2006. **65**(2): pp. 528–34.

60. Neustadter, D. and B. Corn, Analysis of dose to patient, spouse/caretaker, and staff from an implanted trackable radioactive fiducial for use in radiation treatment of pros-tate cancer. *Med Phys,* 2008. **35**(6): pp. 2921.

61. Shchory, T., et al., Static and dynamic tracking accuracy of a novel radioactive tracking technology for target localization and real time tracking in radiation therapy. *Med Phys,* 2008. **35**(6): pp. 2719.

62. Langen, K.M., et al., Correlation between dosimetric effect and intrafraction motion during prostate treatments deliv-ered with helical tomotherapy. *Phys Med Biol,* 2008. **53**(24): pp. 7073–86.

63. Langen, K.M., et al., Dosimetric effect of prostate motion during helical tomotherapy. *Int J Radiat Oncol Biol Phys,* 2009. **74**(4): pp. 134–42.

64. Li, H.S., et al., Dosimetric consequences of intrafraction prostate motion. *Int J Radiat Oncol Biol Phys,* 2008. **71**(3): pp. 01–12.

65. Ngwa, W., et al., Validation of a computational method for assessing the impact of intra-fraction motion on heli-cal tomotherapy plans. *Phys Med Biol,* 2009. **54**(21): pp. 6611–21.

66. Suh, Y., et al., Four-dimensional IMRT treatment planning using a DMLC motion-tracking algorithm. *Phys Med Biol,* 2009. **54**(12): pp. 3821–35.

67. Suh, Y., et al., A deliverable four-dimensional intensity-modulated radiation therapy-planning method for dynamic multileaf collimator tumor tracking delivery. *Int J Radiat Oncol Biol Phys,* 2008. **71**(5): pp. 1526–36.

68. Santhanam, A., et al., Modeling simulation and visualiza-tion of conformal 3D lung tumor dosimetry. *Phys Med Biol,* 2009. **54**(20): pp. 6165–80.

2

Ultrasound-Guided Radiation Therapy

Janelle A. Molloy
University of Kentucky

2.1 Introduction

The integration of three-dimensional conformal radiation therapy (3DCRT) and intensity-modulated radiation therapy (IMRT) into routine clinical practice precipitated the era in which our ability to localize radiation dose distributions exceeded our ability to localize patient anatomy. This paradigm shift prompted the development of improved methods of tumor localization, including patient immobilization devices and image-guidance techniques.[1]

While 3DCRT developed, radiotherapy for prostate cancer gained widespread attention, as the technology and methods for interstitial brachytherapy became well-developed. Implantation of radioactive sources was performed under ultrasound (US) guidance, which provided good soft tissue contrast and real-time feedback. Radiation oncologists and medical physicists were integrally involved in these procedures and gained a high level of skill and comfort with US imaging.[2] It was in this context that US imaging for external beam radiation therapy (EBRT) was introduced.

In this chapter, we will discuss the basic physics of US image formation, review the conditions under which US imaging works well, and describe image artifacts and limitations. Use of US imaging as a localization modality for EBRT will be discussed, including a description of clinical and quality-assurance procedures, use in an interimaging modality environment, and comparison to other localization methods in EBRT.

2.2 Physics of Ultrasound Formation

US propagates via the compression and rarefaction of the medium through which it travels. It obeys the laws of wave mechanics, possessing frequencies of 3–10 MHz, and is subject to reflection and refraction at tissue interfaces. The magnitude of this perturbation depends on the difference in acoustic impedance of the two media, which is defined as

$$Z = c \times \rho \qquad (2.1)$$

where c is the speed of sound in the medium and ρ is its density. The acoustic properties of relevant media are listed in Table 2.1.

US is produced through the excitation of piezoelectric crystals contained in the transducer, which serve as both transmitters and receivers. Transducers are generally categorized as linear or curvilinear, depending on the shape of the transducer surface. The former are used for applications in which the anatomy of interest is located at a shallow depth, and they offer approximately uniform spatial resolution as a function of depth, although at the expense of a limited field of view. In contrast, curvilinear transducer arrays produce a wider, fan-shaped field of view.

Spatial information within the medium of interest is revealed by detecting the time-of-flight between transmitted and received impulses. This information, coupled with assumptions regarding the speed of sound in the tissue of interest, combines to yield the spatial location of tissue interfaces.

TABLE 2.1 The Acoustic Properties of Relevant Tissue Types are Listed

	Density (kg/m³)	Sound Speed (m/s)	Acoustic Impedance (kg/m² s)
Water	1000	1480	1.48
Muscle	1070	1542–1626	1.65–1.74
Liver	1060	1566	1.66
Lung	400	650	0.26
Kidney	1040	1567	1.62
Fat	920	1446	1.33
Brain	1030	1505–1612	1.55–1.66
Bone	1380–1810	2070–5350	3.75–7.38
Blood	1060	1566	1.66
Air	1.2	333	0.0004

Note: Reflections at tissue interfaces depend on differences in acoustic impedance of the adjacent tissue types.

The US pressure amplitude, P, attenuates exponentially with depth (x), with an attenuation coefficient, α, that is inversely proportional to frequency (f). This is described as

$$P(x, f) = P_0\, e^{-\alpha(f)x}. \qquad (2.2)$$

As such, higher frequency US beams are less penetrating than lower frequency beams. US wavelengths are on the order of 0.1–1 mm, and the spatial resolution is proportional to frequency. Thus, the choice of frequency is a compromise between penetration depth and spatial resolution.

The spatial accuracy of a US image relies on several assumptions, which include a constant and known speed of sound. The value most typically assumed is 1540 m/s, which is derived from an average of the speed of sound in muscle, fat, and water. As shown in Table 2.1, this value can vary by as much as ±100 m/s for soft tissues. Bone and air possess markedly different acoustic impedances than soft tissue. As such, bone and air interfaces with soft tissue present effectively infinite acoustic impedances. Such interfaces can lead to image artifacts including shadowing beyond the tissue boundary and mirror image artifacts that are caused by multiple reflections from an object of interest and the tissue boundary.

Speckle noise is characteristic of US imaging and is caused by constructive and destructive interferences within the sinusoidal US pressure field resulting from reflections of multiple microscopic scatterers. This interaction produces the grainy, black and white speckled appearance characteristic of US imaging. This noise can be reduced through the use of spatial compounding, wherein the region of interest is interrogated from multiple angles and the images averaged. This reduces the speckle noise while preserving spatial detail of the objects of interest.

US fields for diagnostic imaging are focused to provide enhanced signal intensity at the depth of interest. This is most commonly achieved electronically by differing the pulse timing across the transducer surface, thereby producing regions of constructive and destructive interference patterns. This technique can be used for both focusing and steering of the US beam. The physics of US propagation and image formation is a well-described topic, and the reader is referred to other texts for more detail.[3,4]

2.3 Image-Guided Prostate Brachytherapy

Prostate brachytherapy is the most common radiation therapy application for which US image guidance is used. This technique gained widespread popularity with patients and physicians in the 1990s. A large part of this was attributable to the availability of low-energy interstitial isotopes (Iodine-125 and Palladium-103). Because the low-energy characteristic x-rays emitted by these sources had a relatively low-penetration depth in tissue, the radiation protection considerations were relaxed and the procedure could be performed on an outpatient basis. Detailed descriptions of this procedure exist within the literature, and as such, only a brief and focused description is provided here.[5,6]

Imaging is used for prostate brachytherapy during the planning, implantation, and postimplantation evaluation processes. As is true for all radiotherapy image-guidance systems, the image data set must be accurately registered to a relevant spatial coordinate system. This is achieved by rigidly attaching the US transducer to a mechanical stepping system and integrated, registered needle insertion template. The US transducer is inserted into the patient's rectum, positioning the needle template over the perineum. The endorectal transducer yields axial and sagittal image sets via two integrated and orthogonal transducer element arrays.

US imaging is well suited for this procedure due, in part, to its unique ability to distinguish soft tissue boundaries. In Figure 2.1, we compare images of a patient's prostate using transrectal US (TRUS), planar kV, and CT imaging. One form of planar kV imaging, fluoroscopy, is often used in the implant suite to verify needle and seed placements. CT imaging is often used following the implant to assess the dose coverage of the implanted seed distribution, which varies from the planned distribution due to the finite accuracy with which the seeds can be placed. The prostatic boundary is visible on the US image, whereas the planar kV image is only able to differentiate boney anatomy. The CT image provides improved, but imperfect, differentiation of local soft tissue detail.

Image data sets can be categorized in terms of their dimensionality, with two- and three-dimensional (2D and 3D) data sets being most commonly used for routine clinical applications. The first three dimensions refer to spatial dimensions, with higher order dimensionality referring typically to time or biophysical function. TRUS and CT imaging are similar, in that 3D data sets are constructed through the acquisition and reconstruction of multiple, parallel 2D images. The acquisition time, anatomical range, and total file size are directly correlated with the number of 2D images acquired. Planar kV imaging is advantageous

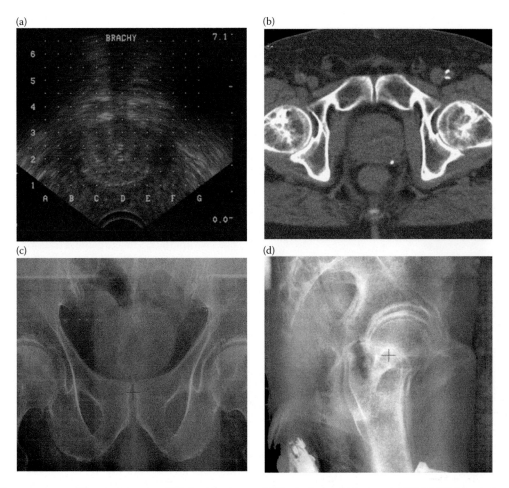

FIGURE 2.1 The appearance of the prostate using differing imaging modalities is shown: (a) transrectal US, (b) CT, (c) anterior planar kV imaging, (d) lateral planar kV imaging. Soft tissue detail is different on the transrectal US and CT images and is not meaningfully present on the kV planar images.

because of its rapid acquisition time and large anatomical field of view. It achieves this, however, through an intrinsic averaging of 3D data, which necessarily reduce its ability to distinguish soft tissues.

It is instructive in this context to note a series of publications that studied differences in prostate volumes determined via US, CT, and MR. These were prompted by observations obtained during clinical practice in which the prostate volume determined via US prior to implant differed markedly from that determined via CT following the implant. Narayana et al. found that the difference in prostate volume between preimplant TRUS and preimplant CT was typically 47%, thus describing intermodality variations.[7] Similarly, Roach et al. compared prostate volumes using noncontrast CT and MR imaging. They found that, on average, the CT-derived prostate volumes were larger than the MR-defined volumes by 32%.[8] This difference may arise due to difficulties in visualizing the prostatic capsule embedded in the surrounding soft tissue matrix. Badiozamani et al. demonstrated that agreement could be achieved by excluding the puborectalis muscles and venous plexis.[9] Notwithstanding,

the differentiation of the prostatic capsule from the surrounding plexus is challenging and requires imaging systems with superior low contrast resolution.

This point is illustrated in Figure 2.2, in which a CT scan (a) is compared to an artist's rendering of the relevant anatomy (c).[10] The prostate contour drawn by the physician is shown in (b). Note that the exact location of the prostate boundary is drawn without the aid of any differentiating gray scale information within the plexus and is therefore inherently subjective.

2.4 US for External Beam Radiation Therapy Image Guidance

The use of US imaging for EBRT guidance requires accurate spatial registration of the transducer and imaging plane. Commercial systems use an articulating arm, infrared (IR) cameras and reflective markers, or an optical camera mounted directly to the transducer. The spatial accuracy of these systems has been measured to be on the order of 1–5 mm.[11–14]

(a)

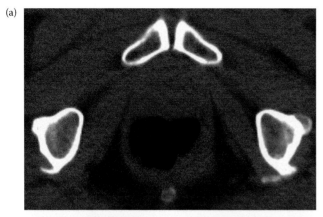

(b)

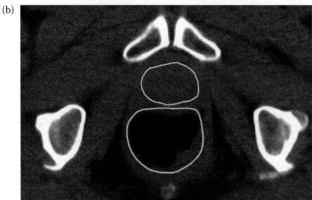

(c)

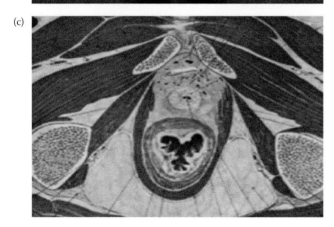

FIGURE 2.2 A CT scan of a patient's prostate (a) with the CTV and rectum drawn in (b). An artist's rendering (c) shows the prostate capsule embedded in the surrounding plexus. CT imaging differentiates between the fat and musculature but is not able to reveal the prostate capsule. Contouring is done using clinical experience and can be subjective. (J. A. Molloy, S. Srivastava, and B. F. Schneider, *Med Phys.*, 31, 433–442, 2004)

2.4.1 General Calibration Techniques

Development of spatially registered US imagery requires transformation of the coordinates in the image plane frame of reference to the treatment room isocenter coordinate system. This requires multiple hardware components that attach rigidly

to the US transducer, treatment room, or accelerator gantry. The various manufacturers of US systems for EBRT guidance use different hardware strategies for achieving communication between the moving US transducer and the fixed treatment room isocenter coordinate system. These are subsequently described in detail.

All systems require certain components that will be described generally as transducer calibration hardware (TCH) and room calibration hardware (RCH). The TCH is the mechanical component that attaches rigidly and reproducibly to the US transducer. It possesses some method for communicating its location and orientation to the RCH. The RCH is rigidly attached to the treatment room (either directly or indirectly) and is therefore considered stationary. The physical location of a pixel within the US image plane is transformed into treatment room coordinates by applying a series of transformation matrices.

$$
\begin{bmatrix} x_{ISO} \\ y_{ISO} \\ z_{ISO} \\ 1 \end{bmatrix} = {}^{ISO}T_{RCH} \times {}^{RCH}T_{TCH} \times {}^{TCH}T_{IP} \times \begin{bmatrix} s_x & s_y & 0 & 1 \end{bmatrix} \times \begin{bmatrix} x_{IP} \\ y_{IP} \\ 0 \\ 1 \end{bmatrix} \quad (2.3)
$$

where,

x_{IP}, y_{IP} = a point with coordinates in the image plane coordinate system

s_x, s_y = image plane scale factors (mm/pixel)

${}^{TCH}T_{IP}$ = transformation matrix from image plane coordinates to transducer hardware coordinates

${}^{RCH}T_{TCH}$ = transformation matrix from transducer hardware coordinates to RCH coordinates

${}^{ISO}T_{RCH}$ = transformation matrix from RCH coordinates to isocenter coordinates

$x_{ISO}, y_{ISO}, z_{ISO}$ = coordinates of the point in the isocenter coordinate system.

The process of deriving the spatial location of an object within the US image plane requires multiple steps. First, the relative spatial position of the pixels within the image plane must be known. This is provided as an integral assumption of the diagnostic US unit and is most commonly verified by interrogating a phantom containing test objects at known spatial locations. The US unit's native ruler tool can be used to verify proper spatial calibration.

Next, one must derive the translational and rotational matrices that transform the location of an image pixel into room coordinates. This process is shown schematically in Figure 2.3. These matrices contain the Euler angles described by classical mechanics and possess a total of 6 degrees of freedom, 3 rotational and 3 translational. A body of literature exists,

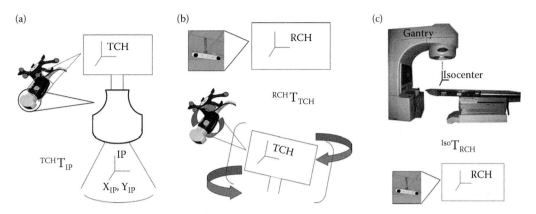

(a)   (b)   (c)

FIGURE 2.3 Transformation matrices need to be determined to spatially register the elements within the US image plane into the treatment room isocenter coordinate system. The transformation from the image plane (IP) to TCH is shown in (a). In (b), the transformation from the TCH to the RCH coordinate system is shown and illustrates the dynamic character of this transformation. Real-time data transmission from the TCH to the RCH is what allows for the accurate superposition of US image data onto the static reference CT (or US) image data set. In (c), the transformation from the RCH to the isocenter (ISO) coordinate system is shown.

describing the methods for deriving the matrix elements.[15–17] These rely on the acquisition of multiple images of the same test object(s) over a range of interrogation angles, followed by the application of computerized optimization routines.

Clinically, it is not necessary for the physicist to derive each matrix independently. Verification of the integrity of the matrix values supplied by the manufacturer is performed by placing a calibration phantom at the treatment room isocenter position. By acquiring and comparing a US image to treatment planning contours of the phantom test objects, the spatial calibration can be verified or adjusted. This process is shown in Figure 2.4.

2.4.2 Device-specific Spatial Calibration

Each manufacturer uses a unique hardware strategy and associated calibration procedure. These can be categorized as articulating arms, IR camera-based systems, and optical camera systems. The calibration processes and hardware components are compared schematically in Figure 2.5.

2.4.2.1 Arm Technology

The B-mode acquisition and targeting (BAT®) system was the first US system introduced to the market for EBRT localization (NOMOS, Cranberry Township, PA, now BEST Medical). Positional feedback was provided by an articulating arm that incorporated optical encoders embedded into each "elbow" joint (shown in Figure 2.6). By rigidly attaching the US transducer to the arm, its location and orientation were accurately known. Its user interface allowed the comparison of the US image to the CT-derived contours in two, quasiorthogonal planes.[18,19]

2.4.2.2 Infrared Camera-based Systems

The Sonarray® US system was introduced to the market by Zmed (now Varian Medical Systems) and differed from the BAT system primarily in two ways.[20] The 3D image data are acquired by sweeping the US image plane across the volume of interest

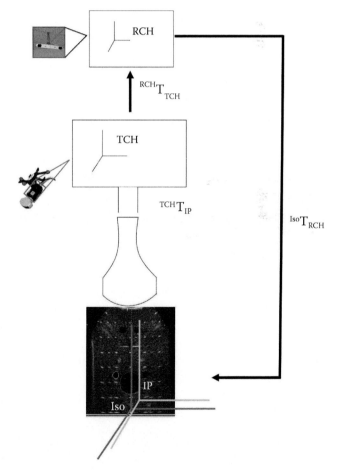

FIGURE 2.4 Multiple transformations are required to calibrate the US image plane with respect to the treatment room isocenter coordinate system. In clinical practice, the integrity of the transformation matrix components is adjusted and verified by comparing a US image of a phantom placed reproducibly at isocenter, with CT-derived contours that correspond to the isocenter coordinate system.

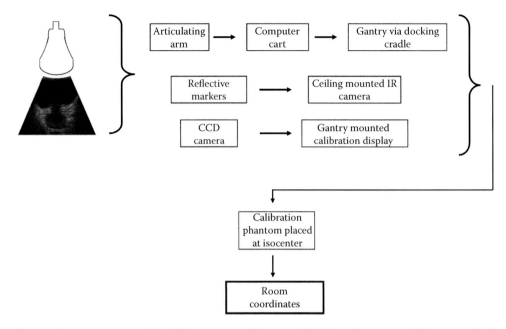

FIGURE 2.5 A schematic diagram comparing the calibration steps and associated hardware for various calibration methods is shown.

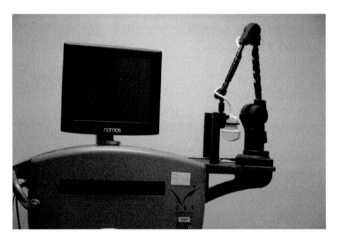

FIGURE 2.6 The BAT® system's early versions used an articulating arm for spatial registration of US images. A docking cradle mounted to the gantry tray slot provides a frame of reference to room coordinates.

and the data reconstructed in three dimensions. The transducer's position and orientation were measured using a ceiling-mounted IR camera system and reflective markers rigidly attached to the transducer. This offered improved positional flexibility over the articulating arm technology and was later incorporated into the BAT system.

The Clarity system (Resonant Medical, now Elekta, Montreal, CA) also provides US guidance via IR camera-based spatial registration.[21,22] This system is integrated into the simulation process as well as the treatment delivery verification process. Spatial registration to the room isocenter is achieved by installing an additional camera into the CT simulation suite and through the application of relevant calibration procedures and software tools. Automated segmentation routines can be used to

define a reference target structure (acquired during simulation) and during daily alignment. The camera and reflective markers for the Clarity system are shown in Figure 2.7.

2.4.2.3 Optical Camera Technology

Optical camera technology is incorporated into CMS's IBeam® system. A small CCD camera is mounted directly onto the US transducer, and an optical calibration plate is mounted to the linear accelerator gantry. This plate possesses geometric patterns that are captured by the camera, as shown in Figure 2.8. The relative positions within the camera's field of view are de-convolved to generate the position and orientation of the US transducer.

2.4.3 User Interface

Commercial systems used for radiotherapy image guidance incorporate user interfaces that present the US image planes in the context of other relevant spatial information. This typically includes CT-derived structure contours and isocenter coordinates. An example from the BAT interface is shown in Figure 2.9. The interface allows simulation of a translation of the patient coordinates to affect a match between the structures of interest.

2.4.4 Clinical Process Flow

The clinical process flow typically begins with a CT-based simulation, including contouring of the structures of interest (e.g., prostate, rectum, bladder) and establishment of the treatment isocenter location within the patient's anatomy. The treatment planning process then proceeds, which yields the linear accelerator input parameters required to affect the desired isodose configuration. The isocenter coordinates, CT-derived structure contours, and, in some cases, CT image data are then transferred to the US guidance system. This transfer process

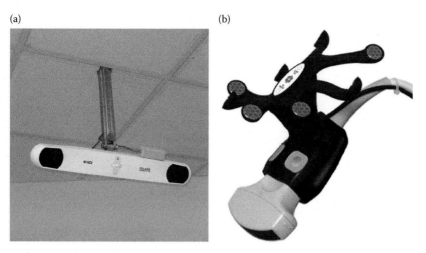

FIGURE 2.7 A ceiling-mounted infrared camera system is shown in (a). The associated US transducer and reflective markers are shown in (b). (Illustration courtesy of Elekta Medical Systems.)

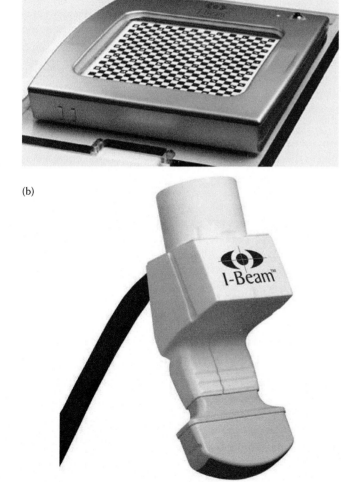

FIGURE 2.8 The calibration grid for the CMS I-beam system (a) is positioned in the gantry tray slot. An image of the geometric pattern is acquired by the transducer-mounted camera (b) and automated pattern recognition algorithms confirm the spatial calibration of the US transducer. (Illustration courtesy of Computerized Medical Systems (CMS).)

typically utilizes a standardized radiotherapy data transfer protocol, such as RTOG or DICOM. These file formats contain the spatial registration information for the isocenter, structures, and CT data that will be required to register the US image information during the localization process.

At the initiation of treatment, the patient is positioned on the linear accelerator support table and aligned to the in-room lasers. The US localization system is used to acquire images of the prostate or other tissues of interest, which are then compared to the reference contours. The user simulates a patient translation using the US guidance system's user interface until the daily US images and reference anatomy are appropriately aligned. The treatment table is then translated by the required amount, and an additional set of US verification images can be acquired if desired.

2.4.5 Clinical Use Issues

Air interfaces effectively present infinite acoustic impedance for diagnostic US imaging systems. As such, good acoustic coupling between the US transducer and patient surfaces must be maintained. This is achieved by applying a coupling gel to the patient surface and maintaining firm pressure to exclude air during image acquisition. Temporary tissue displacement resulting from this pressure has the potential to introduce systematic errors into the localization process.

This issue was studied during the early adoption of US image guidance.[13,23–27] Multiple methods were used to assess prostatic displacement including implantation of fiducial markers and planar x-ray, CT, or MR imaging. In general, these studies found that typical levels of pressure result in displacements of 0–5 mm. The interpretation of these results in terms of clinical impact varies among potential users of these systems. Some regard these displacements to be unacceptable. Others embrace a practice in which users apply only moderate amounts of probe pressure and regard the displacements to be relatively small and acceptable in the context of the improved target visualization and localization. It should be noted that target displacement

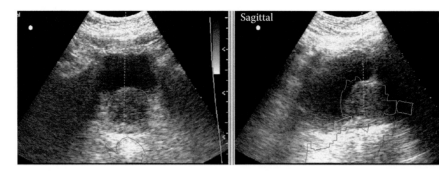

FIGURE 2.9 (See color insert)   The user interface displays quasiorthogonal US images with the isocenter indicators (blue lines) and CT-derived contours of the prostate (orange), urethra (green), rectum (red), and seminal vesicles (yellow). (J. A. Molloy, S. Srivastava, and B. F. Schneider, *Med Phys.*, 31, 433–442, 2004. With permission.)

is inherent in the verification studies of the accuracy of these systems, which suggests that, under typical clinical conditions, the overall displacement and targeting uncertainty remains less than 5 mm.

Appropriate applications of US imaging are limited to anatomical sites for which there exists an acoustic window, that is, an acoustically unobstructed view of the areas of interest. Obstructions are most commonly produced by bone, air, or excessive soft tissue depth. For prostate localization, the acoustic window consists of the region superior to the pubic arch and passing through the bladder. Because of this pathway, insufficient bladder filling can cause a marked decrease in the visibility of distal structures. In clinical practice, patients are typically instructed to arrive for their radiotherapy treatments with a moderately full bladder.

2.4.5.1 Interuser Variability

The interpretation of anatomical information on US imaging is nonintuitive to inexperienced users. This fact prompted several investigations into interuser variability of US alignment. The results and interpretation of these studies vary, with some studies showing only very limited improvement in alignment[28] and others showing US guidance to result in improved target alignment with much lower levels of interuser variability.[29–31] These studies used differing approaches when accounting for user training and indicated a positive correlation between user experience and interobserver consistency. These data underscore the importance of training, experience, and continued assessment during implementation and clinical use.

2.4.5.2 Contouring

Commercial US localization systems incorporate a user interface that presents an outline of manually entered structure contours superimposed onto the daily US images (see Figure 2.9). These contours are used to determine patient repositioning parameters. Within this context, one must consider that the target and OARs are typically contoured for the purpose of dosimetric treatment planning. Asymmetric planning target volume (PTV) margins are often applied around the clinical target volume (CTV) to yield rectal or bladder sparing. For example, the posterior PTV

margin surrounding the prostate CTV is often 3 mm, whereas the PTV margin in the other directions is 5–10 mm. If the PTV contours are used directly for US-guided patient alignment, care must be taken to position the prostate in the same relative location as was intended during the treatment planning process (e.g., closer to the posterior contour boundary). An alternative approach is to create a set of "alignment" contours that do not possess potentially confounding asymmetric margins. Use of a reference US image acquired at the time of simulation also has the potential to reduce systematic errors associated with contouring uncertainties.

2.4.5.3 Intermodality Issues

Additional ambiguity can arise in the US alignment process due to the introduction of interimaging modality differences in the appearance of the structures of interest. This was illustrated qualitatively in Figure 2.2. The Clarity system addresses this issue directly by supplying US guidance systems for both the simulation and treatment suites. In comparing cross-modality (i.e., US/CT) to intramodality (i.e., US/US) alignment, Cury et al. discovered a significant systematic difference between the two methods.[32] Intermodality variations can be caused by differing appearance, contouring issues (described earlier), and tissue deformation.

2.4.6 US Guidance in the Era of Gold Seed Localization

The introduction of gold marker seed localization strategies for prostate radiotherapy prompted a series of studies comparing that method to US localization.[33] Use of gold marker seeds represents an appealing alternative to US localization, due primarily to ease of use and reproducibility. The seeds are, in general, visible using electronic portal imaging devices (EPIDs) and have small interuser variability compared to US localization. The literature[33] comparing prostate positioning using marker seeds and US has revealed discrepancies between the two methods that have raised concerns over the use of US.

While marker seeds *may* (or may not) produce superior daily localization, the literature published to date has not addressed potential sources of error in the seed positioning strategy and has to a large degree regarded the marker seed positions as unquestionable surrogates for the prostate position. Numerous potential sources of error exist in marker seed positioning strategies, including DRR resolution, patient motion, edema-induced seed migration (particularly if the planning CT was performed shortly following the seed implant), and prostate deformation. In addition, marker seeds are indicators of the center of mass of the prostate and do not reveal information regarding local soft tissue deformation, as is often present at the bladder and rectal wall interfaces. Indeed, the US matching process can include an assessment of the positions of these soft tissue interfaces, in addition to the prostate center of mass. The alignment task presented to the user of US guidance is more complex and certainly contributes to interuser variability and discrepancies with seed matching techniques.

2.4.7 US Imaging in the Era of Online Cone-Beam CT Imaging

Cone-beam CT imaging (CBCT) is an alternative imaging modality that can be applied to prostate and other radiotherapy localization tasks. Multiple linear accelerator vendors integrate this technology into their treatment machine platforms. An amorphous silicone flat panel imaging detector and kV x-ray source are mounted onto the linear accelerator gantry. The orientation of the resultant kV imaging plane is orthogonal to therapeutic x-ray beam. By rotating the gantry during image acquisition, a 3D CBCT image data set is acquired. The image data sets are intrinsically spatially registered to room coordinates by mounting the source and image acquisition hardware directly to the accelerator gantry and applying an appropriate calibration protocol.

Online CBCT imaging can be applied to prostate localization, as this imaging modality provides a much wider field of view (compared to US imaging) and good spatial fidelity. Localization can be achieved using adjacent soft tissue anatomy, although the differentiation of the actual prostate capsule is elusive, as already discussed for diagnostic CT imaging.[34] Daily application of this technology, however, results in increased radiation exposure to surrounding normal tissues.[35-37] CBCT has a limited field of view compared to diagnostic CT imaging, and as such, localization of very laterally positioned targets is cumbersome and requires multiple repositioning of the patient support table. In one study, US localization using the BAT system was assessed in comparison to CBCT using fiducial markers and was found to have residual errors of less than 1 mm in all three dimensions.[38]

2.5 Quality Assurance

To date, quality assurance procedures have derived primarily from vendor recommendations. Recently, Tome and Orton described a quality assurance program for US imaging systems for target localizations (UISTLs).[39] They advised that a comprehensive quality assurance program should include training and performance monitoring, as well as prescreening of patients who may not be good candidates for US localization. Professional guidance documents exist for diagnostic US imaging and prostate brachytherapy US systems.[40,41] While these documents do not directly address US guidance systems for external beam radiotherapy applications, they describe relevant principles in terms of image quality and spatial accuracy assessment. The American Association of Physicists in Medicine (AAMP) has charged Task Group 154 with creating a guidance document that focuses exclusively on US image guidance systems for EBRT applications.[42]

Analysis of the potential for error propagation in the US imaging localization chain includes the following components:

CT simulation—Laser alignment, image quality, and scan resolution, particularly in the superior/inferior dimension, will affect system accuracy.

Contouring—Differentiation of the prostate capsule within the surrounding parenchyma is tenuous using CT imaging. Delineation of the CT-derived target volume is user dependent. In addition, since contouring is typically performed on axial CT slices, the continuity and accuracy of the contours can suffer in the superior/inferior dimension. Consistency must be applied when contouring treatment planning structures that usually have asymmetric margins. One method for avoiding confusion during daily patient alignment is to provide separate contours that are designed specifically for target alignment.

Mechanical/spatial calibration—System components include the US transducer coupling to the spatial registration device (i.e., articulating arm or reflective markers), docking cradle or camera, and software calibration parameters.

Image interpretation—Intermodality imaging differences, marginal US image quality, and deformable anatomy all contribute to the potential for alignment discrepancies.

Patient immobilization—Patient motion following US aligment will directly affect accuracy.

A typical quality assurance program may include the following components:
Geometric/spatial accuracy
Daily tests:

- Laser alignment: (1 mm), treatment room and simulator suite, daily
- Positioning constancy: (2 mm), use stationary phantom, daily
- IR camera verification (if applicable): 60-min warm-up, mechanical stability, daily

Monthly tests:

- Positioning constancy: (2 mm), performed by physicist, includes overt camera calibration (if applicable)

- Phantom offset test: (2 mm), offset phantom in three dimensions and verify that system returns it to proper position
- Laser offset test: (1 mm), in simulation suite if applicable; verifies accurate functioning of movable lasers and integration into localization process

Quarterly tests:
- Phantom stability: desiccation, mechanical stability

Annual tests:
- End–end testing: (2 mm), acquire reference CT of phantom, contour structures, set-up, alignment, test for objects near and distant to isocenter

Image quality
Semiannual: (All criteria are compared to baseline)

- Spatial resolution
- Low contrast resolution
- Sensitivity
- Hardware degradation

2.6 Other Applications

2.6.1 Partial Breast Radiotherapy

Partial breast radiotherapy (PBRT) is an emerging application of 3D US guidance. Resonant Medical integrated components into its Clarity® US guidance system designed to support localization for PBRT using EBRT. This clinical scenario utilizes US imaging in the context in which it performs optimally. In comparison to prostate applications, the relatively superficial location of most breast seromas eases the difficulty imposed by US's limited penetration depth. In addition, US is fundamentally a soft tissue differentiator and is well suited for the task of distinguishing the seroma cavity from the surrounding tissues. CT imaging can lack the low contrast resolution necessary for this imaging task, particularly for patients with dense breast parenchyma.[43,44] The additional radiation dose associated with daily CBCT imaging is prohibitive to some clinicians. Figure 2.10 illustrates a potential difference between target delineation based on US imaging versus CT imaging of surgical clips. Use of daily US imaging for patient alignment also has the potential to illuminate changes in the seroma volume that may occur over the course of treatment (see Figure 2.11).

The PBRT module on the Clarity system replaces the standard curvilinear transducer with a linear one. Spatial calibration to the simulation and treatment room isocenters is achieved using the same methods as described for the prostate localization technologies. In addition, the Clarity system incorporates a tracing stylus that is spatially registered using the system's optical guidance technology. This stylus can be used to trace the edges of an electron boost field, compared to the US imaging set. The clinical process flow includes acquisition of a 3D US data set at the time of CT simulation for use as a reference image. This reference image set can be used for target definition during treatment planning and to provide an intramodality reference for subsequent daily localization. Tissue deformation due to probe pressure must be managed in this clinical setting. Use of the reference US image, acquired at the time of simulation and used for treatment planning, can reduce systematic errors.

2.6.2 Upper Abdominal Malignancies

Application of US image guidance for abdominal malignancies is a promising area, given that the target structures and organs at risk are soft tissues. The acoustic window in these scenarios is wide, as there are only minimal boney obstructions, although air pockets within the region can present limited, but unpredictable, obstructions. The complex anatomy within the region requires users with specific confidence in abdominal US. However, CT-derived contours that are presented during the US guidance process can aid in structure recognition.

Mechanistically, the procedures for abdominal US image guidance do not vary significantly from those used for prostate localization. The process includes initial CT simulation and contouring of the target, avoidance, and matching structures. These structures are exported to the US guidance system and used for daily alignment. Abdominal applications differ, however, in that the anatomy of interest is generally only partly differentiated by US imaging, where distinct and complete tissue boundaries are elusive.

Fuss et al. studied the potential of US-guided localization for reducing daily positioning uncertainty, PTV margins, and clinical feasibility for applications in the upper abdomen.[45,46] They used local vascular anatomy as guidance structures to compensate for the limited visibility of the target volumes and organs at risk. Specifically, for hepatic targets, the branches of the portal vein, hepatic artery, and dilated bile ducts were found to be useful guidance structures. For other retroperitoneal sites, the aorta, celiac trunk, superior mesenteric artery, and extra-hepatic aspects of the portal vein system were used as anatomical fiducials. Comparison to control CT scans on 15 patients revealed setup error reduction in 93% of the patients, with a residual setup error of 4.6 ± 3.4 mm. Relative to skin marks, the mean daily shift magnitude was 11.4 ± 7.6 mm.

2.7 Summary and Conclusions

US imaging has been shown to improve target localization for EBRT of the prostate and certain other cancers. The recent introduction of other online imaging modalities such as planar kV, gold seed alignment, and CBCT has precipitated scrutiny of US imaging and reduced its use for EBRT localization. Effective use of US image guidance requires careful attention to related clinical processes.

Use of a reference US image set, acquired during the simulation process, can reduce systematic errors. Such errors may occur as a result of probe-pressure-induced target displacement or from interuser variability resulting from image

(a) (b)

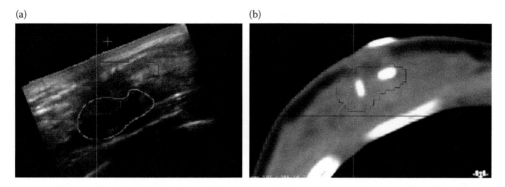

FIGURE 2.10 (See color insert) The potential difference in target definition for a breast seroma as indicated by US imaging (a) (green contour) versus CT imaging and surgical clips (b) (red contour) is illustrated. Soft tissue differentiation on the CT image is not feasible and reliance on surgical clips can produce a systematic positioning error. The seroma cavity is readily identifiable on the US image. (Illustration courtesy of Elekta Medical Systems [formally Resonant].)

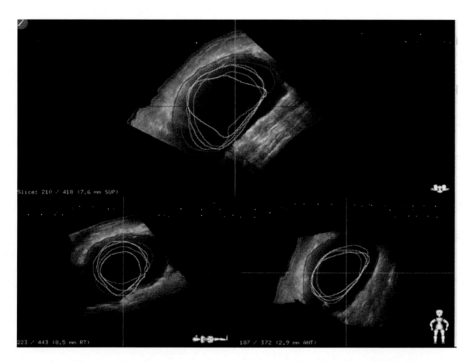

FIGURE 2.11 (See color insert) Changes in seroma volume over the course of treatment may be appreciated via daily US guidance. The various colored contours represent the seroma volume as determined via daily US. (Illustration courtesy of Resonant Medical.)

interpretation differences. Acquisition of a US reference image set during simulation also provides the opportunity to screen for patients who do not image well and allows for alternative image-guidance strategies to be administered if necessary.

If CT data sets are used for target delineation, then they must be acquired with appropriate spatial resolution, particularly in the superior/inferior dimension. Course spatial resolution results in target segmentation and, therefore, alignment uncertainties. In addition, the goals of the target alignment should be communicated to all staff participating in patient treatment, for example, whether to align the prostate/bladder interface or the prostate center-of-mass.

Careful attention to total quality assurance must be applied. This includes accuracy and consistency of laser alignment between the simulation and treatment suites, routine mechanical calibration verification, and sufficient user training.

US imaging possesses excellent soft tissue differentiation and does not contribute to unnecessary low levels of ionizing radiation dose. It is highly cost-effective and portable. In addition to its traditional role in prostate localization, US imaging has promise for other treatment sites, including the breast and upper abdomen. Applications for partial breast irradiation appear particularly promising, given the shallow depth of most of these lesions and the need to differentiate soft tissues in this context.

Acknowledgments

The author acknowledges the contributions of Doug Pfieffer for providing technical details regarding US imaging physics and Ali Bodager for assistance with illustrations and editing. Thanks also to Martin Lachaine from Resonant Medical and members of AAPM Task Group 154, Bill Salter, Alex Markovic, Shawn McNeeley, Wolfgang Tome, and Gordon Chan.

References

1. D. A. Jaffray and J. W. Wong, Managing geometric uncertainty in conformal intensity-modulated radiation therapy, *Semin Radiat Oncol* **9**, 4–19 (1999).
2. J. C. Blasko, P. D. Grimm, and H. Ragde, Brachytherapy and organ preservation in the management of carcinoma of the prostate, *Semin Radiat Oncol* **3**, 240–249 (1993).
3. *Medical CT and Ultrasound: Current Technology and Applications*, L. Goldman and J. Fowlkes, eds. (Advanced Medical Publishing, Madison, WI, 1995).
4. N. Hangiandreou, "B-mode US: basic concepts and new technology," *RadGrap* **23**, 1019–33 (2003).
5. Y. Yu, L. L. Anderson, Z. Li, D. E. Mellenberg, R. Nath, M. C. Cchell, F. M. Waterman, A. Wu, and J. Blaski, Permanent prostate seed implant brachytherapy: report of the American Association of Physicists in Medicine Task Group No. 64, *Med Phys* **26**(10), 2054–76 (1999).
6. H. Holm, N. Juul, J. Pedersen, H. Hansen, and I. Stroyer, Transperineal 125 Iodine seed implantation in prostatic cancer guided by transrectal ultrasonography, *J Urol* (Baltimore) **130**(2), 283–6 (1983).
7. V. Narayan, P. L. Roberson, A. T. Pu., R. J. Winfield, and P. W. McLaughlin, Impact of differences in ultrasound and computed tomography volumes on treatment planning of permanent prostate implants, *Int J Radiat Oncol Biol Phys* **37**, 1181–5 (1997).
8. M. Roach III, P. Faillace-Akazawa, C. Malfatti, J. Holland, and H. Hricak, Prostate volumes defined by magnetic resonance imaging and computerized tomographic scans for three-dimensional conformal radiotherapy, *Int J Radiat Oncol Biol Phys* **35**, 1011–18 (1996).
9. K. R. Badiozamani, K. Wallner, W. Cavanagh, and J. Blasko, Comparability of CT-based and TRUS-based prostate volumes, *Int J Radiat Oncol Biol Phys* **43**, 375–8 (1999).
10. B. L. Carter, J. Morehead, S. M. Wolpert, S. B. Hammerschlag, H. J. Griffiths, and P. C. Kahn, *Cross Sectional Anatomy: Computed Tomography and Ultrasound Correlation* (Appleton-Century-Crofts, New York, 1977), Section 41.
11. J. Lattanzi, S. McNeeley, W. Pinover, E. Horowitz, I. Das, T. Schultheiss, and G. E. Hanks, A comparison of daily CT localization to a daily ultrasound-based system in prostate cancer, *Int J Radiat Oncol Biol Phys* **43**, 719–25 (1999).
12. J. Lattanzi, S. McNeeley, A. Hanlon, T. Schultheiss, and G. E. Hanks, Ultrasound-based stereotactic guidance of precision conformal external beam radiation therapy in clinically localized prostate cancer, *Urology* **55**, 73–8 (2000).
13. C. F. Serago, S. J. Chungbin, S. J. Buskirk, G. A. Ezzell, A. C. Collie, and S. A. Vora, Initial experience with ultrasound localization for positioning prostate cancer patients for external beam radiotherapy, *Int J Radiat Oncol Biol Phys* **53**, 1130–8 (2002).
14. J. A. Molloy, S. Srivastava, and B. F. Schneider, A method to compare supra-pubic ultrasound and CT images of the prostate: technique and early clinical results, *Med Phys* **31**, 433–42 (2004).
15. L. Mercier, T. Lango, F. Lindseth, and L. D. Collins, A review of calibration techniques for freehand 3D ultrasound systems, *Ultrasound Med Biol* **31**, 143–65 (2005).
16. L. G. Bouchet, S. L. Meeks, G. Goodchild, F. J. Bova, J. M. Buatti, and W. A. Friedman, Calibration of three-dimensional ultrasound images for image-guided radiation therapy, *Phys Med Biol* **46**, 559–77 (2001).
17. S. Dandakar, Y. Li, J. A. Molloy, and J. Hossack, A phantom with reduced complexity for spatial 3D ultrasound calibration, *Ultrasound Med Biol* **8**, 1083–93 (2005).
18. D. S. Mohan, P. A. Kupelian, and T. R. Willoughby, Short-course intensity-modulated radiotherapy for localized prostate cancer with daily transabdominal ultrasound localization of the prostate gland, *Int J Radiat Oncol Biol Phys* **46**, 575–80 (2000).
19. J. Morr, T. DiPetrillo, J.-S. Tsai, M. Engler, and D. E. Wazer, Implementation and utility of a daily ultrasound-based localization system with intensity-modulated radiotherapy for prostate cancer, *Int J Radiat Oncol Biol Phys* **53**, 1124–9 (2002).
20. W. A. Tome, S. L. Meeks, N. P. Orton, L. G. Bouchet, and F. J. Bova, Commissioning and quality assurance of an optically guided three-dimensional ultrasound target localization system for radiotherapy, *Med Phys* **29**, 1781–88 (2002).
21. S. Wan, L. Stillwaugh, H. Prichard, J. Bowen, and D. Provost, Evaluation of a 3D ultrasound system for image-guided radiation therapy for prostate cancer, *Int J Radiat Oncol Biol Phys* **72**, S555 (2008).
22. C. Mark, A. Chang, F. DeBlois, F. Cury, T. Vuong, T. Falco, and F. Verhaegen, Monte Carlo dose calculation in prostate patients aided by 3D ultrasound imaging, *Med Phys* **32**, 1935 (2005).
23. J. P. McGahan, J. Ryu, and M. Fogata, Ultrasound probe pressure as a source of error in prostate localization for external beam radiotherapy, *Int J Radiat Oncol Biol Phys* **60**, 788–93 (2004).
24. B. Dobler, S. Mai, C. Ross, et al., Evaluation of possible prostate displacement induced by pressure applied during transabdominal ultrasound image acquisition, *Strahlenther Onkol* **182**, 240–6 (2006).

25. S. McNeeley, M. Buyyounouski, R. Price, et al., Prostate displacement during transabdominal ultrasound, *Med Phys* **29**, 1341 (2002).

26. X. Artignan, M. H. Smitsmans, J. V. Lebesque, D. A. Jaffray, M. van Her, and H. Bartelink, Online ultrasound image guidance for radiotherapy of prostate cancer: impact of image acquisition on prostate displacement, *Int J Radiat Oncol Biol Phys* **59**, 595–601 (2004).

27. B. J. Salter, B. Wang, M. Szegedi, J. D. Tward, and D. C. Shrieve, Prostate displacement during and after transabdominal US guidance, monitored by a real-time tracking system, *Int J Radiat Oncol Biol Phys* **72**, S146–S147 (2008).

28. K. Langen, J. Pouliot, C. Anezinos, et al., Evaluation of ultrasound-based prostate localization for image-guided radiotherapy, *Int J Radiat Oncol Biol Phys* **57**, 635–44 (2003).

29. W. A. Tomé, S. L. Meeks, N. P. Orton, et al., Patient positioning in radiotherapy using optical guided 3-D ultrasound techniques, in *New Technologies in Radiation Oncology*, W. Schlegel, T. Bortfelde, and A. Grosu, eds. Springer Verlag, Berlin (2005), Chapter 12, pp. 151–164.

30. N. P. Orton, H. A. Jaradat, and W. A. Tomé, Clinical Assessment of three-dimensional ultrasound prostate localization for external beam radiotherapy, *Med Phys* **33**, 4710–17 (2006).

31. M. Fuss, S. X. Cavanaugh, C. Fuss, D. A. Cheek, and B. J. Salter, Daily stereotactic ultrasound prostate targeting: inter-user variability, *Technol Cancer Res Treat* **2**, 161–70 (2003).

32. F. L. B. Cury, G. Shenouda, L. Souhami, M. Duclos, S. L. Faria, M. David, F. Verhaegen, R. Corns, and T. Falco, Ultrasound-based image guided radiotherapy for prostate cancer—comparison of cross-modality and intramodality methods for daily localization during external beam radiotherapy, *Int J Radiat Oncol Biol Phys* **37**, 1562–7 (2006).

33. C. F. Serago, S. J. Buskirk, T. C. Igel, A. A. Gale, N. E. Serago, N. E., and J. D. Earle, Comparison of daily megavoltage electronic portal imaging or kilovoltage imaging with marker seeds to ultrasound imaging or skin marks for prostate localization and treatment positioning in patients with prostate cancer, *Int J Radiat Oncol Biol Phys* **65**, 1585–92 (2006).

34. E. A. White, K. K. Brock, D. A. Jaffray, C. N. Catton, Inter-observer variability of prostate delineation on cone beam computerised tomography images, *Clin Oncol* (Royal College of Radiologists) **21**(1), 32–8 (2009).

35. J. R. Perks, J. Lehmann, A. M. Chen, C. C. Yang, R. L. Stern, and J. A. Purdy, Comparison of peripheral dose from image-guided radiation therapy (IGRT) using kV cone beam CT to intensity-modulated radiation therapy (IMRT), *Radiother Oncol* **89**(3), 304–10 (2008).

36. G. X. Ding and C. W. Coffey, Radiation dose from kilovoltage cone beam computed tomography in an image-guided radiotherapy procedure, *Int J Radiat Oncol Biol Phys* **73**(2), 610–7 (2009).

37. J. C. Chow, M. K. Leung, M. K. Islam, B. D. Norrlinger, and D. A. Jaffray, Evaluation of the effect of patient dose from cone beam computed tomography on prostate IMRT using Monte Carlo simulation, *Med Phys* **35**(1), 52–60 (2008).

38. J. Boda-Heggemann, F. M. Kohler, B. Kupper, D. Wolff, H. Wertz, S. Mai, J. Hesser F. Lohr, and F. Wenz, Accuracy of ultrasound-based (BAT) prostate-repositioning: a three-dimensional on-line fiducial-based assessment with cone-beam computed tomography, *Int J Radiat Oncol Biol Phys* **70**(4), 1247–55 (2008).

39. W. A. Tome and N. P. Orton, Quality assurance of ultrasound imaging systems for target localization and online setup corrections, *Int J Radiat Oncol Biol Phys* **71**, S53–S56 (2008).

40. M. M. Goodsitt, P. L. Carson, S. Witt, D. L. Hykes, and J. M. Kofler, Real-time B-mode ultrasound quality control test procedures: report of AAMP Ultrasound Task Group No. 1, *Med Phys* **25**, 1385–406 (1998).

41. D. Pfeiffer, S. Sutlief, W. Feng, H. M. Pierce, and J. Kofler, AAPM Task Group 128: quality assurance tests for prostate brachytherapy ultrasound systems, *Med Phys* **35**, 5471–89 (2008).

42. J. A. Molloy, G. Chan, A. Markovic, S. McNeeley, D. Pfeiffer, B. Salter, and W. Tome, Quality assurance of ultrasound-guided radiotherapy: AAPM Task Group 154, *Med Phys* **38**(2), 857–871 (2011).

43. T. S. Berrang, P. T. Truong, C. Popescu, L. Drever, H. A. Kader, M. L. Hilts, T. Mitchell, S. Y. Soh, L. Sands, S. Silver, and I. A. Olivotto, 3D ultrasound can contribute to planning CT to define the target for partial breast radiotherapy, *Int J Radiat Oncol Biol Phys* **73**, 375–83 (2009).

44. R. P. Petersen, P. T. Truong, H. A. Kader, E. Berthelet, J. C. Lee, M. L. Hilts, A. S. Kader, W. A. Beckham, and I. A. Olivotto, Target volume delineation for partial breast radiotherapy planning: clinical characteristics associated with low interobserver concordance, *Int J Radiat Oncol Biol Phys* **69**, 41–8 (2007).

45. M. Fuss, B. J. Salter, S. X. Cavanaugh, C. Fuss, A. Sadeghi, C. D. Fuller, A. Ameduri, J. M. Hevezi, T. S. Herman, and C. R. Thomas, Jr., Daily ultrasound-based image-guided targeting for radiotherapy of upper abdominal malignancies, *Int J Radiat Oncol Biol Phys* **59**, 1245–56 (2004).

46. M. Fuss, A. Wong, C. D. Fuller, B. J. Salter, C. Fuss, and C. R. Thomas, Jr., Image-guided intensity-modulated radiotherapy for pancreatic carcinoma, *Gastrointest Cancer Res* **1**, 2–11 (2007).

3

In-Room CT System for IGRT

James R. Wong
Morristown Medical Center

Minoru Uematsu
UAS Oncology Center

Zhanrong Gao
Morristown Medical Center

3.1 Introduction

In the past few decades, the radiation oncology field has been transformed by computers—similar to what has happened in our societies. The increase in computing power has led to better computerized treatment planning software, enabling higher quality and more precise delivery of radiation treatments. For example, linear accelerator-based stereotactic radiation therapy (SRT) or stereotactic radiosurgery (SRS) has been made possible, not merely because of advances in head fixation and beam collimation technologies but also because of improvements in software for computer-based treatment planning and delivery. Another important development in the radiation arena is that of intensity-modulated radiation therapy (IMRT), where the fluence intensity of each beam is spatially modulated and regulated (Brahme 1988; Carol et al. 1996; Webb 1992; Yu 1995). Using inverse planning algorithms, each radiation field is broken into multiple small beamlets, allowing optimization of the radiation dose to the target and minimization of the dose to the adjacent critical tissues (Eklof et al. 1990; Kooy and Barth 1990).

A natural progression of the aforementioned advancements for more precise radiation treatments requires verification that the radiation delivered is indeed hitting the target intended, that the radiation delivered to the target is not only precise but also accurate. In fact, such quest for verification of radiation delivery has been an ongoing process—the use of port films to check bony landmarks can be viewed as a rudimentary form of image-guided radiation therapy (IGRT).

In the following sections, we will review the history of in-room CT with regard to IGRT. From the very first type of in-room CT IGRT to the present form, we will see that this particular IGRT approach is dynamic and undergoes constant evolution, and hence, its strength is in adapting to the radiation therapy needs of the future. We will see this system's ability for incorporating the incremental improvements of radiation treatment machines with that of future imaging modalities.

3.2 Early History—The 1990s

In the early 1990s, Uematsu et al. (1996), in their quest to perform SRT or SRS easily without an uncomfortable cranially fixated stereotactic frame, developed a dual computed tomography (CT) linear accelerator unit. This unit, first unveiled at the National Defense Medical College at Saitama, Japan, consists of a linear accelerator, CT scanner, and a motorized table common to both devices. The linear accelerator and the CT are located at opposite ends and share the motorized table as shown in Figure 3.1. The axis of the linear accelerator gantry is coaxial with that of the CT scanner. As such, the isocenter of the treatment target volume, once identified and planned by the CT, can be matched easily with the linear accelerator's gantry axis. This alignment is achieved by rotating the table around the C2 axis. Because SRT and SRS often require radiation to be delivered via noncoplanar arcs, the table in this set up can be rotated around the C1 axis, thus, allowing noncoplanar radiation beams to be delivered.

For the delivery of SRT or SRS, it is very important that the isocenter of the target, as determined by the CT, even after table rotation to the linear accelerator end, can be precisely matched by the isocenter of the linear accelerator. Uematsu et al. demonstrated the precision of this set up by phantom studies illustrated in Figures 3.2–3.4. A metallic target (5 mm

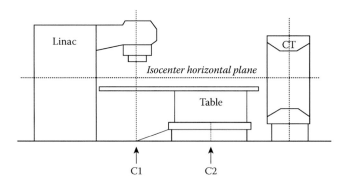

FIGURE 3.1 Diagram of the dual CT-linac treatment unit. The table has two rotational axes; C1 is for isocentric rotation to make noncoplanar arcs and C2 is for rotation between the CT and linac. The gantry axis of the linac is coaxial with that of the CT scanner. (From Uematsu, M., et al., *Int. J. Radiat. Oncol. Biol. Phys.*, (35) 3: 587–592, 1996. With permission.)

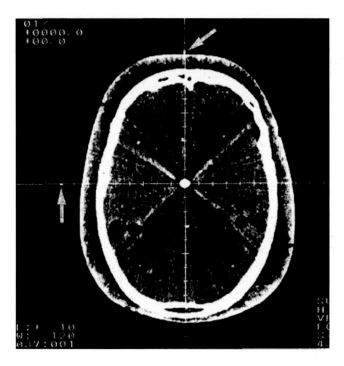

FIGURE 3.2 Final positioning in the phantom examination. (From Uematsu, M., et al., *Int. J. Radiat. Oncol. Biol. Phys.*, (35) 3: 587–592, 1996. With permission.)

in diameter) was put in the phantom and initially scanned with 5-mm slice thick images from the CT scanner. After roughly identifying the target, tiny metallic balls (0.4 mm) were employed to localize the isocenter using 2-mm slice thick images (Figure 3.3). Following this identification of the isocenter, the table was rotated around the C2 axis to match the isocenter of the linear accelerator. Portal films were then obtained with collimator films using a circular aperture (Figure 3.4). At each step, the matching of the isocenter was further confirmed by the assistance of room-mounted lasers. From the portal film

confirmation, it was found that the table rotation error between the CT scanner and the linear accelerator was less than 0.5 mm. Error for the linear accelerator gantry rotation was also within 0.5 mm. Thus, this unit is very accurate and able to treat within a 1-mm isocenter variation.

Treatments of cancers in the brain, liver, and lung using this so-called FOCAL unit (**F**usion **o**f **C**T **a**nd **L**inac) were started in 1994 in Japan. For the treatment of intracranial tumors, survival and tumor control results for patients treated with the FOCAL unit were comparable to published results with conventional SRS- or SRT-treated patients by Gamma Knife or by linac-based, cranially fixated frames (Uematsu et al. 2001).

3.3 From Intracranial to Extracranial Lesions

SRS and SRT have been demonstrated as useful tools for dose escalation in the treatment of intracranial targets. The treatment results for small brain metastasis are excellent, including those metastases from nonsmall-cell lung cancers (NSCLC). The local control rate for these lesions treated by SRS or SRT in the brain is usually around 90%, comparable to that accomplished by surgical resection (Uematsu et al. 2001). These results suggest that small primary lesions of NSCLC may be similarly effectively controlled by high-dose precision radiation therapy to the well-defined targets in the lung (Uematsu et al. 2001). In SRT treatment of brain lesions, multiple radiation beams often pass through many critical neurological pathways to converge at the tumor target. It is not unusual that the tumor target may be closely opposite or adjacent to critical brain structures such as the brainstem or optic pathways. Despite these critical structure limitations, SRT and/or SRS have been shown to be safe and effective for lesions in the brain. In comparison, in the treatment of small lung cancers (≤3 cm), the ratio of high-dose radiation volume to low-dose radiation volume should be smaller than that seen in the treatment of brain tumors. This is because that the overall lung volume is significantly larger than the average brain volume, while the target is of similar size in the brain or the lung for this group of patients studied (both ≤ 3 cm). Moreover, limited volumes of radiation damage in the lung are not likely to cause severe adverse symptoms compared with those in the brain because unlike the brain, tumors in the lung are not always located closely to critical structures and "eloquent" neural tissue, such as the brain stem or major blood vessels. Instead, lung tumor can be at a distance (e.g., 5 cm) from normal structures, and additionally, there is a pulmonary reserve that is usually quite large. Although the adjacent lung tissue to the tumor is destroyed by the radiation, few side effects have been reported using this technique (Uematsu et al. 2001). Thus, small and well-circumscribed lung tumors should be controlled well with focal high-dose radiation therapy. However, it is not easy to administer such highly accurate treatment to targets in the lung. Unlike intracranial targets that can be fixed easily once the bony structure is immobilized by a stereotactic frame, lung targets move

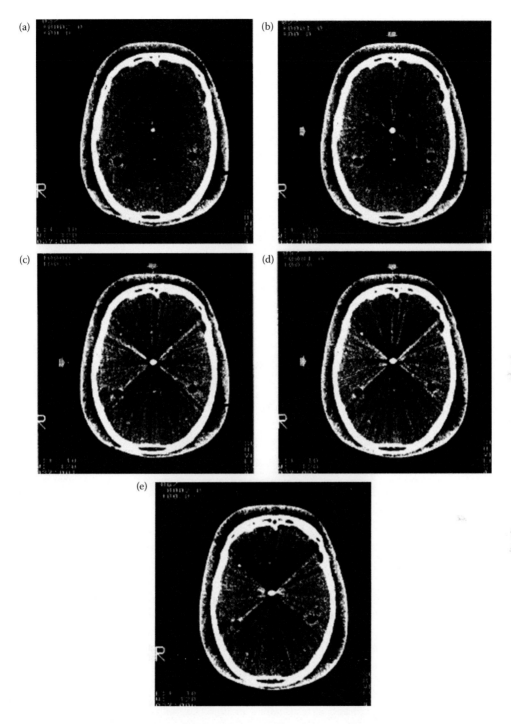

FIGURE 3.3 The phantom examinations. (a) 2 mm cranial from the center; (b) 1 mm cranial from the center; (c) the center of the target; (d) 1 mm caudal from the center; and (e) 2 mm caudal from the center. Two tiny metallic balls are clearly seen in (c), smaller in (b) and (d), and not seen in (a) and (e). (From Uematsu, M., et al., *Int. J. Radiat. Oncol. Biol. Phys.*, (35) 3: 587–592, 1996. With permission.)

and may not be able to be reproducibly positioned despite the fixation of the bony structures (Uematsu et al. 2001).

However, the difficulties in targeting and localization of these moving lung lesions can be overcome by using the FOCAL unit for IGRT. The in-room CT scanner enables the lung tumor to be visualized at the time of radiation therapy. This type of real-time, CT-guided treatment provides extreme precision for tumor localization while providing visualization of the normal lung tissues for maximal dose sparing. With the FOCAL unit, the key concept for treating a moving lung target is executed mainly by isocenter confirmation using CT image acquisition during reduced shallow respiration. Shallow breathing is achieved with 100% oxygen delivered through an oxygen mask (3,000–5,000 cc/min). While the patient is oxygenated, shallow breathing

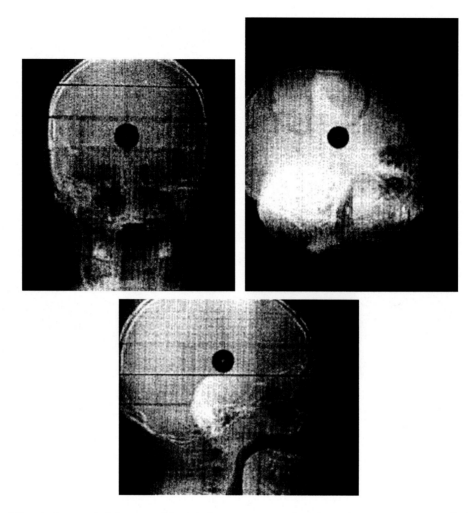

FIGURE 3.4 Portal films in three typical directions following the positioning in Figure 3.2. The errors are very small after the rotation of the table and gantry rotation of the linac. (From Uematsu, M., et al., *Int. J. Radiat. Oncol. Biol. Phys.*, (35) 3: 587–592, 1996. With permission.)

CT scan images are obtained at 4 seconds/slice (with each scan including 2–3 respiratory strokes), and the paradoxical images obtained at inhalation and exhalation extremes are eliminated. The isocenter of the lung tumor is localized by the use of repeat CT scanning and is marked by small metallic markers (placed on the skin) (Uematsu et al. 2000, 2001). The intrafractional lung tumor movements were measured by repeat CT scans prior to and post irradiation delivery (in Figure 3.5) and were usually very small and less than 10 mm. The result of this study is shown in Table 3.1. Various groups have pointed out the uncertainties in CT planning of moving tumors (Balter et al. 1996; Ross et al. 1990), especially with free-breathing image-acquisition schemes and the resulting, observable partial volume effects on individual CT image slices. However, with the use of shallow breathing as described, such uncertainties are minimized.

Using the FOCAL unit, Uematsu and colleagues reported in 2001 (Uematsu et al. 2001) a series of patients with pathologically proven stage 1 NSCLC treated between October 1994 to June 1999. In this series, there were 50 patients with T1-2N0M0

NSCLC, with 33 adenocarcinoma, 13 squamous carcionomas, and 4 Nonsmall-cell carcinomas that were not specified. There were 21 patients judged to be medically inoperable and 29 patients who were medically operable but refused surgery. There were 24 patients with T1 lesions and 26 patients with T2 lesions. Tumor size ranged from 0.8 to 5.0 cm, with a median diameter of 3.2 cm. SRT was given in 5–10 Gy per fraction to a total dosage of 50–60 Gy, with 5 fractions per week. For patients with larger tumors, conventional radiation (2 Gy per fractions to a dosage of 40–60 Gy) was used to reduce tumor size prior to SRT.

The follow up for these patients ranged from 22 to 66 months. Chest CT scans were performed every 3 months for the first 2 years and then every 4–6 months subsequently. Local control was defined as when the tumor showed no local progression on follow-up CT images. With a median follow up of 36 months, few acute or late adverse effects were observed. Two patients had late effects of bony rib fractures, and both had tumors that were initially adjacent to the rib cage, with the bony structures covered in the 80% isodose regions of the SRT. Six patients who

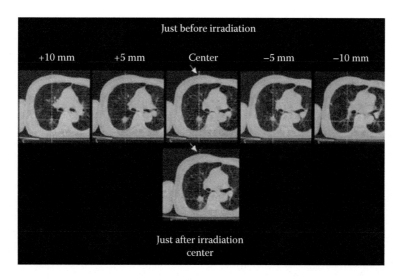

FIGURE 3.5 Evaluation of the intrafractional positioning errors using CT images. Upper five images are obtained before irradiation (110 mm, 15 mm, center position, 25 mm, and 210 mm). After irradiation, the center position is rescanned (lower panel) and is compared with the five upper images. In this series, the errors in the *x*- and *y*-axes are judged to be zero, and the lower center image is very similar to the upper center image and quite different from the other four images. Finally, the positioning error in the *z*-axis is judged to be negligible (0–5 mm), and the total error is also negligible. (From Uematsu, M., et al., *Int. J. Radiat. Oncol. Biol. Phys.*, (72) 1: S37, 2008. With permission.)

TABLE 3.1 Intrafractional Tumor Position Errors

	0 mm	1–3 mm	4–6 mm	Negligible (≤5 mm)	Small (6–10 mm)	Not small (>10 mm)
24 upper lung tumors						
X-axis	22/24	2/24	0			
Y-axis	16/24	8/24	0			
Z-axis				24/24	0	0
Total						
14 lower lung tumors						
X-axis	9/14	5/14	0			
Y-axis	6/14	8/14	0			
Z-axis				10/14	4/14	0
Total				7/14	7/14	0
12 liver tumors						
X-axis	7/12	5/12	0			
Y-axis	4/12	8/12	0			
Z-axis				5/12	7/12	0
Total				3/12	9/12	0

Source: Uematsu, M., et al., *Int. J. Radiat. Oncol. Biol. Phys.*, (72) 1: S37, 2008. With permission.

received both SRT and conventional RT had mild and temporary pleural pain, which did not require any medical interventions or nacrotics. On follow-up CT scans, small regions of atelectasis or lung fibrosis were seen in most patients who received both SRT and conventional RT. However, such changes were rarely observed in patients who received SRT alone. No patients developed symptomatic respiratory deteriorations, including the five patients who had significant chronic obstructive pulmonary disease.

Of all patients studied, 30 were alive without any relapses, 3 were alive with disease, 6 died of disease, and 11 died intercurrently of other causes. The 3-year overall and cause-specific survival rates were 88% and 66%, respectively. The 5-year actuarial overall and cause-specific survivals were 81% and 55%, respectively (Figure 3.6). Three patients had local failure, 5 patients had distant metastasis, and 2 patients had both nodal and distant failure (Table 3.2). Local control, based on CT imaging, was achieved in 94% (47/50) of patients.

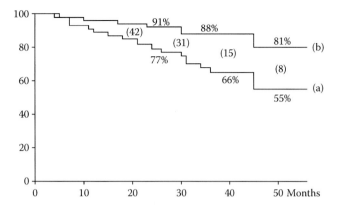

FIGURE 3.6 Actuarial overall (a) and cause-specific (b) survival of all 50 patients. The numbers in parentheses indicate the number of patients at risk beyond those points. (From Uematsu, M., et al., *Int. J. Radiat. Oncol. Biol. Phys.*, (51) 3: 666–670, 2001. With permission.)

TABLE 3.2 Patterns of Failure (Final Status) ($n = 50$)

Isolated local failure	3*
Isolated nodal failure	0
Isolated distant failure	5†
Nodal and distant failure	2‡

Source: Uematsu, M., Shioda, A., Suda, A., et al., *Int. J. Radiat. Oncol. Biol. Phys.*, (51) 3: 666–670, 2001. With permission.

* One alive with disease; 1 dead of disease; 1 dead of other causes (bacterial pneumonia).

† Two alive with disease, 3 dead of disease.

‡ Two dead of disease.

Although the number of patients in the above study was only 50 and the median follow-up period was only 36 months, the authors concluded that image-guided SRT treatment using the FOCAL unit results in a much higher cure rate and fewer side effects than conventional radiation therapy for early-stage lung cancers (Uematsu et al. 2001).

Long-term results for this group, with additional lung cancer patients treated at the same institution, were updated in a follow-up report in 2008 (Uematsu et al. 2008). In this report, 131 patients with clinically stage I and pathologically proven NSCLC were treated from 1994 to 2004 by CT-guided hypofractionated SRT using the FOCAL unit. Half of these patients were judged to be medically inoperable, and the other half were medically operable but refused surgery. In most patients, SRT doses were (50–60 Gy) delivered in 5–10 fractions over 1–2 weeks. Twenty-eight patients, similar to the earlier study, received conventional radiotherapy of 40–60 Gy to shrink the tumor volume prior to receiving SRT. The median follow-up period was 90 months (range: 38–150 months). Local progression on follow-up CT scans was found for five patients. The 5- and 10-year overall survival rates were 54% and 48%, respectively. The 5- and 10-year cause-specific survival rates were 78% and 74%, respectively. The 5- and 10-year overall survival rates of the medically operable patients were 72% and

65%, respectively. Treatment complications were acceptable, and about 20% of patients complained of some chest pain; however, most did not need any medical treatment. One patient suffered treatment-related mortality with fistula formation between the left pulmonary vein and main bronchus. Two patients developed symptomatic pneumonitis, and three patients had minor bone fractures. These long-term results are comparable with results for patients treated by surgical resection and imply that, for well selected patients, IGRT using the FOCAL unit and its in-room CT technique may be a viable alternative to surgical resection.

3.4 Second Generation of In-Room CT: CT on Rails

The initial combination of in-room CT and linear accelerator was developed for the treatment of small lesions intra- and extracranially using SRS or SRT (Uematsu et al. 1996). As IMRT became available in the late 1990s, it was possible to design a tight isodose curve around irregularly shaped and larger lesions (lesions that are 3 cm or more in some of the dimensions). Such lesions were usually not optimally treated by conventional SRT or SRS techniques using noncoplanar arcs. With this in mind, two of us (JRW and MU) approached, collaborated, and assisted Siemens Medical Solutions System (Concord, CA, USA, and Forheim, Germany) in the development of an advanced version of the in-room CT and linear accelerator combination that would accommodate this new type of radiation treatment (IMRT) with image guidance (Wong et al. 2001). The design was a "CT-on-Rail" system coupled with the linear accelerator and commercially known as the "Primatom" (Siemens Medical Systems). The first Primatom was installed at the Morristown Memorial Hospital, NJ, USA. The uniqueness of this system lies in the fact that both the CT scanner and the linear accelerator share a common, isocentric treatment table top, which is made of 4.5-cm thick carbon fiber. But unlike conventional CT scanners where scanning is performed by advancing the patient couch through the CT imaging aperture, the CT-on-rail scanner obtains its images by precision motion of the CT scanner along a pair of rails while the patient and treatment (imaging) table remain stationary. Repeat measurements of table coordinates, electronic readouts, and actual travel distance with projection of an alignment ruler showed that the CT-on-rail system has a mechanical positioning accuracy within 0.5 mm (Wong et al. 2001; Cheng et al. 2003). The system effectiveness and accuracy were tested with a Rando phantom study using comparisons of phantom anatomy on the CT slices containing the treatment beam central axis for CT images obtained on a CT-simulator and the CT-on-rails (Wong et al. 2001). Anatomical differences were assessed by the radiation oncologist using hardcopy printouts to determine the central axis planes in the anterior–posterior (AP), left–right (LR), and cephalic–caudal directions (CC). Unknown to the radiation oncologist, the central axis planes were deliberately displaced by a known amount from small metallic markers placed on the surface of the phantom to indicate the "treatment isocenter." The radiation oncologist was able to determine the displacements of the radio-opaque markers to within 2 mm of the actual isocenter in multiple repeated experiments (Wong et al. 2001).

Kuriyama and colleagues described a similar CT-on-rails system in a 2003 report (Kuriyama et al. 2003). The positional accuracy of the common couch was 0.2, 0.18, and 0.39 mm in the lateral, longitudinal, and vertical directions, respectively. The scan-position accuracy of the CT gantry was within 0.4 mm in all directions.

Thieke et al. (2006) described the advantages of the linac-CT-on rail combination as follows: (1) By using a CT gantry mounted on rails, image acquisition is accomplished without couch or patient movements, thus eliminating two sources of reduced accuracy. (2) The kilovoltage CT scanner enables diagnostic image quality with high soft-tissue contrast. This high-fidelity imaging allows for detection of soft-tissue target deviations even when bony landmarks are repositioned correctly. (3) The CT data set can be used without transformation for treatment planning and dose calculation. Because of these advantages, the in-room CT-on-rails unit is well suited for target verification, set up error corrections, detection of interfraction target movements, as well as recalculation of actual dose delivered. Systematic changes of the patient's anatomy while under therapy, such as weight loss and tumor mass shrinkage, can be considered, and radiation treatment plans can be redesigned or reoptimized as necessary.

Reoptimization of the treatment plan interfractionationally lays the ground work for adaptative radiation treatment and should be easily achievable with the in-room CT-on-rails scanner.

3.5 Treatment of Prostate Cancers Using CT-on-Rails

Prostate cancer treatment by various IGRT methods have been extensively studied (Falco et al. 2002; Fiorino et al. 2008; Grigorov et al. 2003; Kupelian et al. 2006; Lattanzi et al. 2000; Ramsey et al. 2007; Wong et al. 2001; Wong et al. 2005; Wong et al. 2008), including prostate IGRT using the in-room CT approach (Cheng et al. 2008; Gao et al. 2007; Merrick et al. 2008; Wong et al. 2008).

One of the earliest and largest studies on the CT-on-rails for treatment of prostate cancers was reported by the group at Morristown Medical Center (Wong et al. 2005). They reported 108 patients with biopsy-proven prostate cancer who were treated using the Primatom CT-on-rails between May 2000 to January 2001. The clinical stages were T1c–T3; the Gleason scores were 5–8; and the prostate-specific antigen levels were 2.5–239 ng/ml. The treatment technique using the CT-on-rails was as follows: the patient was first placed on the treatment couch according to tattoo marks on the skin, which had been determined at the time of CT-simulation and delineated the target isocenter. Metallic BB markers were then placed over these tattoo marks. The treatment couch was then rotated 180° for the verification CT scan. After the CT-on-rails images were obtained and the images generated, the clinical target volume (CTV) and rectum were identified on each slice and subsequently plotted on the beam's eye view. In both the treatment planning CT and the in-room CT scans, the central axis plane of the prostate was established as the middle CT cut between the most superior cut and the most inferior cut of the prostate. The isocenter cut from the in-room CT was compared with the isocenter cut that was established at treatment planning and marked on the skin with the metallic BBs. This comparison, in turn, established the superior and inferior direction changes. The corresponding in-room CT slice images superior and inferior to the central planes were plotted and compared with those from the baseline treatment planning CT scan. Thus, the change in the shape and position of the CTV was determined for the daily in-room CT images compared to the CT-simulation images. A beam's eye view of the overlay of the current or treatment day's prostate position with that of the treatment plan's prostate position is shown in Figure 3.7. The couch was then rotated 180° back to the treatment position. The BB locations were checked against the lasers to ensure that no patient movements had occurred.

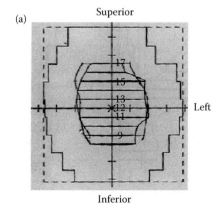
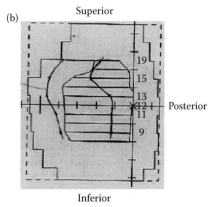

FIGURE 3.7 Beam's eye view of prostate positions as plotted from computed tomography AP scans. Area with horizontal line represents prostate position on day of simulation. Area without horizontal lines represents prostate position on day of treatment. (a) Evaluation of LR movement. (b) Evaluation of AP movement. (From Wong, J. R., et al., *Phys. Med.*, (XVII) 4: 272–276, 2001. With permission.)

The position of the isocenter was adjusted if necessary, and radiation treatment was delivered immediately afterward. This whole procedure added approximately 20 min to the regular treatment time. It was found that, for some patients, significant variations in the prostate and rectum positions occurred from day to day (Wong et al. 2005). A representative example of these variations in position is shown in Figure 3.8. It can be seen that during the course of five consecutive days, the rectum varied significantly in size and the prostate was also in different positions. From their evaluation of 540 consecutive daily CT images acquired during the last part of the cone down treatment, they found that for AP–PA isocenter adjustments, 46% of the 540 scans required no new isocenter adjustment, 10% required a shift of 3–4 mm, 29% required a shift of 5–9 mm, and 15% required a shift of ≥ 10 mm. In the superoinferior direction, 2% required a shift of 3–4 mm, 21% required a shift of 5–9 mm, and 4% required a shift of ≥ 10 mm. In the right–left direction, 10% required a shift of 3–4 mm, 19% required a shift of 5–8 mm, and 5% required a shift of ≥ 10 mm. Dosimetric calculations using IMRT with 5-mm margin coverage from the clinical target volume (prostate gland) was performed for a representative patient. With a posterior shift of 10 mm for the prostate, the dose coverage dropped from 95–107% to 71–100% coverage.

Frank and colleagues studied 15 patients who had undergone IMRT for prostate carcinoma (Frank et al. 2008). Patients had one pretreatment planning CT scan followed by three in-room CT scans per week using a CT-on-rails system. The prostate, bladder, rectum, and pelvic bony anatomy were contoured in 369 CT images. Volumetric and positional changes were analyzed. It was found that the mean systematic internal prostate and seminal vesicles variation was 0.1 ± 4.1 mm and 1.2 ± 7.3 mm in the AP axis, −0.5 ± 2.9 mm and −0.7 ± 4.5 mm in the superior–inferior axis, and 0.2 ± 0.9 mm and −0.9 ± 1.9 mm in the LR axis, respectively. The mean magnitude of the three-dimensional displacement vector was 4.6 ± 3.5 mm for the prostate and 7.6 ± 4.7 mm for the seminal vesicles. The rectal and bladder volume changes during treatment correlated with the anterior and superior displacement of the prostate and seminal vesicles.

Because of the excellent soft-tissue images provided by the diagnostic-quality CT images, Knight and colleagues examined the changes in bladder and rectal volumes as well as the prostate shift with the CT-on-rails throughout an entire course of radiation treatment for 25 prostate cancer patients (Knight et al. 2006). With 816 pretreatment verification CTs obtained, 82 online corrections (10%) were performed. Patient

set-up uncertainty was found to be greatest in the AP direction. Daily fluctuations in organ volume were observed (8–516% and 27–342% of the planned bladder and rectum volumes, respectively). Large volumes at the time of planning were strongly associated with large systematic errors. Organ motion was greatest in the AP direction and was significantly correlated with rectal volume.

Wong and colleagues reviewed 349 patients with CT scans obtained during image-guided radiotherapy using CT-on-rails (Wong et al. 2008). Five to 10 CT scan images were obtained per patient. In total, 1,870 CT scans were collected and analyzed just prior to the delivery of daily radiation treatment, and 5,610 interfractional prostate shifts were reviewed. It was found that for the AP direction 44% required no setup adjustments (if the target shift from planned position was < 3 mm, no adjustment was performed), 14% had shifts of 3–5 mm, 29% had shifts of 6–10 mm, and 13% had shifts of > 10 mm. In the superior–inferior direction, 81% had no setup adjustments (i.e., shift < 3 mm), 2% had shifts of 3–5 mm, 15% had shifts of 6–10 mm, and 2% had shifts of > 10 mm. In the LR direction, 65% had no setup adjustment, 13% had shifts of 3–5 mm, 17% had shifts of 6–10 mm, and 5% had shifts of > 10 mm. The authors further simulated the effect of isocenter adjustments by a composite plan, to include all 15 daily target shifts or without isocenter adjustments into the dose calculation. Figure 3.9 compares the composite dose distributions for a prostate irradiation with and without such isocenter adjustments, as determined from in-room, CT-on-rails daily imaging. The composite dose distribution is calculated by summing dose distributions over 15 fractions with beam shifts simulating corresponding target shifts. As shown in Figure 3.9, the dose gradient at the interface between rectum and prostate is sharp with IGRT daily fraction adjustments, whereas without correcting for target shifts the dose gradient becomes broader, with an increase in the volume of rectum irradiated with a high dose.

Peng et al. reviewed daily in-room CT-on-rail images for 10 prostate cancer patients treated with CT-guided repositioning (Peng et al. 2008). For each of the patients' planning CT scans, prostate-PTV contours were generated with margins of 0, 2, 4, and 6 mm. The plans were then applied to the daily CT image sets by aligning the centers of mass (COM) of the daily and planning prostate volumes (closely replicating the actual practice of IGRT with CT-on-rails). The amount of organ deformation was quantified in terms of maximum overlap ratio between the planning and treatment prostate volumes. Their results indicate that the optimum margin with the current

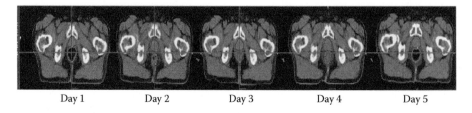

| Day 1 | Day 2 | Day 3 | Day 4 | Day 5 |

FIGURE 3.8 (See color insert)   Prostate and rectum position for five consecutive treatment days. Prostate outlined in red; rectum in green. (From Wong, J. R., et al., *Phys. Med.*, (XVII) 4: 272–276, 2001. With permission.)

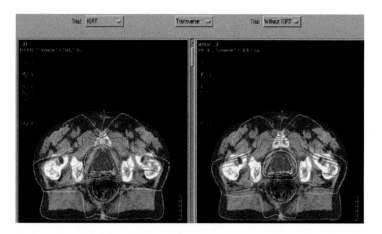

FIGURE 3.9 (See color insert) Dose comparison for treatment with and without image-guided intensity-modulated radiotherapy (IGRT). (From Wong, J. R., et al., *Int. J. Radiat. Oncol. Biol. Phys.*, (75) 1: 49–55, 2009. With permission.)

standard of repositioning using in-room imaging is between 0 mm and 2 mm. The optimum margins in the directions of the bladder and rectum were the same. For most patients, the optimum margin was < 2 mm. When a 0 mm margin (no margin) was used, daily underdosing was common (minimum dose was < 80% of planned dose for 20% of the treatment days), and the accumulative minimum dose was 80–85% for patients with large deformations of the target volume. They estimated that the use of the optimum margin reduces the underdosing and may lead to a 4–11% higher therapeutic ratio.

3.6 Treatment of Extracranial Cancers Other Than Prostate Cancers

3.6.1 Treatment of Breast Cancers

Morrow et al. enrolled patients with prone breast irradiation to be treated on a linac and CT-on-rails combination (Morrow et al. 2008). Patients were selected who could fit through the bore of the CT and had surgical clips placed in the lumpectomy cavity at time of surgery. The CT images were acquired for five consecutive fractions. Rotation of the torso and rotation/distortion of breast tissue are easily seen in the CT-on-rails images and any misalignments are corrected if necessary. The distortion of the breast tissue affects position of the clips and surgical cavity. The magnitude of the daily shifts varied for each of the patients, with the smallest average shift of 0 ± 3 mm and the largest of –18 ± 3 mm. The shifts determined from CT registration and from portal images were strongly correlated ($r = 0.8$ for vertical and $r = 1.0$ for longitudinal directions). It was found that the surgical clips were not identifiable on the portal films and thus could not serve as surrogates for cavity identification.

3.6.2 Treatment of Esophageal Cancers

Sasidharan and colleagues studied interfraction esophagus motion with IGRT using the CT-on-rails (Sasidharan et al. 2005). They analyzed the daily shift of the esophagus in 6 IGRT lung patients, using 78 sets of diagnostic quality CT images. Comparisons were made by fusion of the primary and the daily CT-on-rails image series using specialized commercial software (Coherence Adaptive Radiotherapy Workstation, Siemens Medical Systems). Each patient's spine was used as a base reference and the shift was measured at the following three locations: a CT slice close to the gastro-esophageal (GE) junction (location 1, L1), a point 10 slices above the GE junction (location 2, L2), and a final point 15 slices above the GE junction (location 3, L3). The center point of the esophagus cross section was taken as the origin for measurements. Measurements corresponding to each patient's left, right, posterior, and anterior directions were obtained. They found that all patients had esophageal motions. The greatest levels of motion are found in the anterior direction and toward the patient's left. The highest levels of motion are found mostly in the regions around the gastro-esophageal junction. The average daily shift and the maximum observed shifts are summarized in Table 3.3. While all patients have esophageal motion, the amount of motion does not appear to be clinically significant so long as an appropriate Internal Target Volume (ITV) is considered.

3.6.3 Treatment of Paraspinal Tumors

Tumors in the paraspinal regions pose a critical challenge for radiotherapy because unintended spinal cord overdosage can lead to severe consequences such as para- or tetraplegia. However, insufficient dose may increase chance of local recurrence. As such, ultra-precise dose applications have been devised for the treatments of paraspinal tumors (Lohr et al. 1999; Shiu et al. 2003; Kriminski et al. 2008). Intrafractional motion has been shown to be minor in studies that used pre- and post-treatment CT scans. To compensate for interfractional patient motion, Stoiber and colleagues at the German Cancer Research Center and University Clinic Heidelberg explored the use of CT-on-rails for a simple target-point correction that was implemented by movements of the treatment table (Stoiber et al. 2009). Eighty-two patients with paraspinal tumors were treated with image-guided IMRT between 2002 and 2006. Thirty-seven of these patients were excluded and 45 patients were analyzed. Eleven patients had cervical, 21 had thoracic, and 13 had lumbar paraspinal tumors. Thirty-seven patients had primary and 8 patients had metastatic spinal tumors.

Every patient was immobilized with an individually customized fixation device as seen in Figure 3.10. During the fractionated treatment course, the patients received localization CT-on-rails scanning at least once per week with some critical cases receiving daily CT scanning for

localizations. The scanned volume included the whole target volume plus margins of at least 1 cm above and below; the reconstructed slice thickness was 3 mm. Altogether, a total of 321 CT studies were obtained. Image registrations were performed with the control CT scans stereotactically correlated with the respective planning CT scan (in Figure 3.11). All 321 control CT scans were evaluated. The rotational errors were negligible. Translational errors were smallest for cervical tumors (−0.1 ± 1.1, 0.3 ± 0.8, and 0.1 ± 0.9 mm along the LR, AP, and superior–inferior axes), followed by thoracic (0.8 ± 1.1, 0.3 ± 0.8, and 1.1 ± 1.3 mm) and lumbar tumors (−0.7 ± 1.3, 0.0 ± 0.9, and 0.5 ± 1.6 mm). The residual deviations of the

TABLE 3.3   Percent of Patients with CTV0 Bias

	−15 mm	−10 mm	−5 mm	0 mm	5 mm	10 mm	15 mm
CTVapex	1.6%	3.1%	18.1%	55.2%	15.2%	4.7%	1.7%
CTVmid	0%	0.3%	12.7%	61.5%	20.9%	4.2%	0.3%
CTVbase	0.1%	1.4%	1.6%	63.2%	17.4%	1.4%	0.3%

Source: Sasidharan, S., et al., *Int. J. Radiat. Oncol. Biol. Phys.*, 63, S91–S92, 2005. With permission.

The 0 mm bin contains those patients with −2.5 to 2.5 mm bias. The 5 mm bin contains those with 2.5 to 7.5 mm bias. etc.

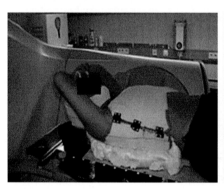
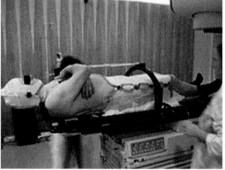

FIGURE 3.10   Patient fixation with body cast and head mask. Left: Fixation for cervical and thoracic paraspinal tumors. Right: Fixation for lumbar tumors (with stereotactic localizers attached). (From Stoiber, E. M., et al., *Int. J. Radiat. Oncol. Biol. Phys.*, (75) 3: 933–940, 2009. With permission.)

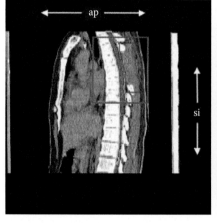
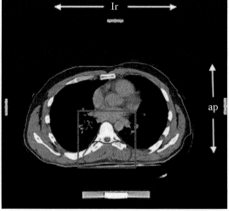

FIGURE 3.11 (See color insert)   Example case with a thoracic paraspinal tumor. Outlined are the target and boost volume (magenta), the spinal cord (yellow), and the registration box (green) in sagittal view (left) and axial view (right). lr = left–right axis; ap = anterior–posterior axis; si = superior–inferior axis. (From Stoiber, E. M., et al., *Int. J. Radiat. Oncol. Biol. Phys.*, (75) 3: 933–940, 2009. With permission.)

three subsections were < 1 mm. The results of the analysis are summarized in Table 3.4. The measured setup uncertainties are in agreement as reported by other institutions (Guckenberger et al. 2007; Yenice et al. 2003). The additional dose delivered to the patient by the CT-on-Rails scanning was negligible (< 1 cGy per scan). Because the in-room CT scanner meets diagnostic standards, the image quality is excellent, with even lower doses required for each scan acquired compared to both kilovoltage and megavoltage cone-beam CT (Stutzel et al. 2008). On the basis of the presented data, the authors felt that relying on the stereotactic positioning device alone might be insufficient for some cases and daily CT image guidance is recommended in all patients treated for paraspinal lesions with high doses (Stoiber et al. 2009).

3.7 CT-on-Rails and Treatment of Obese Patients

Obesity is a major health problem in developed and some developing countries. Recent data indicate that obese patients may have higher incidence of radiation treatment failures (Efstathiou et al. 2007; Strom et al. 2006; Stroup et al. 2007). From their review of patients with prostate cancers treated by external beam radiation therapy, Strom et al. (Stroup et al. 2007) showed that the probability of 10-year biochemical failure-free survival for obese patients is 20–25% lower than that for the normal weight, over weight, and mildly obese patient groups (62–65%). However, the cause of this phenomenon was not explicitly concluded in their study, and they suggested that there may be intrinsic reason for the obesity causing higher radiation failures in these patients. The patients described in their study (Stroup et al. 2007) were not treated with image guided techniques and as such, is it possible that these patients' increased failures are a result of uncertainties of treatment set up secondary to the lack of image guidance (Wong et al. 2009). The treatment of large patients with prostate cancer is challenged by a large abdominal girth. When lying flat on the treatment couch, the anterior and the LR skin marks of these patients may not remain stationary relative to the alignment lasers in the treatment room. This is especially true for the anterior marker because of the large amount of fatty tissues in the abdomen as shown in Figure 3.12. Thus, daily setup in the LR direction is difficult and may result

TABLE 3.4 Systematic and Random Positioning Errors for Paraspinal Tumors Located in the Cervical, Thoracic, and Lumbar Spine

Location	3D Displacement (mm)	Translational Error (mm)			Rotational Error (°)		
		LR Axis	AP Axis	SI Axis	LR Axis	AP Axis	SI Axis
Cervical (*n* = 11)	2.6 ± 1.0	–0.1 ± 1.1	0.3 ± 0.8	0.1 ± 0.9	–0.3 ± 0.5	0.0 ± 0.4	0.1 ± 0.6
Thoracic (*n* = 13)	3.8 ± 1.3	0.8 ± 1.1	0.3 ± 0.8	1.1 ± 1.3	–0.1 ± 10.6	0.1 ± 0.4	0.2 ± 0.4
Lumbar (*n* = 13)	4.0 ±1.5	–0.7 ± 1.3	0.0 ± 0.9	0.5 ± 1.6	–0.2 ± 0.3	0.0 ± 0.4	0.0 ± 0.4

Source: Stoiber, E. M., et al., *Int. J. Radiat. Oncol. Biol. Phys.*, (75) 3: 933–940, 2009. With permission.

3D, three-dimensional; LR, left; AP, anterior-posterior; SI, superior-inferior.

Values are mean (systematic) ± standard deviation (random). Three-dimensional displacement per patient is also given.

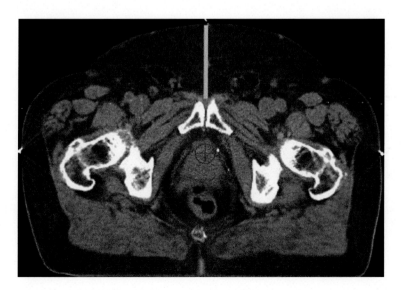

FIGURE 3.12 CT scan images of an obese patient. Note the significant amount of subcutaneous adipose-tissue thickness as indicated by the white solid line. Anterior tattoo marks on the skin in this location are subjected to set up uncertainties. (From Wong, J. R., et al., *Int. J. Radiat. Oncol. Biol. Phys.*, (72) 5: 1396–1401, 2008. With permission.)

in large day-to-day variation of skin markers relative to bony structure. Wong et al. undertook an analysis of 117 patients with 1,465 in-room CT-on-rails scans obtained with IGRT for prostate cancer between January 2005 and April 2007 (Wong et al. 2009). The standard deviations (SDs) of prostate shifts for all patients, along with patient weight, body mass index (BMI), and subcutaneous adipose-tissue thickness (SAT), were determined. Patients were classified as normal weight (26.5%), overweight (48.7%), mildly obese (17.9%), and moderately to severely obese (6.9%). Notably, 1.3, 1.5, 2.0, and 21.2% of the respective shifts were greater than 10 mm in the left-right (LR) direction for the four patient groups, whereas in the anterior-posterior (AP) direction the shifts greater than 10 mm were 18.2, 12.6, 6.7, and 21.0%, respectively. Strong correlations were observed between SAT, BMI, patient weight, and SDs of daily shifts in the LR direction ($p < 0.01$). Figure 3.13a–c plots the cumulative probability of daily shift as a function of shift magnitude for the four patient groups in the AP, LR, and radial or superior-inferior (SI) directions, respectively. When the BMI increased from < 25 to > 35, there was a progression of the SDs of the shifts in the LR direction (in Table 3.5), from 3.0 mm (normal weight), to 3.4 mm (overweight), to 3.8 mm (mildly obese), and finally to 8.9 mm (severely obese). On the other hand, for the AP direction, the corresponding SDs of the isocenter shifts are 7.0, 6.1, 4.7, and 7.4 mm, respectively, which basically indicates no clinically relevant difference among the various groups. Similarly, for the SI direction, the corresponding SDs of the isocenter shifts are 2.2, 1.4, 1.1, and 2.3 mm, respectively; these differences are probably not clinically significant.

From the above data, Wong et al. (2009) concluded that the higher biologic/biochemical failure observed by Strom et al. for obese patients maybe explained by target miss, as these patients were treated without image guidance, and that image guidance for the treatment of obese patients is desirable because it can

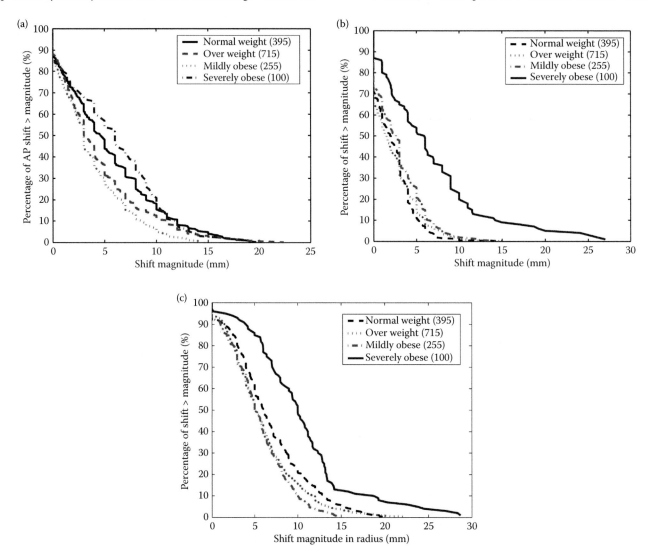

FIGURE 3.13 (a) Percent AP shift in magnitude for the four patient groups. (b) Percent LR shift in magnitude for the four patient groups. (c) Percent radius shift in magnitude for the four patient groups. (From Wong, J. R., et al., *Int. J. Radiat. Oncol. Biol. Phys.*, (72) 5: 1396–1401, 2008. With permission.)

TABLE 3.5 Standard Deviation (SD) of Target Displacement from Planned Positions for each Patient Group

Direction	Normal Weight (BMI ≤25) N = 31 (mm)	Over Weight (BMI 25 to ≤30) N = 57 (mm)	Mildly Obese (BMI 30 to ≤35) N = 21 (mm)	Severely Obese BMI > 35 N = 8 (mm)	Entire Population N = 117 (mm)
AP	7.0	6.1	4.7	7.4	6.3
LR	3.0	3.4	3.8	8.9	4.0
SI	2.2	1.4	1.1	2.3	1.7

AP, anterior–posterior; BMI, body mass index; LR, lift-right; SAT, suncutaneous adipose-tissue thickness; SI, superior-interior

correct target displacement before radiation delivery. In fact, this observation may be generalized to treatment of cancers other than prostate.

Most current image-guided techniques are not well suited for severely obese patients. Ultrasonographic guidance is limited by image quality, which is especially worse with increased distance from the abdominal surface to the bladder (Serago et al. 2002). Kilovoltage CT, megavoltage CT, and megavoltage portal images using Electronic Portal Imaging Devices produce adequate images for patients with normal and overweight BMI, but image quality deteriorates with increasing BMI because of increased photon scatter and attenuation. For patients with higher BMI, these onboard imaging devices may require implanted fiducial markers to detect any shifts of the target. IGRT using the CT–on-rails system, especially with a large-bore diagnostic-quality CT scanner (84 cm aperture) produces excellent image quality even for patients with high BMI values and hence maybe especially useful.

3.8 Future Directions and Conclusions

In the previous sections, various groups have demonstrated the usefulness of the in-room CT in combinations with the linear accelerator. System capabilities and functions are constantly evolving and are able to meet new challenges and incorporate new treatment techniques. The strength of the system is that many components are readily available and upgradable. The first installation of the in-room CT with linear accelerator was designed for easy reproducible, noninvasive SRT/surgery. The next installation of CT-on-rails allowed the applications of real-time imaging technology to conventional radiation therapy such as 3D conformal RT, and then subsequently IMRT. One drawback of the in-room CT is the geometrical limitation that no real-time imaging is possible during actual radiation delivery. However, by using real-time tumor-tracking devices such as fiducial implants with fluoroscopic tracking systems (Ebe et al. 2004) or radio-frequency transmitter implants (McGary 2004), the change or movement of target location intrafractionally can be readily determined. In-room CT, with its accompanying high-quality CT images (as currently used for simulation treatment planning), is especially suitable for future, efficient software that would enable real-time treatment planning. Moreover, with the future arrival of molecular or physiologic CT imaging, the in-room CT scanner may find new use for treatments incorporating biological parameters.

Acknowledgments

We thank our colleagues at Morristown Medical Center (MMC) and Siemens Medical Solutions whose support over the years has been and continue to be invaluable. They include but are not limited to the following people: Scott Merrick, Dennis Falkenstein, Chris Amies, Mark Lauterbach, Shmuel Aharon, Mona Karim, Jackie Vizoso, Liz Rodriquez, and Teri Rizzolo.

References

Balter, J. M., Ten Haken, R. K., Lawrence, T. S., Lam, K. L., & Robertson, J. M. 1996, Uncertainties in CT-based radiation therapy treatment planning associated with patient breathing, *Int. J. Radiat. Oncol. Biol. Phys.,* vol. 36, no. 1, pp. 167–174.

Brahme, A. 1988, Optimization of stationary and moving beam radiation therapy techniques, *Radiother. Oncol.,* vol. 12, no. 2, pp. 129–140.

Carol, M., Grant, W. H., III, Pavord, D., Eddy, P., Targovnik, H. S., Butler, B., Woo, S., Figura, J., Onufrey, V., Grossman, R., & Selkar, R. 1996, Initial clinical experience with the Peacock intensity modulation of a 3-D conformal radiation therapy system, *Stereotact. Funct. Neurosurg.,* vol. 66, no. 1–3, pp. 30–34.

Cheng, C., Wong, J. R., Merrick, S., Langley, B., & Gao, J. Z. 2008, Predicting isocenter shift due to prostate motion and selecting patient specific posterior margin for IGRT in the external beam treatment of prostate cancer, *Int. J. Radiat. Oncol. Biol. Phys.,* vol. 72, no. 1, p. S563.

Cheng, C. W., Wong, J., Grimm, L., Chow, M., Uematsu, M., & Fung, A. 2003, Commissioning and clinical implementation of a sliding gantry CT scanner installed in an existing treatment room and early clinical experience for precise tumor localization, *Am. J. Clin. Oncol.,* vol. 26, no. 3, p. e28–e36.

Ebe, K., Shirato, H., Hiyama, A., Kanzaki, R., Tsukamoto, K., Ariga, M., Karino, Y., Mukae, H., Matsumoto, T., & Matsunaga, N. 2004, Integration of fluoroscopic real-time tumor-tracking system and tomographic scanner on the rail in the treatment room, *Int. J. Radiat. Oncol. Biol. Phys.,* vol. 60, no. 1, p. S604.

Efstathiou, J. A., Chen, M. H., Renshaw, A. A., Loffredo, M. J., & D'Amico, A. V. 2007, Influence of body mass index on prostate-specific antigen failure after androgen suppression and radiation therapy for localized prostate cancer, *Cancer*, vol. 109, no. 8, pp. 1493–1498.

Eklof, A., Ahnesjo, A., & Brahme, A. 1990, Photon beam energy deposition kernels for inverse radiotherapy planning, *Acta Oncol.*, vol. 29, no. 4, pp. 447–454.

Falco, T., Shenouda, G., Kaufmann, C., Belanger, I., Procaccini, C., Charrois, C., & Evans, M. 2002, Ultrasound imaging for external-beam prostate treatment setup and dosimetric verification, *Med. Dosim.*, vol. 27, no. 4, pp. 271–273.

Fiorino, C., Alongi, F., Broggi, S., Cattaneo, G. M., Cozzarini, C., Di Muzio, N., Maggiulli, E., Mangili, P., Perna, L., Valdagni, R., Fazio, F., & Calandrino, R. 2008, Physics aspects of prostate tomotherapy: planning optimization and image-guidance issues, *Acta Oncol.*, vol. 47, no. 7, pp. 1309–1316.

Frank, S. J., Dong, L., Kudchadker, R. J., De Crevoisier, R., Lee, A. K., Cheung, R., Choi, S., O'Daniel, J., Tucker, S. L., Wang, H., & Kuban, D. A. 2008, Quantification of prostate and seminal vesicle interfraction variation during IMRT, *Int. J. Radiat. Oncol. Biol. Phys.*, vol. 71, no. 3, pp. 813–820.

Gao, Z., Wong, J., Merritt, S., Uematsu, M., & Cheng, C. 2007, A novel method of image guided radiation treatment of prostate cancer using a quasi-adaptive margin and evidence based isocenter shift, *Int. J. Radiat. Oncol. Biol. Phys.*, vol. 69, no. 3, pp. S366–S367.

Grigorov, G., Kron, T., Wong, E., Chen, J., Sollazzo, J., & Rodrigues, G. 2003, Optimization of helical tomotherapy treatment plans for prostate cancer, *Phys. Med. Biol.*, vol. 48, no. 13, pp. 1933–1943.

Guckenberger, M., Meyer, J., Wilbert, J., Baier, K., Bratengeier, K., Vordermark, D., & Flentje, M. 2007, Precision required for dose-escalated treatment of spinal metastases and implications for image-guided radiation therapy (IGRT), *Radiother. Oncol.*, vol. 84, no. 1, pp. 56–63.

Knight, K. A., Cox, J., & Duchesne, G. 2006, 2276: daily image guided radiation therapy for prostate cancer: an assessment of treatment plan reproducibility. *Int. J. Radiat. Oncol. Biol. Phys.*, vol. 66, no. 3, pp. S363-S364.

Kooy, H. M. & Barth, N. H. 1990, The verification of an inverse problem in radiation therapy, *Int. J. Radiat. Oncol. Biol. Phys.*, vol. 18, no. 2, pp. 433–439.

Kriminski, S. A., Lovelock, D. M., Seshan, V. E., Ali, I., Munro, P., Amols, H. I., Fuks, Z., Bilsky, M., & Yamada, Y. 2008, Comparison of kilovoltage cone-beam computed tomography with megavoltage projection pairs for paraspinal radiosurgery patient alignment and position verification, *Int. J. Radiat. Oncol. Biol. Phys.*, vol. 71, no. 5, pp. 1572–1580.

Kupelian, P. A., Langen, K. M., Zeidan, O. A., Meeks, S. L., Willoughby, T. R., Wagner, T. H., Jeswani, S., Ruchala, K. J., Haimerl, J., & Olivera, G. H. 2006, Daily variations in delivered doses in patients treated with radiotherapy for localized prostate cancer, *Int. J. Radiat. Oncol. Biol. Phys.*, vol. 66, no. 3, pp. 876–882.

Kuriyama, K., Onishi, H., Sano, N., Komiyama, T., Aikawa, Y., Tateda, Y., Araki, T., & Uematsu, M. 2003, A new irradiation unit constructed of self-moving gantry-CT and linac, *Int. J. Radiat. Oncol. Biol. Phys.*, vol. 55, no. 2, pp. 428–435.

Lattanzi, J., McNeeley, S., Donnelly, S., Palacio, E., Hanlon, A., Schultheiss, T. E., & Hanks, G. E. 2000, Ultrasound-based stereotactic guidance in prostate cancer—quantification of organ motion and set-up errors in external beam radiation therapy, *Comput. Aided Surg.*, vol. 5, no. 4, pp. 289–295.

Lohr, F., Debus, J., Frank, C., Herfarth, K., Pastyr, O., Rhein, B., Bahner, M. L., Schlegel, W., & Wannenmacher, M. 1999, Noninvasive patient fixation for extracranial stereotactic radiotherapy, *Int. J. Radiat. Oncol. Biol. Phys.*, vol. 45, no. 2, pp. 521–527.

McGary, J. E. 2004, Theoretical foundation for real-time prostate localization using an inductively coupled transmitter and a superconducting quantum interference device (SQUID) magnetometer system, *J. Appl. Clin. Med. Phys.*, vol. 5, no. 4, pp. 29–45.

Merrick, S. A., Wong, J., Cheng, C., & Gao, J. 2008, Dosimetric analysis of treatment plan degradation after large shift corrections during image guided radiation therapy (IGRT) for the treatment of prostate cancer, *Int. J. Radiat. Oncol. Biol. Phys.*, vol. 72, no. 1, pp. S552–S553.

Morrow, N. V., White, J., Rownd, J. J., & Li, X. A. 2008, IGRT with CT-on-rails for prone breast irradiation, *Int. J. Radiat. Oncol. Biol. Phys.*, vol. 72, no. 1, p. S522.

Peng, C., Ahunbay, E., Godley, A., Lawton, C. A., & Li, X. 2008, PTV margin to account for deformation during prostate IGRT, *Int. J. Radiat. Oncol. Biol. Phys.*, vol. 72, no. 1, p. S570.

Ramsey, C. R., Scaperoth, D., Seibert, R., Chase, D., Byrne, T., & Mahan, S. 2007, Image-guided helical tomotherapy for localized prostate cancer: technique and initial clinical observations, *J. Appl. Clin. Med. Phys.*, vol. 8, no. 3, p. 2320.

Ross, C. S., Hussey, D. H., Pennington, E. C., Stanford, W., & Doornbos, J. F. 1990, Analysis of movement of intrathoracic neoplasms using ultrafast computerized tomography, *Int. J. Radiat. Oncol. Biol. Phys.*, vol. 18, no. 3, pp. 671–677.

Sasidharan, S., Allison, R., Jenkins, T., Wolfe, M., Mota, H., & Sibata, C. 2005, Interfraction esophagus motion study in image guided radiation therapy (IGRT), *Int. J. Radiat. Oncol. Biol. Phys.*, vol. 63, pp. S91–S92.

Serago, C. F., Chungbin, S. J., Buskirk, S. J., Ezzell, G. A., Collie, A. C., & Vora, S. A. 2002, Initial experience with ultrasound localization for positioning prostate cancer patients for external beam radiotherapy, *Int. J. Radiat. Oncol. Biol. Phys.*, vol. 53, no. 5, pp. 1130–1138.

Shiu, A. S., Chang, E. L., Ye, J. S., Lii, M., Rhines, L. D., Mendel, E., Weinberg, J., Singh, S., Maor, M. H., Mohan, R., & Cox, J. D. 2003, Near simultaneous computed tomography image-guided stereotactic spinal radiotherapy: an emerging paradigm for achieving true stereotaxy, *Int. J. Radiat. Oncol. Biol. Phys.*, vol. 57, no. 3, pp. 605–613.

Stoiber, E. M., Lechsel, G., Giske, K., Muenter, M. W., Hoess, A., Bendl, R., Debus, J., Huber, P. E., & Thieke, C. 2009, Quantitative assessment of image-guided radiotherapy for paraspinal tumors, *Int. J. Radiat. Oncol. Biol. Phys.*, vol. 75, no. 3, pp. 933–940.

Strom, S. S., Kamat, A. M., Gruschkus, S. K., Gu, Y., Wen, S., Cheung, M. R., Pisters, L. L., Lee, A. K., Rosser, C. J., & Kuban, D. A. 2006, Influence of obesity on biochemical and clinical failure after external-beam radiotherapy for localized prostate cancer, *Cancer*, vol. 107, no. 3, pp. 631–639.

Stroup, S. P., Cullen, J., Auge, B. K., L'Esperance, J. O., & Kang, S. K. 2007, Effect of obesity on prostate-specific antigen recurrence after radiation therapy for localized prostate cancer as measured by the 2006 Radiation Therapy Oncology Group-American Society for Therapeutic Radiation and Oncology (RTOG-ASTRO) Phoenix consensus definition, *Cancer*, vol. 110, no. 5, pp. 1003–1009.

Stutzel, J., Oelfke, U., & Nill, S. 2008, A quantitative image quality comparison of four different image guided radiotherapy devices, *Radiother. Oncol*, vol. 86, no. 1, pp. 20–24.

Thieke, C., Malsch, U., Schlegel, W., Debus, J., Huber, P., Bendl, R., & Thilmann, C. 2006, Kilovoltage CT using a linac-CT scanner combination, *Br. J. Radiol.*, vol. 79, no. 1, p. S79–S86.

Uematsu, M., Fukui, T., Shioda, A., Tokumitsu, H., Takai, K., Kojima, T., Asai, Y., & Kusano, S. 1996, A dual computed tomography linear accelerator unit for stereotactic radiation therapy: a new approach without cranially fixated stereotactic frames, *Int. J. Radiat. Oncol. Biol. Phys.*, vol. 35, no. 3, pp. 587–592.

Uematsu, M., Fukui, T., Tahara, K., Sato, N., Shiota, A., & Wong, J. 2008, Long-term results of computed tomography guided hypofractionated stereotactic radiotherapy for stage I non-small cell lung cancers, *Int. J. Radiat. Oncol. Biol. Phys.*, vol. 72, no. 1, p. S37.

Uematsu, M., Shioda, A., Suda, A., Fukui, T., Ozeki, Y., Hama, Y., Wong, J. R., & Kusano, S. 2001, Computed tomography-guided frameless stereotactic radiotherapy for stage I non-small cell lung cancer: a 5-year experience, *Int. J. Radiat. Oncol. Biol. Phys.*, vol. 51, no. 3, pp. 666–670.

Uematsu, M., Shioda, A., Suda, A., Tahara, K., Kojima, T., Hama, Y., Kono, M., Wong, J. R., Fukui, T., & Kusano, S. 2000, Intrafractional tumor position stability during computed tomography (CT)-guided frameless stereotactic radiation therapy for lung or liver cancers with a fusion of CT and linear accelerator (FOCAL) unit, *Int. J. Radiat. Oncol. Biol. Phys.*, vol. 48, no. 2, pp. 443–448.

Webb, S. 1992, Optimization by simulated annealing of three-dimensional, conformal treatment planning for radiation fields defined by a multileaf collimator: II. Inclusion of two-dimensional modulation of the x-ray intensity, *Phys. Med. Biol.*, vol. 37, no. 8, pp. 1689–1704.

Wong, J. R., Cheng, C. W., Grimm, L., & Uematsu, M. 2001, Clinical implementation of the world's first primatom, a Combination of CT scanner and linear accelerator, for precise tumor targeting and treatment, *Phys. Med.*, vol. XVII, no. 4, pp. 272–276.

Wong, J. R., Gao, Z., Merrick, S., Wilson, P., Uematsu, M., Woo, K., & Cheng, C. W. 2009, Potential for higher treatment failure in obese patients: correlation of elevated body mass index and increased daily prostate deviations from the radiation beam isocenters in an analysis of 1,465 computed tomographic images, *Int. J. Radiat. Oncol. Biol. Phys*, vol. 75, no. 1, pp. 49–55.

Wong, J. R., Gao, Z., Uematsu, M., Merrick, S., Machernis, N. P., Chen, T., & Cheng, C. W. 2008, Interfractional prostate shifts: review of 1870 computed tomography (CT) scans obtained during image-guided radiotherapy using CT-on-rails for the treatment of prostate cancer, *Int. J. Radiat. Oncol. Biol. Phys.*, vol. 72, no. 5, pp. 1396–1401.

Wong, J. R., Grimm, L., Uematsu, M., Oren, R., Cheng, C. W., Merrick, S., & Schiff, P. 2005, Image-guided radiotherapy for prostate cancer by CT-linear accelerator combination: prostate movements and dosimetric considerations, *Int. J. Radiat. Oncol. Biol. Phys.*, vol. 61, no. 2, pp. 561–569.

Yenice, K. M., Lovelock, D. M., Hunt, M. A., Lutz, W. R., Fournier-Bidoz, N., Hua, C. H., Yamada, J., Bilsky, M., Lee, H., Pfaff, K., Spirou, S. V., & Amols, H. I. 2003, CT image-guided intensity-modulated therapy for paraspinal tumors using stereotactic immobilization, *Int. J. Radiat. Oncol. Biol. Phys.*, vol. 55, no. 3, pp. 583–593.

Yu, C. X. 1995, Intensity-modulated arc therapy with dynamic multileaf collimation: an alternative to tomotherapy, *Phys. Med. Biol.*, vol. 40, no. 9, pp. 1435–1449.

4

Megavoltage Fan Beam CT IGRT

Gustavo Hugo Olivera
21st Century Oncology

Thomas Rockwell
Mackie
University of Wisconsin

4.1 Introduction to Helical Tomotherapy

Helical tomotherapy is the combination of an intensity-modulated radiotherapy (IMRT) device and a helical computed tomography (CT) scanner. Figure 4.1 contains diagrams of the main components of the machine, which is commercialized as the Hi-Art™ Helical Tomotherapy machine (TomoTherapy, Madison, WI).

In this device the beam from a 6-MV linear accelerator is collimated to a fan beam by a primary jaw pair that is made of tungsten and is 23 cm thick. The setting of the jaw pair creates a fan beam that can vary from 1 to 5 cm wide at the isocenter. Integrated x-ray shielding has been designed to produce a field leakage of 0.01% (Ramsey et al., 2006), which is a factor of 10 less than IEC (International Electromechanical Commission) guidelines. There is no field-flattening filter, and hence, the intensity at the central axis is higher than the intensity away from the central axis. Thin filters are placed in the beam before and after the monitor chamber for low energy x-ray removal. While the intensity varies across the field, the beam quality is nearly invariant because there is no differential hardening caused by a flattening filter. The distance from the source to the center of rotation is 85 cm, which is less than the 100 cm typical of a linac. The distance from the source to the detector is 132 cm. The diameter of the bore is 85 cm, which is comparable to a large bore CT simulator.

The 6-MV fan beam is modulated by a binary multileaf collimator containing 64 leaf pairs that define 64 beamlets, each 0.625 cm wide at the rotation center. Pneumatic pistons retract leaves from the beam. The delivery is broken up into 51 arc projections for each rotation of the gantry. The time interval that a leaf is retracted is proportional to

the energy fluence through one beamlet of the fan beam. Collimator leaves are made of high-purity tungsten and are 10 cm tall, with leakage on the order of 0.3 to 0.5 percent. This low leakage is by design because the device was created for dedicated IMRT, which typically requires higher monitor units for delivery compared to non-IMRT, open-field radiotherapy. Opposing the linac there is an exit detector arc that intercepts the fan beam and is used for several purposes, including generation of CT images for image guidance, device quality assurance (QA), and dose reconstruction (*in-vivo* dosimetry), for a record of the dose delivered to the patient during treatment. This exit detector is relatively efficient at high megavoltage (MV) beams (Judy et al., 1977; Keller et al., 2002; Ruchala et al., 1999) because most of the photons interact in the tungsten septa that separate the xenon detector channels. The CT detector is used for many purposes; the more important are the generation of CT for image guidance, QA of the machine, and dose reconstruction (*in-vivo* dosimetry), which is the generation of the dose that was delivered to the patient during treatment.

Behind the CT detector, there is a beam stop that attenuates the exiting radiation, thereby reducing the room structural shielding needed for the machine installation. The beam stop is also used to balance the gantry.

There are two delivery modes on the tomotherapy unit, helical tomotherapy and topotherapy. Helical delivery means that when the machine is rotating, the couch also moves simultaneously, creating a helical trace of the radiation source as the patient table continuously moves through the device aperture. The ratio between the distance traveled by the couch per rotation and the treatment field (or slice) width is called the "pitch" (see Figure 4.2).

Figure 4.3 is a representation of the multileaf collimator (MLC) for two projections. Each one of these projections delivers some

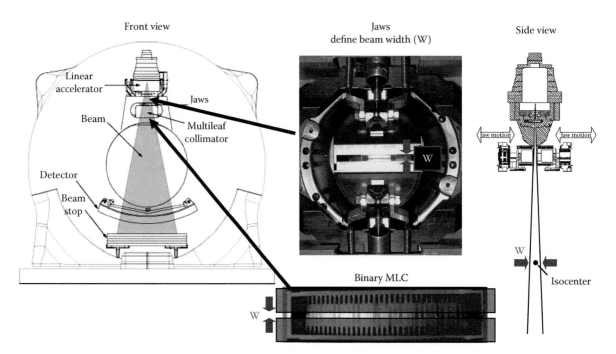

FIGURE 4.1 Schematic views and main components of a Hi-Art™ (TomoTherapy Inc., Madison WI) helical tomotherapy machine.

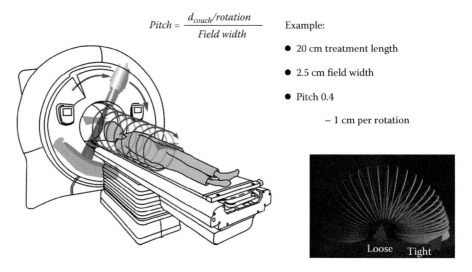

$$Pitch = \frac{d_{couch}/rotation}{Field\ width}$$

Example:

- 20 cm treatment length
- 2.5 cm field width
- Pitch 0.4
  - 1 cm per rotation

FIGURE 4.2 Representation of helical delivery and illustration of the meaning of pitch. During the helical delivery the MLC controls the amount of time that radiation is reaching the patient.

amount of energy fluence to the patients when their MLC leaves are open. The time that each leaf is open is represented by a 2D array called a "sinogram", which is used to represent the delivery pattern. The time that each leaf is open corresponds to a certain gray value on the sinogram representation (the longer the leaves are open, the higher the radiation intensity, and the whiter the color displayed).

A recently introduced mode of delivery, topotherapy, was designed to deliver high-quality treatments to simple cases such as node-negative tangential breast treatments. Topotherapy uses a fixed gantry while the couch and MLC move to produce an intensity-modulated field from a single direction. Each field is delivered with full compensation and has an intensity-modulated

field from a single direction. Each field that is delivered with full compensation has the inferior and superior borders nearly parallel. Both the tomotherapy and topotherapy modes are capable of irradiating a field that is 40 cm wide and 160 cm long.

The system is integrated as shown in Figure 4.4. A central database holds all patient treatment and record/verify information. The database is connected to an operator station (OS), which is used to control the CT scan, to register the CT image set to the original planned CT set, and to deliver treatment to the patients. The OS can also be used in physics mode to perform QA operations. Also connected to the database are planning stations that are used to generate (optimize) the plans that will be delivered as well as perform and analyze patient

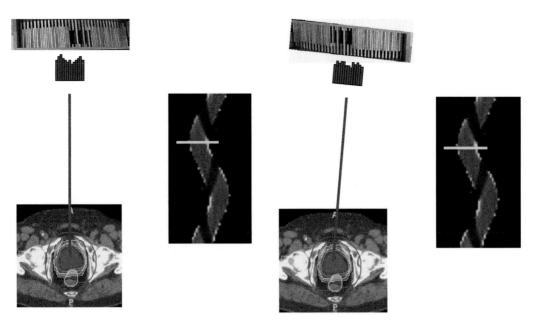

FIGURE 4.3 Representation of treatment delivery in a helical tomotherapy machine for two neighboring projections of a prostate therapy treatment, including sinograms of intensity modulation.

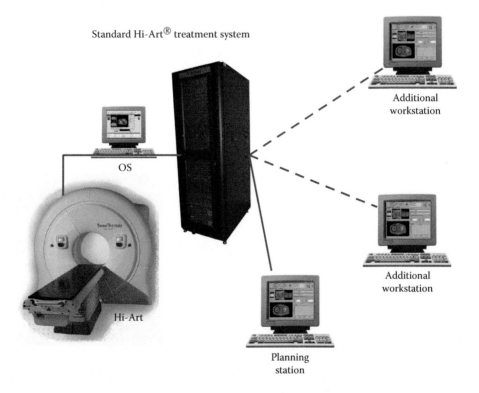

FIGURE 4.4 Component diagram of the integrated tomotherapy system.

QA. dose calculations are performed in a cluster of computers using the convolution/superposition algorithm. The convolution/superposition is very well suited to be used as dose calculation for an IMRT machine such as tomotherapy since the fan beam is not hardened by a field-flattening filter, and it is well suited for calculating the dose for nonuniform intensity beamlets.

4.2 Tomotherapy Workflow

The integrated tomotherapy system allows for a very simple workflow. During the treatment planning phase, a plan is optimized to generate the irradiation pattern to deliver to the patient. Typically, the beamlets that compromise the treatments are precomputed automatically for each case before optimization. The plan is optimized by the user, indicating the allowed tradeoff for each anatomical structure. Once the beamlets are computed, plan optimization takes typically from 5 to 15 min depending on the complexity. When the plan is accepted, it can be delivered to a phantom for QA or to the patient. Phantom QA can be performed using film, ionization chamber, or other adequate electronic reader device.

During a typical treatment session, the patient is placed on the couch with the same fixation/immobilization restraint devices typically used in radiotherapy. An MVCT is obtained using a detuned MV energy, to verify the daily anatomy and position. The daily MVCT is registered with the planning CT using the automatic and manual fusion tools available on the OS. Once patient registration is determined, any correcting offset can be applied for the day's treatment. The tomotherapy device can automatically account for 4 degrees of freedom: 3 translations and patient roll about the device axis of rotation. Figure 4.5 illustrates the mean adjustments that were applied in more than 3,800 patient treatments on tomotherapy units at the University of Wisconsin (Schubert et al., 2009). Translation variations are more prevalent in the thorax, abdomen, and pelvis. Nearly simultaneously, similar results were reported by Lin et al. (2009).

Once the patient is located in the desired position, the treatment session can be delivered. The tomotherapy system also has an adaptive module that can be used to check the patient position every day or the amount of dose delivered to the patient during that treatment session. The details of adaptive therapy will be discussed in Section 4.5.

4.3 Details of Image Formation

The linear accelerator used to generate the treatment beam is detuned to a lower MV energy, about 3.5 MV, for CT image acquisition. This imaging modality is referred to as MVCT imaging (Jeraj et al., 2004). Typical spectra for treatment and MVCT beams are presented in Figures 4.6 and 4.7.

The CT detector used in the machine is xenon gas elements that are separated by narrow tungsten septal plates and has been described previously (Judy et al., 1977; Keller et al., 2002; Ruchala et al., 1999). The standard image matrix size is 512 × 512 pixels, and the field of view has a diameter of 40 cm. The image reconstruction is performed using a filtered back-projection (Ruchala et al., 1999).

On the OS, the operator is tasked with the selection of the scan length and the slice thickness (fine, normal, or coarse). Three pitch values (1, 2, and 3) are preprogrammed; these are referred to as fine, normal, and coarse, respectively. The standard jaw setting for the imaging mode is 4 mm, and the preprogrammed pitch values correspond to a nominal slice spacing of 2, 4, and 6 mm. The rotational period during the image acquisition is fixed at 10 s. Using a half-scan reconstruction technique, this translates to an acquisition rate of 1 slice per 5 s. The imaging dose depends on the selected pitch and the thickness of the imaged anatomy, but it is typically in the range of 1–3 cGy (Shah et al., 2008). The total scan time depends on the number of selected slices.

The dose for MVCT is sufficiently low that its use is justified for daily setup. Figures 4.8 and 4.9 show the dose distributions for one MVCT session. Figures 4.8a (breast patient), 4.8b (prostate patient), and 4.8c (lung patient) were acquired using the "normal" setting. The dose would be approximately twice as high for the fine setting and 2/3 as high for the coarse setting.

Figure 4.9 shows the imaging dose distribution (Gy) received during an MVCT session using the normal setting for a craniospinal patient. As can be seen, the dose is minimal, making this imaging approach acceptable for daily patient setup. The maximum dose is at the level of the neck and is on the order of 1 cGy.

4.3.1 Image Noise

Noise is expressed relative to the linear attenuation coefficient of water, μ_{water}, and is corrected for the contrast scale

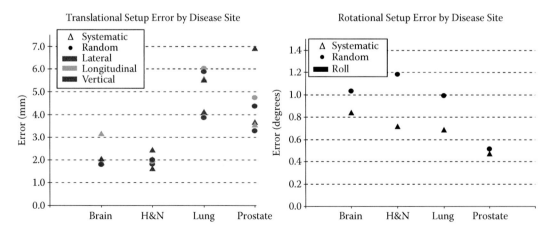

FIGURE 4.5 Translation (left panel) and rotation setup errors (1 S.D. uncertainty) as detected by more than 3,800 daily setup corrections on the helical tomotherapy unit at the University of Wisconsin. (From Schubert LK., et al. *Int J Radiat Oncol Biol Phys.*, 73:1260–9, 2009. With permission.)

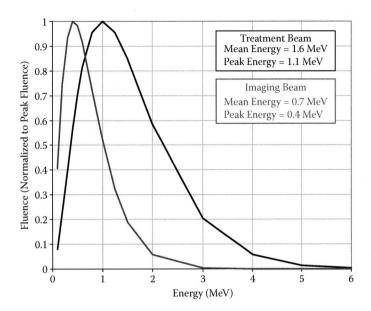

FIGURE 4.6 Photon spectrum for the linac in treatment mode and MVCT modes.

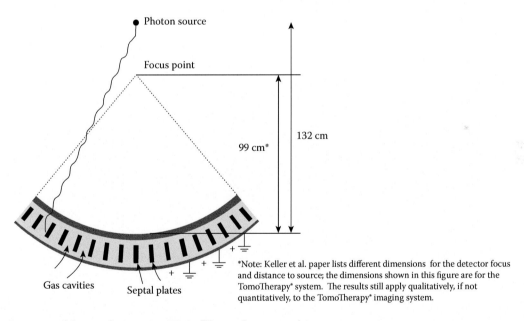

FIGURE 4.7 Geometry of the exit detector in a Hi-Art™ tomotherapy machine.

(CS) of the scanner (Judy et al., 1977). Based on that definition, a noise metric can be obtained in the following way:

$$\text{Noise} = \sigma_{CT} \times CS \times 100/\mu_{water}, \qquad (4.1)$$

where

$$CS = (\mu_{polycarbonate} - \mu_{water})/(HU_{polycarbonate} - HU_{water}). \qquad (4.2)$$

Based on this technique, noise values of 3.7–3.8 have been published for MVCT images (Meeks et al., 2005). This corresponds to a standard deviation of about 35–36 HU in a homogeneous water bath.

4.3.2 Image Uniformity

Uniformity can be determined by the average HU in smaller ROIs (approximately 5 mm in radius). The ROI should be located in the center and periphery of the phantom. The difference between the peripheral HU and the central HU is determined.

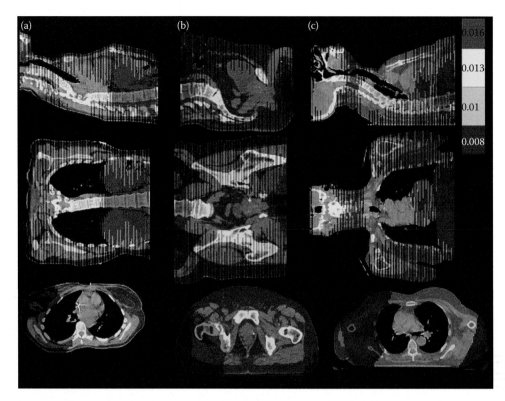

FIGURE 4.8 (See color insert)   MVCT Dose (Gy) for normal setting for different anatomical sites: (a) Breast, (b) Prostate, and (c) lung (courtesy of Sanford Meeks, M.D. Anderson Hospital, Orlando, Florida.)

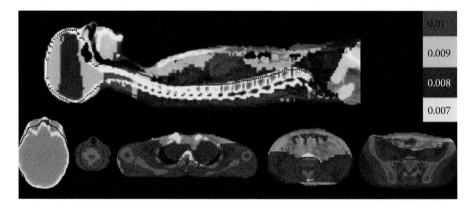

FIGURE 4.9 (See color insert)   MVCT Dose (Gy) for coarse setting for a craniospinal case (Courtesy of Sanford Meeks, M.D. Anderson Hospital, Orlando, Florida.)

The HU difference between peripheral and central water ROIs should be less than 25 HU. A 25 HU difference in water would translate to a 2.5% variation on the calculated density of water.

4.3.3 Image Resolution

Spatial resolution typically is measured with a high-contrast hole pair test pattern, facilitated by use of a resolution plug provided by the vendor. This plug contains a precision-drilled hole pattern and is inserted into a solid water cylindrical phantom (nicknamed the "cheese phantom") that is typically used for determining CT electron density maps.

Figure 4.10 shows an MVCT and a photograph of the high-contrast plug. The smallest resolvable hole pattern indicates that MVCT images that are reconstructed with the typical 512 × 512 pixel matrix allow the resolution of a 1.25-mm high-contrast object (Meeks et al., 2005), which is better than the vendor specification of 1.6 mm for minimum resolution of a high-contrast object.

4.3.4 Use of MVCT for Calculation of Patient Treatment Dose

One of the very desirable features of fan-beam MVCT is that it does not have significant photoelectric absorbance; thus,

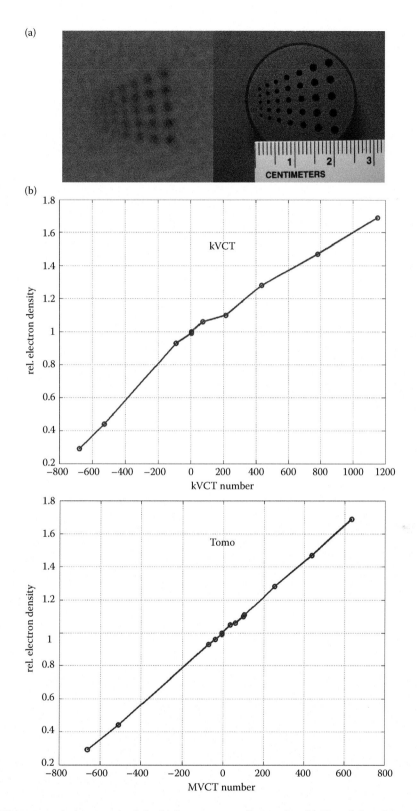

FIGURE 4.10   (a) MVCT image and photograph of the high contrast resolution plug (b) Plot of the relative electronic density against the CT# for a diagnostic kV CT and MVCT. As can be observed, for an MVCT this relationship is linear (Courtesy of Katja Langen, M.D. Anderson Hospital, Orlando, Florida.)

metal artifacts and cupping artifacts in reconstructed images are minimized, and reliable CT numbers are produced that can be used to compute dose. For an MVCT, there is a linear relationship between CT# and electron density. This makes MVCT very useful for processes such as dose reconstruction and adaptive radiotherapy.

Langen et al. (2005) performed extensive studies on the use of MVCT for dose calculation. In that work, the authors conclude "The use of MVCT images for dose calculations can be accomplished with an accuracy that is similar to that of dose computations in kV CT images. The recalculation technique can be used to obtain dose distributions on the daily MVCT image set." If the MVCT images are used for dose calculations, the reproducibility of this calibration curve should be monitored on a monthly basis or after a change to a component of the beamline with a subset of electron density plugs that cover lung-, bone-, and water-like densities. If the calibration differed by 20 HU near water equivalent densities and by up to 50 and 80 HU in lung- and bone-like densities resulted in dosimetric differences of typically 2% or less for tomotherapy treatment plans (Langen et al., 2005). Tomotherapy MVCT images have also been used to provide images largely uncontaminated by metal artifacts for use in planning high-dose-rate brachytherapy (Holly et al., 2009).

4.4 Clinical Utility of Tomotherapy with Daily Image Guidance

4.4.1 IGRT Head and Neck

Tomotherapy can be used for complex dose prescriptions that include dose constraints for target and adjacent normal structures. Head and neck cancer is one such application. Tomotherapy easily enables multiple organs at risk (OAR) to be specified and different dose levels to be prescribed to multiple planning target volumes (PTVs). Moreover, the prescriptions typically are delivered more homogeneously with lower doses to the OARs (Lee et al., 2008; Sheng et al., 2006).

Before image guidance, it was assumed that head and neck treatments were fairly accurate. However, even when using custom immobilization, with CT image guidance, patients often need to be translated by many millimeters for correct set-up (Vaandering et al., 2009; Zeidan et al., 2007). A study of setup variations for a variety of clinical sites including head and neck is shown in Figure 4.5. In addition, head and neck patients can have significant rotational deviations from the original planning CT. These include changes in the position of the head with respect to the neck. When this is seen, the positioning of the patient must be altered and another CT taken. Figure 4.5 illustrates that head and neck patients also have considerable roll around the axis of rotation of the machine. With a tumor position, a long distance from the axis of rotation even one degree of rotation could result in significant movement of the target volume. Such roll corrections can be performed automatically by the tomotherapy unit without adjusting the patient's setup.

How important is daily CT imaging for head and neck cancer? Setup adjustment records on head and neck patients who had received daily image guidance on tomotherapy were analyzed to determine what would be the setup uncertainty if less frequent setups were performed (Zeidan et al., 2007). Figure 4.11 shows that if weekly instead of daily setups had been performed, as compared to daily CT setups, about 55% of patients would have greater than 3 mm setup error and about a quarter of them would have had a setup error greater than 5 mm.

Figure 4.11 indicates that there is a small residual uncertainty that is related to the error in the daily setup process. Using repeat CT scans, it has been shown that tomotherapy has a setup uncertainty of less than 1 mm (Boswell et al., 2006; Woodford et al., 2007), which is sufficient for both head and neck cancer and stereotactic radiosurgery.

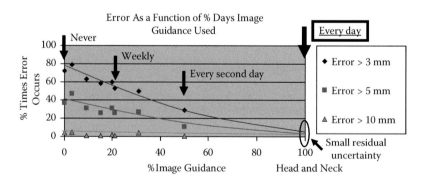

FIGURE 4.11 The effect of imaging schedule on delivery accuracy for head and neck patients. The study was based on tomotherapy treatments that received daily image guidance (100% image guidance) and registration that improved the setup to within a millimeter. The setup results were analyzed to determine what would be the setup error if less frequent image guidance were used. For example, 50% image guidance would be the equivalent of every second day, and 20% image guidance would be imaging once a week. (From Zeidan OA., et al. *Int J Radiat Oncol Biol Phys.* 67:670–77. With Permission.)

4.4.2 IGRT Prostate

Prostate cancer is frequently treated with tomotherapy because the approach is capable of placing a high-dose gradient between the prostate and the rectum, thereby lowering the dose to the rectum and maintaining a homogeneous dose to the prostate. In advanced prostate treatment, nodal tracks can also be targeted concomitantly at a lower dose and still maintain a reasonable dose to the bladder, bowel, and rectum. Cozzarini et al. (2008) found that treatment of advanced high-risk prostate cancer with treatment of the pelvic nodes with tomotherapy resulted in lower than expected grade 1 and 2 toxicities and an absence of gastrointestinal grade 3 toxicity.

Daily image guidance is universally used for prostate radiotherapy with tomotherapy. This is because differential filling of the bladder and rectum can shift the prostate considerably (Kupelian et al., 2006). A tomotherapy MVCT can image the adipose layer around the prostate and allow the wall of the rectum to be visualized, thereby allowing the degree of rectal filling to be assessed (Fiorino et al., 2008). Although marker seeds placed in the prostate may be used, most centers use only the soft tissue anatomy for registering the patient. An example of an MVCT image of the prostate with implanted markers is shown in Figure 4.12.

The imaging and registration processes for prostate radiotherapy are typically 1 to 2 min and 3 to 5 min, respectively, on tomotherapy. A concern has been expressed that peristaltic motion may be significant during the imaging

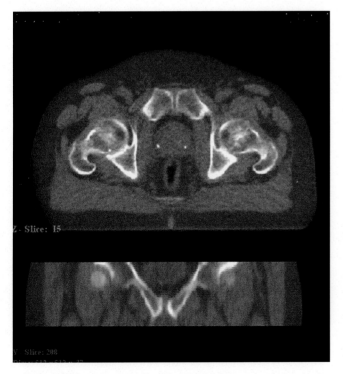

FIGURE 4.12 Example of an MVCT for prostate treatment. It is possible to visualize the prostate and rectal wall. The patient has implanted markers. The markers are clearly visible with no metal artifacts.

and registration. A study using radiofrequency markers (Calypso, Seattle, WA) showed that significant motion, as compared to the tomotherapy MVCT image, of a magnitude greater than 3 mm occurred less than 7% of the time in the anterior–posterior dimension and less than 3% of the time in the superior–inferior dimension (Langen et al., 2009). Similarly, using repeat MVCT scans before and after treatment, Tournel et al. (2008) found that the movement of patients during treatments was limited to 2.5, 2.0, and 1.1 mm in the lateral, longitudinal, and vertical directions, respectively. Systematic errors were limited to <1 mm, justifying few millimeter prostate margins for internal movement.

4.4.3 IGRT Lung

Tomotherapy is a versatile treatment system for lung cancer. In a comparison of 3D conformal radiation therapy (3D CRT) and tomotherapy, it was found that tomotherapy produced a more homogeneous dose distribution and improved high-dose conformity to the lung and esophagus (Cattaneo et al. 2008). Tomotherapy is often used to treat difficult lung tumors such as mesothelioma. Sterzing et al. (2008) reported that tomotherapy provided a more homogeneous coverage to the mesothelioma target volume as compared to step-and-shoot IMRT and could reduce the mean dose to the contralateral lung to below 5 Gy. Tomotherapy is used for stereotactic body radiosurgery for small lung tumors using a few large fractions of radiotherapy. In these treatments, daily image guidance is extremely important to enable each fraction to be setup correctly.

In a protocol of 46 inoperable lung cancer patients with high-stage disease (37/46 were stage III or IV), dose-escalated hypofractionated tomotherapy was used (Adkison et al., 2008). The actuarial 2-year overall survival was calculated to be 47%, with a median survival of 18 months. Survival and local control curves from this study are shown in Figure 4.13. When patients on the protocol were compared stage for stage to patients reported by Mountain (1997), the expected 2-year survival was 21.5%. Furthermore, there was no incidence of grade 3 esophagitis or pneumonitis. Grade 2 pneumonitis was associated with the use of adjuvant chemotherapy. The use of chemotherapy with all forms of IMRT, including tomotherapy, should be carefully considered since IMRT tends to irradiate a larger portion of the normal lung to a lower dose. Adjuvant chemotherapy can add an effective dose to the whole lung that is equivalent to about 10 Gy and gives patients a higher incidence of pneumonitis than they would receive with radiation alone.

There is concern in all forms of IMRT for lung cancer that an interplay effect due to motion of the thorax (more correctly called an "interference" or "aliasing" effect) could result in unplanned hot and cold spots in the target volume and hot spots being produced in the OAR. In a careful set of investigations by Kissick et al. (2005, 2008), they showed that with the usual treatment protocols (2.5 cm jaw width and a sufficient PTV margin to include the breathing excursions) used with tomotherapy, this interference effect is negligible if

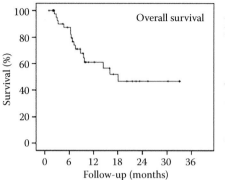
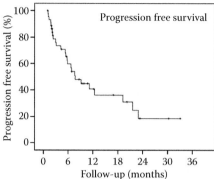

FIGURE 4.13   Survival and progression-free survival for a University of Wisconsin study of dose escalation for advanced lung cancer using helical tomotherapy (From Adkinson JB., et al *Technol Cancer Res Treat.* 7: 441–7). According to Mountain (1997), the expected survival for this cohort of patients was only 21.2 % at two years if conventional doses and 3D CRT were used instead.

the patient breathes relatively regularly even if the magnitude of tidal motion is almost as large as the slice width. The patient needs to be registered to the time-averaged position of the breathing motion.

For the interference effect, respiratory frequency is more important than amplitude. The reason for the robustness to breathing of tomotherapy is that the frequency of respiratory motion (typically 0.2 Hz) is separated well from both the couch movement through the jaws (a frequency of typically 0.02 Hz) and frequency of MLC actuation (an average of about 2 Hz). Therefore, regular motion of the lung blurs the dose distribution created by the much more rapid fluence pattern inherent and specific to tomotherapy. If the breathing is regular, then this blurring will be constant in time as the couch moves through the jaws. The motion blurring will add in quadrature to the beam profile blurring already present. The results become the same as in 3D CRT with the following: a sufficient margin for relatively regular motion on the CTV, some care in setting the treatment parameters to avoid interference, and registration to the time-averaged tumor position. Patients that cannot stop from shifting their time-averaged position should not be treated on a tomotherapy machine or receive any IMRT treatment. In tomotherapy, a cough or gasp may be tolerated if it is much faster than the time it takes for the couch to traverse the beam—the unwanted fast random movement will get corrected by time averaging, if fast enough. A device like BodyFix™ (Medical Intelligence Medizintechnik GmbH, Schwabmtinchen, Germany) may work very well in controlling breathing regularity, increase frequency and lower amplitude slightly, and prevent the patient shifting of the tumor's average position (Siker et al., 2006).

Using MVCT, there is an excellent density contrast between the healthy lung and the tumor. Figure 4.14 shows that the MVCT images can be analyzed to determine the change in the anatomy due to tumor regression. Furthermore, dose can be recomputed on the daily images to determine the actual dose delivered on the anatomy of the day (the methods are discussed more in Section 6). Figure 4.14 indicates that most of the tumor is receiving more than 5% higher dose than planned due to less attenuation in the expanded lung that was previously occupied by tumor. When large changes in the apparent target volume are seen, there is no standard approach for replanning. The physician may choose to change the margins of the tumor and replan the treatment (Ramsey et al., 2006) or to continue to irradiate the newly inflated lung in case there is residual disease still present (Siker et al., 2006).

The CT scanning time on a tomotherapy unit is much longer than for a conventional diagnostic CT scanner. One rotation takes 10 s as compared to subsecond on a diagnostic unit. This results in blurring of the MVCT scan in areas of motion. If these images are used to outline the tumor, then one must remember that there is already motion expressed in the image and hence an additional margin for motion, if any, should be small.

Difficult breast cases can be treated with tomotherapy. Conventional breast cases using a pair of tangential beams are easy to treat with 3D CRT and hence, most simple breast cases are treated on a conventional linac. More difficult cases, such as node-positive disease, left-sided treatment on a funnel-shaped chest wall (see Figure 4.15), or bilateral cancer, are often treated with tomotherapy. Goddu et al. (2009b) has shown that tomotherapy provides better dose distributions than 3D CRT for treatment of node-positive left-sided breast cancer. They reported that the PTV was irradiated more homogeneously and tomotherapy kept the dose to the heart lower than 3D CRT.

On the tomotherapy planning system, it is possible to use some unique structure blocking capabilities to control the dose to the heart and contralateral breast. On tomotherapy, a structure can be declared a partial or fully blocked structure. A partially blocked structure flags the optimizer to allow beamlets to pass through it after it has gone through the PTV, but it does not allow the beamlets to go through the partially blocked structure

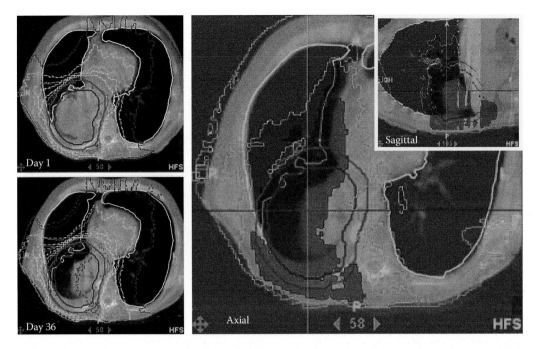

FIGURE 4.14 (See color insert) MVCT scans of the lung on the first and 36th fraction for lung cancer. The computed dose distribution using the MVCT images is also shown. On the left panel, the dose difference color wash is shown. Red are the regions that are 5% high. Light blue is 5% reduced dose. In general the tumor is receiving more dose than planned, but the dose to the cord has not increased.

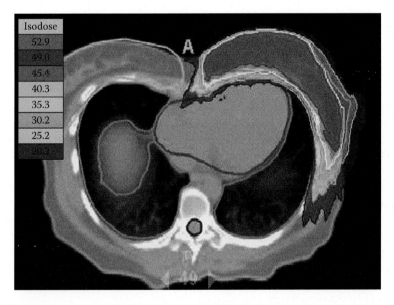

FIGURE 4.15 (See color insert) Treatment using helical tomotherapy of a left-sided breast patient with a funnel-shaped chest wall. (Courtesy of Florian Sterzing, Heidelberg University.)

on its way to the tumor. If the structure is declared fully blocked, the optimizer will not allow beamlets to irradiate that structure at all. It is possible to contour all or part of the heart or lungs as a structure that will be partially or fully blocked.

As stated, a topotherapy treatment mode is available, called TomoDirect™, which uses a fixed gantry and couch movement during treatment to provide compensated or even dynamic IMRT treatments field-by-field.

This mode is particularly useful for tangential breast radiotherapy. Both breast fields are fully compensated, and the setup techniques used for tangential delivery can be used. This mode also supports "breast flash" so that the small movements in the lateral and anterior–posterior direction (typically less than 2 mm) during breathing can be accommodated in each of the fields. Figure 4.16 shows a tangential treatment of a right-sided breast using topotherapy (TomoDirect™) on a tomotherapy unit.

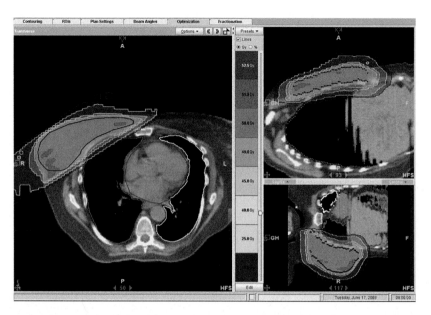

FIGURE 4.16 (See color insert) Planning of a topotherapy treatment mode called TomoDirect™ for tangential treatment of a right breast. The dose is delivered with the gantry fixed and the couch and leaves moving. Each field provides tissue compensation for missing tissue. In this case, the hot spots are only 3% higher than the median dose.

Breast radiotherapy can benefit from daily image guidance (Goddu et al., 2009a). However, there is concern that daily CT guidance may not be clinically warranted for breast cancer and some physicians use MVCT less often than daily. This is because of the worry that extra dose to the contralateral breast might result in an increased probability of a second breast cancer malignancy. The tomotherapy MVCT will add about 1 cGy of dose to the contralateral breast, which is about 20% of the dose that breast will receive due to scatter into the breast from a conventional 3D CRT treatment. Moreover, using conventional IMRT for the treatment instead of tomotherapy will result in more dose to the contralateral breast than the MVCT dose on tomotherapy will. Image-guided setup using a camera system such as the VisionRT™ (Vision RT Ltd., London, UK) system may be as accurate as an MVCT registration for a whole breast treatment. However, for concomitant boosting of the lumpectomy site, CT scanning may provide better setup information depending on when the treatment occurs. If the treatment is only for a few weeks after surgery, the seroma replacing the removed breast tissue is visible on an MVCT image. Eventually after a few months, the lumpectomy site cannot be visualized on an MVCT image.

4.4.5 IGRT Brain

Tomotherapy has been used for treating a variety of novel brain and CNS tumors. Yartsev et al. (2005) compared a variety of modalities for treatment of a variety of cranial tumors: stereotactic radiosurgery, 3D conformal, step-and-shoot IMRT, proton radiotherapy, and helical tomotherapy. They found that tomotherapy provided high-dose conformity

compared with proton radiotherapy and provided slightly lower integral dose as compared with the other photon techniques.

Multiple intracranial metastases can be treated simultaneously with tomotherapy. The reason for this is that there is no need to move a metastasis to the isocenter to treat it. Metastases may be treated anywhere within the brain with the isocenter at the same position as during the planning CT scan. In addition, the whole brain may be treated in addition to treating visible multiple metastases to a higher dose (Bauman et al., 2007). Even more complicated treatments are possible. Illustrated in Figure 4.17, whole brain plus multiple metastases may be treated while sparing the hippocampus (Gutierrez et al., 2007). This treatment is predicted to allow long-term survivors to have fewer memory deficits.

Boswell et al. (2006) showed that MVCT imaging can provide a set-up accuracy within a millimeter for a head phantom test case. For the specific case of setting up a brain tumor, Woodford et al. (2007) demonstrated that setups within 0.5 mm were possible as long as the fine or normal setting was used and if the CT field of view in the longitudinal direction was at least 2 cm long. This accuracy is less than the slice width. This is because multiple images are used with corresponding averaging. Because the brain moves little in the cranium, the automated registration based on bone may be preferred to the setting that uses all of the image data.

Some stereotactic radiosurgery programs based on tomotherapy use MVCT for localization in conjunction with a good immobilization system to ensure that the patient is setup and will remain setup for the extended treatment times that are necessary for high total doses. Immobilization

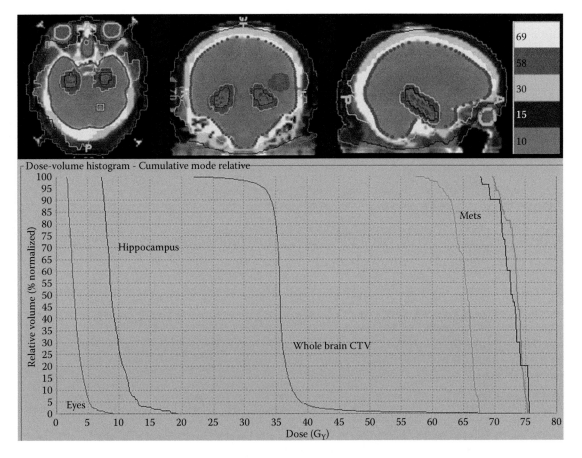

FIGURE 4.17 (See color insert) Whole brain treatment with simultaneous treatment of visible metastases and conformal avoidance of the hippocampus.

systems range from reinforced face masks, to bite-block-based systems, to rigid fixation attached to the skull. A thermal plastic face mask easily fits inside the tomotherapy aperture. If a classic radiosurgical stereotactic frame is used, the CT localization frame may be worn for the setup and treatment on a tomotherapy system. It is possible for the frame to be worn during treatment because the convolution/superposition algorithm is capable of taking into account the attenuation of the frame (and in any case such frames attenuate the beam very little).

4.4.6 IGRT TMI

Total marrow irradiation (TMI) is a new type of treatment pioneered by helical tomotherapy users (Hsieh et al., 2009; Hui et al., 2005; Schultheiss et al., 2007; Shueng et al., 2009; Wong et al., 2006). To prepare for a bone marrow transplant for acute leukemia or multiple myeloma, the treatment irradiates bone marrow continuously for 1.6 m long from the top of the skull to the thighs. Such an irradiation would take 30 to 60 min of beam-on time depending on the slice width and the degree of modulation. The legs are either irradiated by turning the patient around and using the tomotherapy unit, or on a separate linear accelerator unit using conventional AP–PA

fields. Bones that contain marrow are outlined, using sufficient margin for setup variation, and sensitive normal tissue structures are outlined to enable avoidance. Using tomotherapy, it is possible to deliver a more uniform dose to the tumor and a much lower dose to critical tissues as compared to conventional total body irradiation (TBI). Figure 4.18 illustrates a typical dose distribution for a TMI treatment.

Wong et al. (2006) have an ongoing clinical trial to safely raise the prescription dose to the bone marrow to 16 Gy using helical tomotherapy delivered TMI. This trial is predicated on the finding of a previous dose escalation study that raised the dose from 12 to 15.75 Gy (Clift et al., 1998) using TBI. As shown in Figure 4.19, Clift et al. (1998) found that the higher dose reduced the disease relapse rate significantly; however, early deaths due to radiation toxicity increased proportionately so that there was no net survival benefit. As shown in Figure 4.20, the TMI dose escalation trial will seek to reduce the relapse rate without increasing the toxicity of the radiation. In fact, at 16 Gy, the toxicity should be equivalent to the toxicity at 10 Gy.

TMI also uses CT image guidance; rather than taking a CT scan throughout the entire 1.6 m irradiation length, three separate scans are typically used to align the patient: one through the head and neck, one through the thorax and abdomen, and one in the pelvis. The registration results are

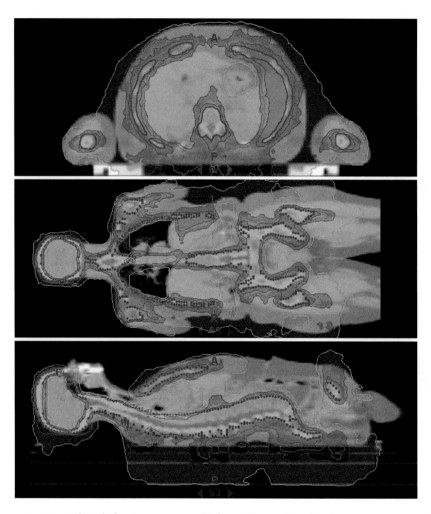

FIGURE 4.18   Total marrow treatment (TMI) plan to prepare a multiple myeloma patient for a bone marrow transplant. The prescribed dose was 10 Gy in 10 fractions of 2 Gy delivered twice a day for one week.

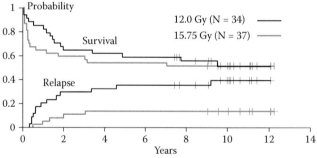

Fig 1. Kaplan-Meier estimates of survival and cumulative incidence of relapse for patients conditioned for HLA-identical marrow transplantation by 120 mg/kg cyclophosphamide and 12.0 Gy or 15.75 Gy of fractionated TBI. Results are updated to February 1998.

FIGURE 4.19   Survival and relapse rates for a clinical trial the used 12 Gy or 15.75 Gy delivered with total body irradiation (TBI). The relapse rate for the higher dose arm is much less than for the lower dose arm;   however, the higher dose arm had far more early toxicity. From Clift et al. (1998).

compared and, if consistent, the results are averaged. There is some differential couch sag between a tomotherapy unit and a typical CT scan. For example, a tomotherapy couch has less sag as it is extended than a GE Discovery LS. This means that it is expected that the vertical displacement will vary systematically between the three couch sites. The differences in vertical displacement are accounted for in the PTV margin in the vertical direction. Note that it would be ideal if the tomotherapy unit had the same sag as the diagnostic CT scanner. This means that the differential sag between a

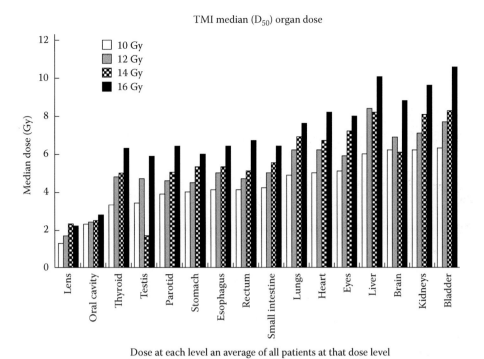

TMI median (D$_{50}$) organ dose

Dose at each level an average of all patients at that dose level

FIGURE 4.20 Normal tissue median doses for a clinical trial to raise the prescribed dose from 10 Gy to 16 Gy. The median doses at 16 Gy are less than or equal to the median doses that would be received to these tissues from total body irradiation at 10 Gy. (From Wong Jy., et al *Int J Radiar Oncol BIrl phys.* 73: 273–9).

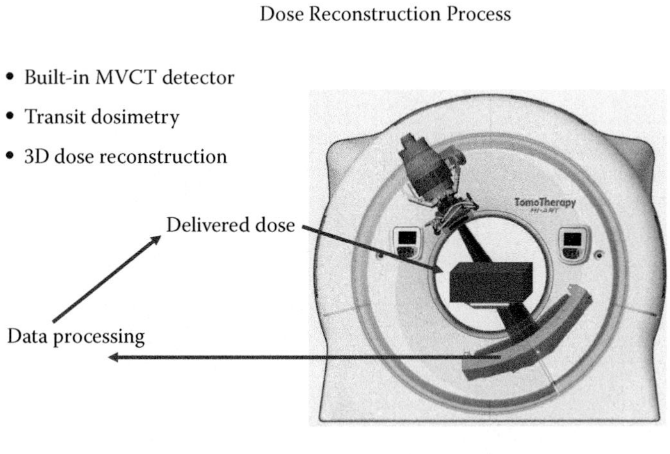

Dose Reconstruction Process

- Built-in MVCT detector
- Transit dosimetry
- 3D dose reconstruction

Delivered dose

Data processing

FIGURE 4.21 The dose reconstruction process, based on the principle of transit dosimetry.

conventional linac couch and a CT scanner would be worse and not better than a tomotherapy unit. The issue of sag on a conventional linac is not noticed because such long treatment fields are never done with lateral fields on a conventional linac.

4.5 Dose Reconstruction and Advanced Adaptive Radiotherapy

Delivery verification by replanning based on the daily CT scan has been commercially released in the Hi-Art™ unit since 2007. This section will describe other image-guided

features that are works in progress but which have been in pilot release at a few clinical sites.

4.5.1 Dose Reconstruction

Dose reconstruction is the process by which the dose deposited to the patient can be inferred from data obtained just before or during delivery (see Figure 4.21). The needed data are the CT patient representation, exit detector data, and the couch speed. Dose reconstruction provides a more accurate representation of dose deposited in the patient just before treatment. By contrast, standard patient QA just verifies the dose deposited to a phantom at a time different than treatment. Different approaches to dose reconstruction can be developed depending on the data and the accuracy of the data available.

Dose reconstruction can be used in different fashions. For instance, a technique can be advised where the dose is reconstructed on just few points of interest and is presented to the operator just after treatment. Such a technique will be very useful for the therapists to detect (flag) possible errors or inconsistencies and could then immediately advise a physicist or physician.

One implementation of such a technique is depicted in Figures 4.22–4.24 and will be referred as *online dose reconstruction*. Figure 4.22 is a representation of the planning station where the user (in this case for a head and neck case) will select points of interest for which they would like to know the dose deposited during treatment. In this case, points in the PTV, parotids, and spinal cord are selected. Figure 4.23 is a representation of the OS where results of the dose reconstruction for the selected points are displayed seconds after the treatment is performed. Trending can be observed for each one of the structures selected as function of the fraction number. A color code—green, yellow, or red—is used to indicate regions in, borderline, or out of tolerance, respectively. Also the difference between plan and delivered dose for the point of interest on a fraction is also represented.

Figure 4.24 is the representation of the online dose reconstruction for a lung case. As can be observed on the plot, the target dose trends toward the yellow region. This trend is an indication of a change with respect to the original plan. This may or may not be an error, and further investigation is needed. However, the therapists are provided with a quick flag to proceed according to predetermined protocols.

Further investigation of this case shows that the dose difference between plan and delivery is due to anatomical changes, which is weight loss in this case (see Figure 4.25). Therefore, the dosimetrical consequences are probably not important; however, information to make informed decisions based on quantitative data during the course of treatment is very valuable.

As can be observed, the online dose reconstruction technique can detect inconsistencies during a fractionated treatment. However, in many cases, deliveries may be hypofractionated, and in these cases, it may be desirable to know the result at the beginning of the treatment. For these cases, a possible implementation of the online dose reconstruction is to perform a mini-fraction (e.g., 10% of the dose) before the majority (90%) of the dose is delivered. This approach is very valuable for hypofractionated treatments where the room for error is much smaller.

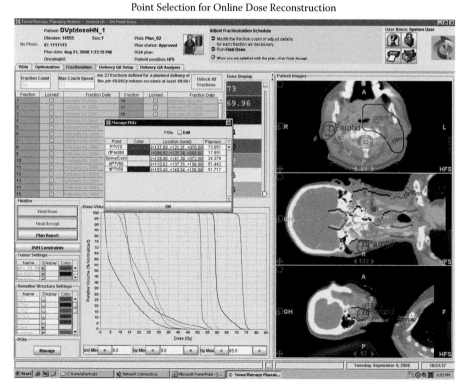

FIGURE 4.22   Point selection on the planning station to perform online dose reconstruction for a head and neck case. A few points in the PTV, parotids, and spinal cord are selected for which to report the dose following treatment.

Point Analysis for Online Dose Reconstruction

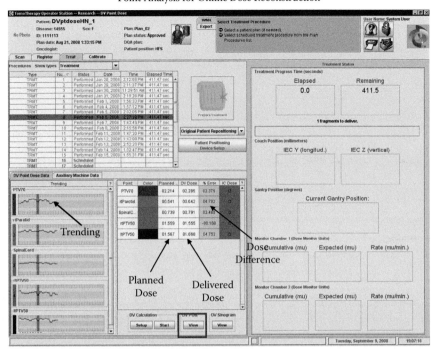

FIGURE 4.23 Online dose reconstruction points generated seconds after treatment. Trending for different fractions as well as the difference between planned and delivered dose for the current fraction are represented.

Online Dose Reconstruction: Lung Case

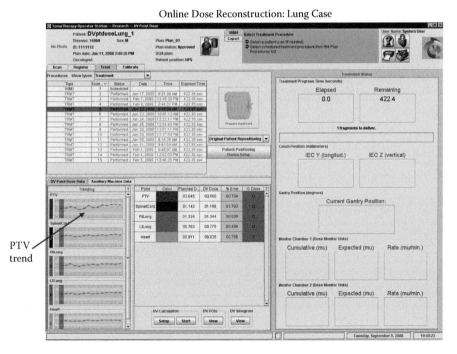

FIGURE 4.24 Online dose reconstruction for a lung case.

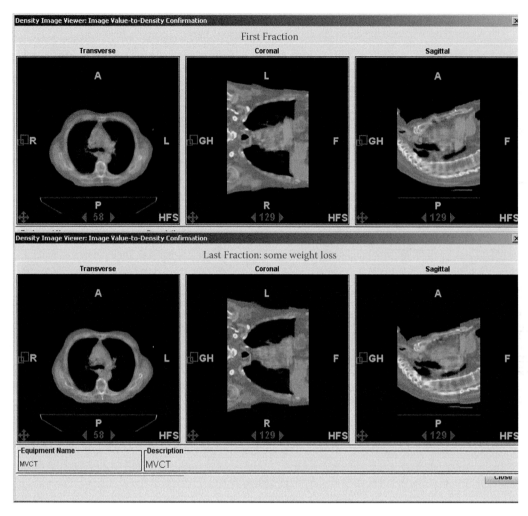

FIURE 4.25 Weight loss for a lung case between first and last fraction for a lung case resulting on difference between plan and delivered dose on the online dose reconstruction technique.

4.5.2 Advanced Adaptive Radiotherapy

The concept of adaptive technique in radiotherapy was introduced first by Di Yan (Yan et al., 1997). As a general definition, adaptive therapy is the use of feedback information to analyze how the treatment is progressing (as compared to the original plan) and take actions if necessary to correct or adapt the course of the treatment.

In the tomotherapy framework, two approaches are possible. One is online for cases such as prostate where variations cannot be predicted beforehand. The second approach is offline where changes are progressive and can be analyzed and/or corrected on periods on the order of one week.

In order for adaptive therapy to be clinically viable, two things are very desirable: (1) it should account for anatomical changes, and (2) it should be fully automatic and produce results in a reasonable time. To account for anatomical changes, techniques such as deformable registration are very useful. Deformable registration techniques (Xing et al., 2007) compare two different image sets and provided a vector map that relates one image set

to the other. Figure 4.26 shows a diagnostic CT (left image) and a daily MVCT (central image). On the central panel, a deformation map is also depicted that should be applied to the image of the center to generate the original CT (2D components of the 3D vector map). The image in the right panel corresponds to application of the deformation map to the center image. The deformation maps are not only useful to map CTs but also can be used to map the planned contours delineated on the diagnostic planning CT to the daily MVCT. As can be observed, the contours on the central panel of Figure 4.26 are mapped from the original physician's contours used as template. Therefore, deformable registration provides an automatic way to generate daily contours from the original contour set.

Deformable registration techniques can also be used to map the dose distribution when the anatomy is changing. Figure 4.27 shows the parotid glands for two instances of time. If we wish to know the cumulative dose for the parotid, then the dose on the locations indicated by the arrow need to be added to obtain the cumulative dose. Therefore, to obtain

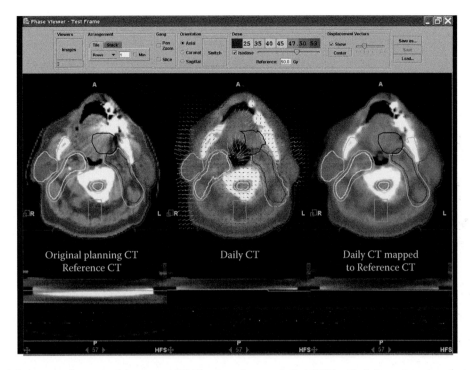

FIGURE 4.26 The left image is the original diagnostic CT. The central image daily MVCT with deformation map obtained from deformable registration of the two images (contours are also obtained by deforming the planned contours). The image on the right corresponds to the daily image applying the deformation map.

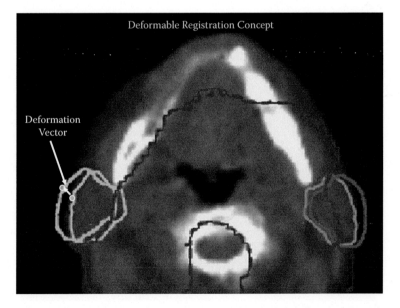

FIGURE 4.27 Two instances of the parotid and the vector that need to be used to add the dose for a single point using deformable registration.

cumulative dose using deformable registration, the dose distribution needs to be mapped to a common framework such as planning CT before it is added.

The process to add dose to obtain cumulative dose using deformable registration is described in Figure 4.28. The daily images are deformably registered with the plan image. Once the deformation maps are obtained, these maps are applied to the daily dose to map that dose to the planning CT. Daily doses are mapped to the planning CT that is used as reference. Daily doses are obtained by dose reconstruction of the daily fraction. On the planning framework, the daily doses are added to generate the cumulative dose. In this way, planned and cumulative doses deposited on the patient can be compared on the same framework.

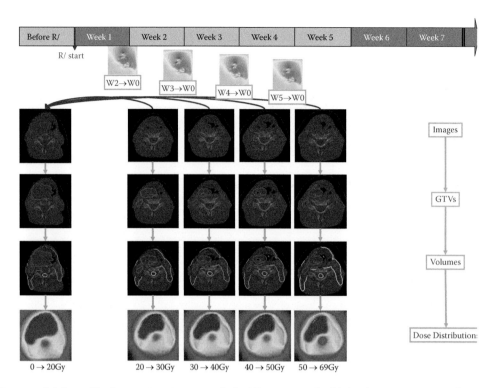

FIGURE 4.28 Process of deformable dose registration using daily CT to map and add the dose in a common framework. (Courtesy of Pierre Cassadot and Vincent Gregoire).

In summary, deformable registration is a key tool for adaptive therapy that allows automatic daily contour generation and generates cumulative doses. Deformable registration is addressed in detail in Chapter 12.

Tomotherapy is well suited to make the adaptive process fully automatic. Once the patient who will undergo adaptive radiotherapy is selected, the process proceeds automatically as follows:

a. Daily CT is generated, and the patient setup is adjusted.
b. A merged image between the planning CT and the daily CT is generated (containing MVCT where available and planning CT on the rest).
c. Deformable registration between the planning CT and the merge image is generated.
d. Dose reconstruction is performed on the merged image.
e. Contours are automatically generated with deformable registration using the planning contours as a template. If desired, the physician may inspect the new contours.
f. Daily dose-volume histograms (DVHs) are obtained.
g. Daily dose is mapped to the planning CT.
h. Dose applied to the planning CT is added to create a cumulative dose.
i. Daily and cumulative data are available for review.

All this process can be done in matter of minutes, allowing the adaptation process to be clinically viable. It is still a matter of research when and how to reoptimize a plan.

A head and neck case is used as an example to demonstrate delivered plan analysis and possible actions for adaptive radiotherapy. Figure 4.29 shows the quick review panels of the adaptive user interface. On this panel (Figure 4.29a), daily and cumulative dose can be analyzed. Also, daily and cumulative DVHs are available to be analyzed. The full line corresponds to the plan, and the dashed line corresponds to the actual delivery. On the next quick review panel (Figure 4.29b), trending values (such as D95%, D50%, volume of parotids, etc.) can be displayed as function of fraction number. Trending lines and DVHs in Figure 4.29b show good target coverage for the whole treatment. A slight increase of the target dose as the fraction number increased is observed. The dose on both parotids was higher at the end of the treatment as compared to the planned dose.

If we analyze the D50% of the parotids as function of the fraction number, we can see a steady increase with some small structures in fractions 17 and 29 (as indicated in Figure 4.30a). In Figure 4.30b, we can observe the volume of the parotids as a function of the number of fractions. A steady decrease of the parotid volumes can be observed as the patient looses weight.

Through data analysis, it is shown that the steady increase of dose and the steady decrease of the parotid volume are both related to patient weight loss. The sudden increases for fractions 17 and 29 (circled data in Figure 4.30a) are related to patient positioning. In order to analyze positioning, we will analyze

(a)

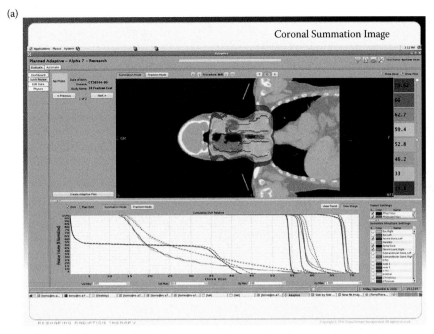

(b)

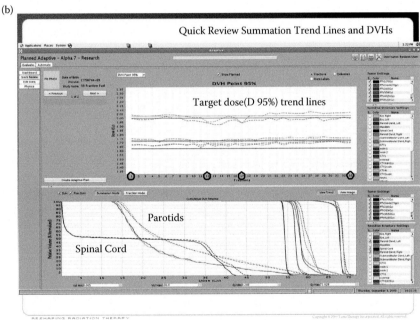

FIGURE 4.29 (a) Quick Review Panel cumulative dose review mode. (b) Quick Review Panel trending mode.

fraction 1, which corresponds to minimum patient weight loss. Figure 4.31a displays the plan and the actual DVH for fraction 1. As can be observed, the plan and delivered doses are in very good agreement. The planned contours and the daily contours are also very similar. This is mainly due to a minimum anatomical change between the planning CT and fraction 1 CT. This can be also observed in Figure 4.31b where, on the fused images between the planning CT and first fraction CTs, there are hardly any differences. In Figure 4.31b, the gray scale image corresponds to the planning CT, and the yellow image is from the daily CT.

For sake of space, we will only analyze fraction 29, but similar conclusions can be drawn using fraction 17. Figure 4.32a corresponds to the daily DVH for fraction 29. The right parotid dose (DVH) is very different from the treatment plan, and the trending plot also shows a deviation. In Figure 4.32b, a considerable weight loss can be observed, comparing the treatment plan imaging and the fraction 29 image. Differences between the planning contours and the daily contours generated with deformable registration are also noticeable. In particular, the parotid volume seems to be small as indicated by the trending plot in Figure 4.30b. Figure 4.33 is an overlay

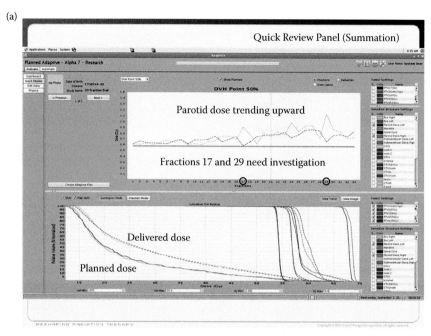

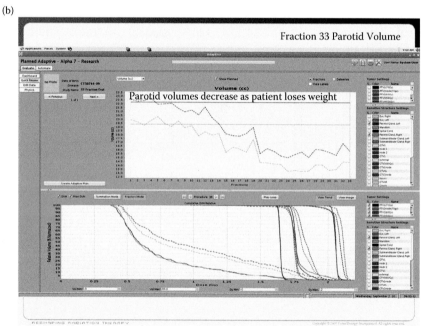

FIGURE 4.30 (a) Quick Review Panel steady increase of the parotid dose as a function of fraction number. (b) Quick Review Panel steady decrease of the parotids volume as function of fraction number. The volume reduction is related to weight loss.

of the plan dose on the planning CT and contours as well as the fraction 29 dose on the fraction 29 CT and contours. It is clear that the dose distribution is covering a bigger portion of the parotids compared to the original plan. By looking at how the patient was aligned during treatment in Figure 4.33b, it can be observed that weight loss is an obvious component impacting the dose distribution; however, there is also a small misalignment impacting the dose. The smooth trending on D50% corresponds to the weight loss components, and the spikes correspond to patient positional misalignments. Figure 4.34 shows that a small correction of 5 mm lateral, 0.12 mm anterior–posterior, and 2 degrees of roll will compensate for this observed weight loss to automatically shift the image until the newly determined PTV best fits into the planned dose distribution.

For this example case, a replanning at the middle of treatment could certainly reduce the parotid dose, as well. It is also interesting to note that unless daily treatments are

(a)

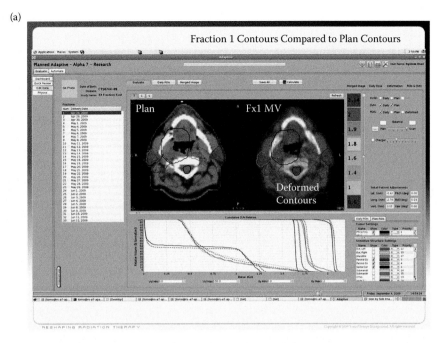

(b)

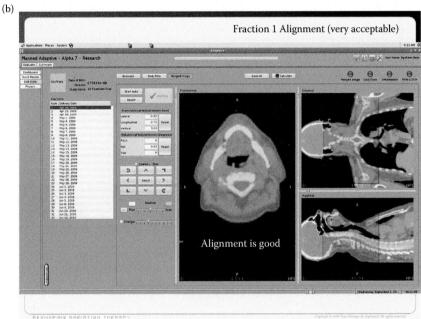

FIGURE 4.31 (a) Plan, fraction 1 contours and DVH. (b) Fusion of plan image (gray-scale image) and daily CT (yellow).

observed and analyzed using the techniques discussed, it is not possible to make quantitatively informed decisions about which treatment fractions are fulfilling the intended plan and which ones are not.

4.6 Summary

Helical tomotherapy and topotherapy are delivery modes using a treatment unit that is the combination of a CT scanner and a radiotherapy treatment device on a CT-like ring gantry. Rather than being an add-on function, CT image guidance was built into the design of the unit. Helical tomotherapy delivers highly modulated intensity-modulated rotational radiotherapy using a binary MLC modulating a fan beam. The same beam system can be used to deliver topotherapy, which has the gantry stationary and the couch moving during the modulated delivery. Because of its degree of modulation and 360 degree delivery, helical tomotherapy can simultaneously produce very uniform dose distributions to the target volume and low doses to

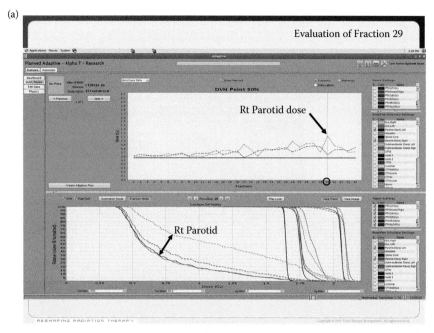

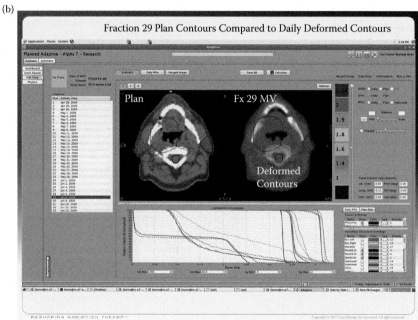

FIGURE 4.32 (a) Daily DVH for Fraction 29 and D50 % parotid trending. (b) Plan and fraction 29 CT and contour comparison.

neighboring sensitive structures. At the clinics in which it is installed, helical tomotherapy is typically used to treat the most complicated cases, such as head and neck, mesothelioma, advanced breast, node-positive prostate, and even TMI. There is clinical evidence that helical tomotherapy can improve patient outcomes (e.g., survival in advanced lung cancer). The newer topotherapy mode was designed to provide fast and quality treatments (all fields are compensated) for simple cases, especially tangential breast, and was designed to compliment helical tomotherapy in single-vault facilities.

Good dose distributions with high gradients cannot produce good outcomes if they cannot be delivered sufficiently accurately. CT image guidance ensures that the patient is set up according to plan, and if there is adequate immobilization at the time of treatment, the treatment will be delivered to the correct anatomical site. Most tomotherapy patients receive daily CT guidance. This is enabled by having a low-dose CT (typically 1 cGy per day) and integrated tools to speed the setup process. The setup verification process enables translation and rotation adjustments but often there are anatomical changes, such as weight loss or tumor shrinkage, which cannot be adjusted by

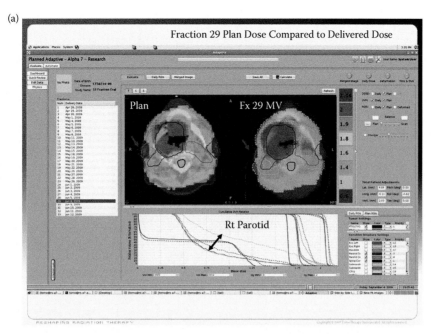

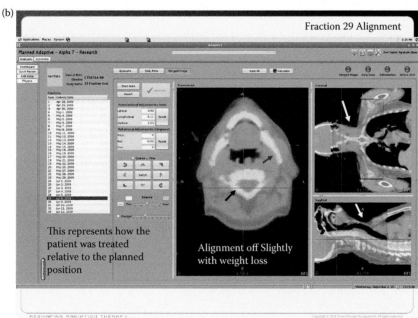

FIGURE 4.33 (a) Plan and daily dose overlay on plan and daily CT and contour, respectively. (b) Patient registration between plan and daily image as the patient was treated.

rigid shifts. Adaptive radiotherapy using dose verification can determine the dose delivered on the daily CT image.

A new form of adaptive radiotherapy is being developed for the tomotherapy system. It uses dose reconstruction and deformable registration to take into account the effect of anatomical changes to the patient. Deformable registration enables the contours to be mapped to the altered CT image set. It also maps the dose to a common anatomical framework so that the actual dose delivered can be accurately compared to the planned doses. This approach enables an accurate basis for replanning the patient instead of just assuming that the dose that was delivered up to that point was correct.

Disclosures

The authors are employees of TomoTherapy Inc., the developer of the Hi-Art™ tomotherapy system. They have equity ownership in the company. They are inventors of systems licensed by TomoTherapy Inc. from the Wisconsin Alumni Research Foundation, which is paying them royalties on the inventions.

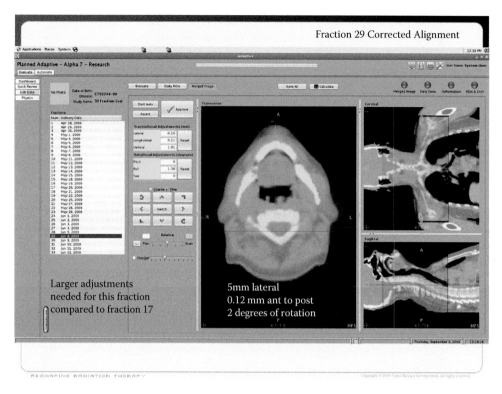

FIGURE 4.34 Patient registration to adjust miss alignment reducing parotids dose.

References

Adkison JB, Khuntia D, Bentzen SM, Cannon GM, Tome WA, Jaradat H, Walker W, Traynor AM, Weigel T, and Mehta MP. (2008). Dose escalated, hypofractionated radiotherapy using helical tomotherapy for inoperable non-small cell lung cancer: preliminary results of a risk-stratified phase I dose escalation study. *Technol Cancer Res Treat.* 7:441–7.

Bauman G, Yartsev S, Fisher B, Kron T, Laperriere N, Heydarian M, and VanDyk J. (2007). Simultaneous infield boost with helical tomotherapy for patients with 1 to 3 brain metastases. *Am J Clin Oncol.* 30:38–44.

Boswell S, Tome W, Jeraj R, Jaradat H, and Mackie TR. (2006). Automatic registration of megavoltage to kilovoltage CT images in helical tomotherapy: An evaluation of the setup verification process for the special case of a rigid head phantom. *Med Phys.* 33:4395–404.

Cattaneo GM, Dell'oca I, Broggi S, Fiorino C, Perna L, Pasetti M, Sangalli G, di Muzio N, Fazio F, and Calandrino R. (2008). Treatment planning comparison between conformal radiotherapy and helical tomotherapy in the case of locally advanced-stage NSCLC. *Radiother Oncol.* 88:310–8.

Clift RA, Buckner CD, Appelbaum FR, Sullivan KM, Storb R, and Thomas ED. (1998). Long-term follow-Up of a randomized trial of two irradiation regimens for patients receiving allogeneic marrow transplants during first remission of acute myeloid leukemia. *Blood.* 92:1455–6.

Cozzarini C, Fiorino C, Di Muzio N, Valdagni R, Salonia A, Alongi F, Broggi S, Guazzoni G, Montorsi F, Rigatti P, Calandrino R, and Fazio F. (2008). Hypofractionated adjuvant radiotherapy with helical tomotherapy after radical prostatectomy: planning data and toxicity results of a Phase I-II study. *Radiother Oncol.* 88:26–33.

Fiorino C, Alongi F, Broggi S, Cattaneo GM, Cozzarini C, Di Muzio N, Maggiulli E, Mangili P, Perna L, Valdagni R, Fazio F, and Calandrino R. (2008). Physics aspects of prostate tomotherapy: planning optimization and image-guidance issues. *Acta Oncol.* 47:1309–16.

Goddu SM, Yaddanapudi S, Pechenaya OL, Chaudhari SR, Klein EE, Khullar D, El Naqa E, Mutic S, Wahab S, Santanam L, Zoberi I, and Low DA. (2009a). Dosimetric consequences of uncorrected setup errors in helical tomotherapy treatments of breast-cancer patients. *Radiother Oncol.* 93:64–70.

Goddu SM, Chaudhari S, Mamalui-Hunter M, Pechenaya OL, Pratt D, Mutic S, Zoberi I, Jeswani S, Powell SN, and Low DA. (2009b). Helical tomotherapy planning for left-sided breast patients with positive lymph nodes: comparison to conventional multiport breast technique. *Int J Radiat Oncol Biol Phys.* 73:1243–51.

Gutierrez AN, Westerly DC, and Tome WA. (2007). Whole brain radiation therapy with hippocampal avoidance and simultaneously integrated brain metastases boost with helical tomotherapy: a planning study. *Int J Radiat Oncol Biol Phys.* 69:589–97.

Holly R, Myrehaug S, Kamran A, Sankreacha R, and Morton G. (2009). High-dose-rate prostate brachytherapy in a patient with bilateral hip prostheses planned using megavoltage computed tomography images acquired with a helical tomotherapy unit. *Brachytherapy*. 8:70–3.

Hsieh CH, Wei MC, Lee HY, Hsiao SM, Chen CA, Wang LY, Hsieh YP, Tsai TH, Chen YJ, and Shueng PW. (2009). Whole pelvic helical tomotherapy for locally advanced cervical cancer: technical implementation of IMRT with helical tomotherapy. *Radiat Oncol*. 4:62.

Hui SK, Kapatoes J, Fowler J, Henderson D, Olivera G, Manon RR, Gerbi B, Mackie TR, and Welsh JD. (2005). Feasibility study of helical tomotherapy for total body or total marrow irradiation. *Med Phys*. 32:3214–224.

Jeraj R, Mackie TR, Balog J, Olivera G, Pearson D, Kapatoes J, Ruchala K, and Reckwerdt P. (2004). Radiation characteristics of helical tomotherapy. *Med Phys*. 31:396–404.

Judy PF, Balter S, Bassano D, McCullough EC, Payne JT, and Rothenberg L. (1977). Phantoms for performance evaluation and quality assurance of CT scanners. Report No. 1, Diagnostic Radiology Committee Task Force on CT Scanner Phantoms. American Association of Physicists in Medicine.

Keller H, Glass M, Hinderer R, Ruchala K, Jeraj R, Olivera G, and Mackie TR. (2002). Monte Carlo study of a highly efficient gas ionization detector for megavoltage imaging and image-guided radiotherapy. *Med Phys*. 29:165–75.

Kissick MW, Flynn RT, Westerly DC, Hoban PW, Mo X, Soisson ET, McCall KC, Mackie TR, and Jeraj R. (2008). On the impact of longitudinal breathing motion randomness for tomotherapy delivery. *Phys Med Biol*. 53:4855–73.

Kissick MW, Boswell SA, Jeraj R, and Mackie TR. (2005). Confirmation, refinement, and extension of a study in intrafraction motion interplay with sliding jaw motion. *Med Phys*. 32:2346–350.

Kupelian PA, Langen KM, Willoughby TR, Wagner TH, Zeidan OA, and Meeks SL. (2006). Daily variations in the position of the prostate bed in patients with prostate cancer receiving postoperative external beam radiation therapy. *Int J Radiat Oncol Biol Phys*. 66:593–6.

Langen KM, Meeks SL, Poole DO, Wagner TH, Willoughby TR, Kupelian PA, Ruchala KJ, Haimerl J, and Olivera GH. (2005). The use of megavoltage CT (MVCT) images for dose recomputations. *Phys Med Biol*. 50:4259–76.

Langen KM, Lu W, Willoughby TR, Chauhan B, Meeks SL, Kupelian PA, and Olivera G. (2009). Dosimetric effect of prostate motion during helical tomotherapy. *Int J Radiat Oncol Biol Phys*. 74:1134–42.

Lee TK, Rosen II, Gibbons JP, Fields RS, and Hogstrom KR. (2008). Helical tomotherapy for parotid gland tumors. *Int J Radiat Oncol Biol Phys*. 70:883–91.

Lin L, Shi C, Eng T, Swanson G, Fuss M, and Papanikolaou N. (2009). Evaluation of inter-fractional setup shifts for site-specific helical tomotherapy treatments. *Technol Cancer Res Treat*. 8:115–22.

Meeks SL, Harmon JF Jr, Langen KM, Willoughby TR, Wagner TH, and Kupelian PA. (2005). Performance characterization of megavoltage computed tomography imaging on a helical tomotherapy unit. *Med Phys*. 32:2673–81.

Mountain CF. (1997). Revisions in the international system for staging lung cancer. *Chest* 111:1710–17.

Ramsey C, Langen K, Kupelian P, Scaperoth D, Meeks S, Mahan S, and Seibert R. (2006). A technique for adaptive image-guided helical tomotherapy for lung cancer. *Int J Radiat Oncol Biol Phys*. 64:1237–44.

Ruchala KJ, Olivera GH, Schloesser EA, and Mackie TR. (1999). Megavoltage CT on a tomotherapy system. *Phys Med Biol*. 44:2597–621.

Siker M, Tome W, and Mehta M. (2006). Tumor volume changes on serial imaging with megavoltage CT for non-small-cell lung cancer during intensity-modulated radiotherapy: how reliable, consistent, and meaningful is the effect? *Int J Radiat Oncol Biol Phys*. 66:135–41.

Schubert LK, Westerly DC, Tome WA, Mehta MP, Soisson ET, Mackie TR, Ritter MA, Khuntia D, Harari PM, and Paliwal BR. (2009). A comprehensive assessment by tumor site of patient setup using daily MVCT imaging from more than 3,800 helical tomotherapy treatments. *Int J Radiat Oncol Biol Phys*. 73:1260–9.

Schultheiss TE, Wong J, Liu A, Olivera G, and Somlo G. (2007). Image-guided total marrow and total lymphatic irradiation using helical tomotherapy. *Int J Radiat Oncol Biol Phys*. 67:1259–67.

Shah AP, Langen KM, Ruchala KJ, Cox A, Kupelian PA, and Meeks SL. (2008). Patient dose from megavoltage computed tomography imaging. *Int J Radiat Oncol Biol Phys*. 70:1579–87.

Sheng K, Molloy J, and Read P. (2006). IMRT dosimetry of the head and neck: a comparison of treatment plans using linac-based IMRT and helical tomotherapy. *Int J Radiat Oncol Biol Phys*. 65:917–23.

Sterzing F, Sroka-Perez G, Schubert K, MSnter MW, Thieke C, Huber P, Debus J, and Herfarth KK. (2008). Evaluating target coverage and normal tissue sparing in the adjuvant radiotherapy of malignant pleural mesothelioma: helical tomotherapy compared with step-and-shoot IMRT. *Radiother Oncol*. 86:251–7.

Shueng P-W, Lin S-C, Chong N-S, Lee H-Y, Tien H-J, Wu L-J, MD, Chen C-A, Lee J.J-S, and Hsieh C-H. (2009). Total marrow irradiation with helical tomotherapy for bone marrow transplantation of multiple myeloma: first experience in Asia. *Tech Can Res Treat*. 8:29–37.

Tournel K, De Ridder M, Engels B, Bijdekerke P, Fierens Y, Duchateau M, Linthout N, Reynders T, Verellen D, and Storme G. (2008). Assessment of intrafractional movement and internal motion in radiotherapy of rectal cancer using megavoltage computed tomography. *Int J Radiat Oncol Biol Phys*. 71:934–9.

Vaandering A, Lee JA, Renard L, and Gregoire V. (2009). Evaluation of MVCT protocols for brain and head and neck tumor patients treated with helical tomotherapy. *Radiother Oncol*. 93:50–6.

Wong JYC, Liu A, Schultheiss T, Popplewell L, Stein A, Rosenthal J, Essensten M, Forman S, and Somlo G. (2006). Targeted total marrow irradiation using three-dimensional image-guided tomographic intensity-modulated radiation therapy: An alternative to standard total body irradiation. *Biol Blood Marrow Trans.* 12:306–15.

Wong JY, Rosenthal J, Liu A, Schultheiss T, Forman S, and Somlo G. (2009). Image-guided total-marrow irradiation using helical tomotherapy in patients with multiple myeloma and acute leukemia undergoing hematopoietic cell transplantation. *Int J Radiat Oncol Biol Phys.* 73:273–9.

Woodford C, Yartsev S, and Van Dyk J. (2007). Optimization of megavoltage CT scan registration settings for thoracic cases on helical tomotherapy. *Phys Med Biol.* 52:N345–N354.

Xing L, Siebers J, and Keall P. (2007). Computational challenges for image-guided radiation therapy: framework and current research. *Semin Radiat Oncol.* 17:245–57.

Yan D, Wong J, Vicini F, et al. (1997). Adaptive modification of treatment planning to minimize the deleterious effects of treatment setup errors. *Int J Radiat Oncol Biol Phys.* 38:197–206.

Yartsev S, Kron T, Cozzi L, Fogliata A, and Bauman G. (2005). Tomotherapy planning of small brain tumours. *Radiother Oncol.* 74:49–52.

Zeidan OA, Langen KM, Meeks SL, Manon RR, Wagner TH, Willoughby TR, Jenkins DW, and Kupelian KA. (2007). Evaluation of image-guidance protocols in the treatment of head and neck cancers. *Int J Radiat Oncol Biol Phys.* 67:670–77.

Kilovoltage Cone-Beam CT Guidance of Radiation Therapy

Jeffrey H. Siewerdsen
Johns Hopkins University

Jan-Jakob Sonke
Netherlands Cancer Institute

5.1 Background, Introduction, and Overview

The development of digital x-ray imaging technologies in the 1990s spurred considerable activity in research, development, and clinical application of image-guided radiation therapy (IGRT) techniques to improve the precision of this proven therapeutic approach. The advent of active matrix flat-panel detectors (FPDs) was the main breakthrough technology in this regard, offering a platform for the development of higher performance megavoltage (MV) electronic portal imaging devices (EPIDs), kilovoltage (kV) radiographic and fluoroscopic imaging systems, and—the focus of this chapter—kV cone-beam CT (kV CBCT) systems for volumetric guidance based on tomographic images acquired at the time of therapy. kV CBCT offered submillimeter spatial resolution combined with soft-tissue contrast resolution potentially approaching that of diagnostic-quality computed tomography (CT) and overcame numerous limitations associated with localization based on projection imaging (orthogonal portal images) and rigid bony anatomy. As a means of reducing patient setup error, the potential of the new technology was clear, and the majority of radiotherapy linear accelerators sold circa 2010 feature the option of on-board kV CBCT integration. A decade after the introduction of this technology in IGRT, it remains an active topic of research in areas of image quality optimization, novel reconstruction techniques, advanced acquisition techniques, and clinical applications.

5.1.1 A Brief Natural History of CBCT for IGRT

The application of CT to radiation therapy traces to the very origin of the imaging modality. Allan Cormack, who shared the 1979 Nobel Prize in Physiology or Medicine with Godfrey Hounsfield for the invention of CT, was motivated at least in part in his formulation of CT by the desire to "reconstruct" the heterogeneous distribution of attenuation coefficients in the body for purposes of radiation dose calculation. By the end of the decade, CT was finding a role in radiation treatment planning (Payne et al., 1978), and through the 1980s, CT would form the basis for what would become 3D and 4D treatment planning for modern radiotherapy (Edwards et al., 1981). The role of this modality has grown over three decades of activity in the diagnosis and staging of cancer, as well as in the planning, guidance, and assessment of radiation therapy response. Such activity includes the evolution of CT from single-slice axial CT to helical CT (Kalender, 1995) and multidetector CT (MDCT) (Taguchi and Aradate, 1998; Hu, 1999), the last of which converges with the topic of this chapter—CBCT—epitomized in diagnostic applications by CT scanners featuring 256, 320, or more detector rows, and in therapy applications by CBCT platforms based on large-area FPDs. A summary timeline of such evolution in CT and CBCT is shown in Figure 5.1.

The enabling technology for high-performance CBCT in the late 1990s was large-area FPDs featuring real-time, distortion-less, digital readout. While such detectors were originally developed in medical applications for 2D radiography, fluoroscopy, and portal imaging, their performance characteristics resolved many of the factors that limited the use of x-ray image intensifiers (XRIIs) in 3D imaging—namely distortion, susceptibility to magnetic fields, veiling glare, and a fairly bulky form factor. With such limitations largely resolved, FPDs enabled high-quality CBCT reconstruction, featuring submillimeter spatial resolution and soft-tissue visibility sufficient for therapy guidance. Their implementation in a variety of CBCT platforms and applications quickly followed (some illustrated in Figure 5.2), including preclinical (small animal) imaging (Wong et al., 2008), ring gantries for 3D angiography (Ning et al., 1999), breast imaging (Boone and Lindfors, 2006; Chen and Ning, 2002), C-arms for interventional guidance (Fahrig et al., 2006; Siewerdsen et al., 2005), and on-gantry implementation for radiotherapy guidance (Jaffray and Siewerdsen, 2000; Jaffray et al., 2002).

For IGRT, the use of FPDs for kV CBCT presented an advance over early embodiments of MV CT (Mosleh-Shirazi et al., 1998) as well as kV CBCT based on XRIIs (Fahrig and Holdsworth 2000) and CCDs (Jaffray et al., 1999). The first decade of the 21st century saw increasingly widespread clinical use of such systems, with a variety of clinical platforms described in sections later in this chapter.

Recognizing the ongoing, rapid evolution of kV CBCT for IGRT in terms of its hardware embodiments, reconstruction techniques, and scope of clinical applications, the state of the art at the time of writing involves a radiographic/pulsed-fluoroscopic x-ray tube and large-area FPD mounted on the accelerator gantry—typically (although not necessarily) oriented orthogonally to the MV treatment beam. The source-detector orbit is circular, ranging from a limited arc (tomosynthesis) to a half-scan (180° + fan angle) or full-scan (360°) orbit. Numerous variations on these themes are being pursued and point to a changing landscape of higher performance kV CBCT technologies in the near future. These include new sources (e.g., multiple focal spots), new detectors (e.g., higher-efficiency, lower-noise, faster, photon-counting, etc.), new hardware platforms (e.g., on-gantry, off-gantry, C-arm, and other configurations), new source-detector orbits (e.g., helical CBCT and other noncircular trajectories), and new reconstruction techniques (e.g., algorithms based on noncircular orbits, iterative reconstruction, and incorporation of prior information).

5.1.2 CBCT Geometry

The geometry of CBCT imaging systems is dictated by the requirements and constraints of the clinical application and has significant influence on every aspect of imaging performance, including spatial resolution, x-ray scatter, field of view (FOV), etc. Figure 5.3 illustrates several pertinent geometric factors and a basic definition of geometric terms.

First, we consider coordinate systems (x,y,z) in the object or reconstruction domain, with origin nominally at isocenter (the center of reconstruction given by the intersection of the axis of rotation with the central axial plane). Similarly, we consider the 2D coordinates (u,v) in the detector (FPD) plane, with origin either in a "corner" pixel or at the center (or piercing point) of the FPD. It is furthermore helpful to distinguish the term "pixel" (the "picture element" on the detector, also variously called the detector element, or "del") from the term "voxel" (the "volume element" in the reconstructed image). Below, the term "pixel" therefore refers to an element in the 2D detector domain (u,v), whereas "voxel" refers to an element in the 3D image domain (x,y,z). The so-called "piercing point" refers to the point in the (u,v) plane containing a ray that is orthogonal to the detector and passes through the x-ray focal spot.

The overall system geometry is determined by the source-to-axis distance (SAD), also called the source-to-isocenter distance, and the source-to-detector distance (SDD). For IGRT systems, a typical scale is approximately SAD ~100 cm and SDD ~150 cm. The corresponding magnification factor is given simply by

$$M = \frac{SDD}{SAD} \qquad (5.1)$$

For a detector of lateral dimension L_u perpendicular to the axis of rotation and longitudinal L_v parallel to the axis of rotation, the corresponding FOV at isocenter is

$$FOV_{xy} = L_u\left(\frac{SAD}{SDD}\right) = \frac{L_u}{M} \text{ (lateral FOV)}, \qquad (5.2)$$

$$FOV_z = L_v\left(\frac{SAD}{SDD}\right) = \frac{L_v}{M} \text{ (longitudinal FOV)} \qquad (5.3)$$

There is a natural one-to-one relationship between the detector pixel size (a_{pix}) and the "natural" voxel size (a_{vox}) of 3D reconstructions implied by this geometry

$$a_{vox} = \frac{a_{pix}}{M} \text{ ("natural" voxel size)}, \qquad (5.4)$$

but it is important to recognize at least two important points: (i) the voxel size is completely arbitrary and may be specified as a free parameter in the reconstruction, greater than or less than a_{vox}, at the whim of the operator (but selected in a manner consistent with clinical requirements); and (ii) the voxel size, a_{vox}, should not be confused with a metric of spatial resolution. As an arbitrary parameter of reconstruction, a_{vox} certainly affects the minimum feature size that might be resolved in the image, but spatial resolution is properly characterized by factors such as the modulation transfer function (MTF) and not the voxel size. On a similar note, the corresponding "size" or format of the 3D reconstruction is

$$N_{voxels-xy} = \frac{FOV_{xy}}{a_{xy}}, \qquad (5.5)$$

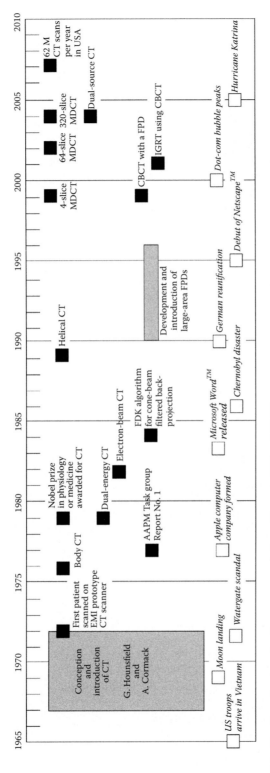

FIGURE 5.1 Timeline of various developments over the last ~50 years of CT and CBCT.

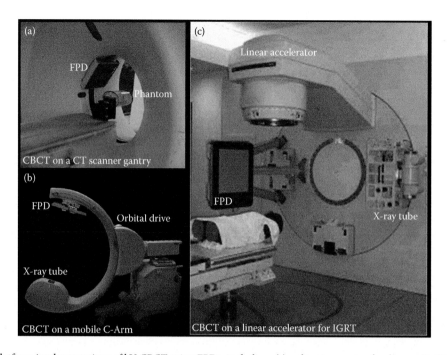

FIGURE 5.2 Early platform implementations of kV CBCT using FPDs, including: (a) a slip-ring gantry for diagnostic CT. Courtesy Dr. R. Ning (University of Rochester, Rochester NY) in association with Ning et al., Medical Imaging 1999: Physics of Medical Imaging, *SPIE* Vol. 3659:192–203, 1999; (b) a mobile C-arm for image-guided surgery Reproduced from the work of Dr. J. H. Siewerdsen et al. (Johns Hopkins University, Baltimore MD) in association with Siewerdsen et al., *Med Phys.* 32:241–254, 2005; and (c) the gantry of a medical linear accelerator for IGRT Courtesy of Dr. D. A. Jaffray (Princess Margaret Hospital, Toronto ON) in association with Jaffray et al., *Int J Radiat Oncol Biol Phys.* 53(5):1337–1349, 2002.

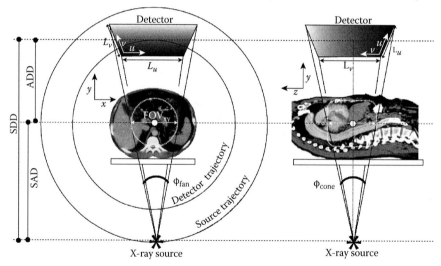

FIGURE 5.3 Illustration of CBCT geometry.

$$N_{\text{voxels}-z} = \frac{\text{FOV}_z}{a_z}, \qquad (5.6)$$

where a_{xy} is the voxel size in the axial (x,y) plane, and a_z is the voxel size in the z-direction (also called the slice thickness). However, neither should the image size (e.g., "256" or "512") be taken as a measure of spatial resolution—it is simply a function of voxel size and FOV, each of which are arbitrary reconstruction parameters and do not describe the underlying physical factors governing spatial resolution.

The system geometry defines two important angular extents—the fan angle (ϕ_{fan}) and the cone angle (ϕ_{cone}). The fan angle is that subtended laterally, as in conventional axial CT

$$\phi_{\text{fan}} = 2\tan^{-1}\left[\frac{L_u}{2\text{SDD}}\right]$$

$$= 2\tan^{-1}\left[\frac{\text{FOV}_u}{2\text{SAD}}\right]. \qquad (5.7)$$

Note that this is the full-fan angle, not to be confused with the half-fan angle sometimes quoted (for example, the half-fan angle properly denoted γ in (Kak and Slaney, 1988)). The fan angle governs the lateral FOV—that is the "width" of the beam and the lateral extent of imaging (and possible lateral truncation effects described below). It also sets the minimum arc requirement for "complete" 3D reconstruction by filtered backprojection from a circular orbit—specifically ($180° + \varphi_{fan}$). Anything less than ($180° + \varphi_{fan}$) constitutes a tomosynthesis acquisition and is not a "complete" 3D reconstruction, suffering primarily from limited resolution in the "depth" direction (denoted y in Figure 5.3). Note also the relationship of φ_{fan} to detector size and FOV_{xy} in Equation 5.7, which determines the minimum source-detector arc for complete 3D reconstruction as a function of detector size and system geometry.

The other pertinent angular parameter in the geometry of Figure 5.3 is the "cone angle," ϕ_{cone}, which governs the longitudinal FOV:

$$\phi_{cone} = 2\tan^{-1}\left[\frac{L_v}{2\text{SDD}}\right]$$

$$= 2\tan^{-1}\left[\frac{\text{FOV}_v}{2\text{SAD}}\right]. \qquad (5.8)$$

Note that this is the full-cone angle, not the half-cone angle sometimes quoted. The cone angle is also related to the so-called "cone-beam artifact" associated with unsampled spatial frequencies (along the z direction)—the so-called "null cone" discussed below in relation to Tuy's condition for exact 3D reconstruction. In its relation to the longitudinal FOV, the cone angle also relates to the "long object problem" associated with an object exceeding the FOV along the z direction (which is almost always the case for human body imaging) and the "chamfer" region that is evident as an incomplete (poor image quality) zone at the top and bottom of 3D reconstructions.

An example will help to put scale and meaning to these simple geometric definitions. Consider a simple CBCT system comprising an x-ray source and a 40 × 40 cm² FPD centered on the x-ray beam with pixel pitch of 0.4 mm, SAD = 100 cm, and SDD = 150 cm. This basic configuration implies

$$M \equiv \frac{150 \text{ cm}}{100 \text{ cm}} = 1.50,$$

$$\text{FOV}_{xy} = \text{FOV}_z = (40 \text{ cm})\left(\frac{100 \text{ cm}}{150 \text{ cm}}\right) = \frac{40 \text{ cm}}{1.5} = 26.7 \text{ cm},$$

$$a_{vox} = \frac{0.4 \text{ mm}}{1.5} = 0.267 \text{ mm},$$

$$N_{voxels-xy} = N_{voxels-z} = \frac{26.7 \text{ cm}}{0.0267 \text{ cm}} = 1,000,$$

$$\phi_{fan} = \phi_{cone} = 2\tan^{-1}\left[\frac{40 \text{ cm}}{2 \times 150 \text{ cm}}\right] = 15.2°.$$

The system therefore gives a 26.7 × 26.7 × 26.7 cm³ cylindrical FOV, which could encompass, for example, a large portion of the head or most internal organs; truncation artifacts (discussed below) are therefore to be expected in imaging of the chest, abdomen, or pelvis. A "natural" voxel size of 0.267 mm is indicated; whether or not the system spatial resolution is sufficient to discern ~0.267 mm features is another matter, related to the intrinsic spatial resolution characteristics as discussed below. The "natural" voxel size implies a (1,000 × 1,000 × 1,000) voxel format reconstruction for the entire FOV, which is likely beyond practical computing and storage limits. The same volume reconstructed at voxel size of ~0.80 mm [(333 × 333 × 333) voxel format] is likely a more practical approach. The fan angle for the system is 15.2°, meaning the minimum arc for complete reconstruction is ~195.2°, and the cone angle is similarly 15.2°, which is certainly within the realm of potentially significant cone-beam artifacts (discussed below) with structures up to ~13 cm off the central plane (depending on the frequency content of the object being imaged).

5.1.3 "Offset Detector" Geometry for Increased FOV

The FOV of the imaging geometry depicted in Figure 5.3 is fundamentally limited by the size of the detector, yielding a cylinder of diameter FOV_{xy} and length FOV_z with conically chamfered caps according to the cone angle. With detector sizes currently applied in CBCT guidance of ~30–40 cm at SDD ~150–160 cm, the typical reconstruction FOV may be adequate for imaging the head and neck region but is too small to image, for instance, the whole pelvis. Local reconstruction in the presence of significant lateral truncation (with solution of "the interior problem") is an important algorithmic approach, discussed briefly below. However, while such an algorithm may restore image quality within the small FOV, applications sometimes simply require a larger FOV. An effective physical means of extending the lateral FOV of a CBCT scanner is to partially displace the detector laterally—the so-called "offset-detector geometry" in which the detector is shifted by up to half its width along the u direction. In doing so, and with a full 360° rotation, different parts of the object are projected in views covering short-scan segments of the full rotation, as illustrated in Figure 5.4. For the partially displaced detector position, the centrally located portion of the object is in the FOV of the imaging system over the full scan, requiring an appropriate data-weighting scheme for image reconstruction (Liu et al., 2003).

5.1.4 CBCT Image Reconstruction

The most prevalent form of CBCT image reconstruction is 3D filtered backprojection, with the first practically implemented algorithm attributed to Feldkamp et al. (1984). The "FDK" algorithm is fundamentally similar to filtered backprojection in axial CT reconstruction from a circular orbit of the source and detector, extended to account for the divergent beam (i.e., φ_{cone} in Figure 5.3)

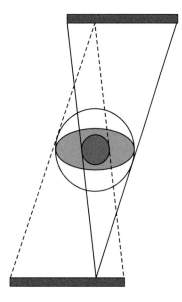

FIGURE 5.4 Schematic representation of the offset-detector scanning geometry. The elliptical object is too large to be encompassed in all projections of the normal "centered-detector" geometry and therefore exceeds the nominal FOV described by Equation 2. By partly displacing the detector laterally, the FOV of the scanner is extended (light gray circle), scanning each side of the object over only a section of a full rotation. Only the central part (small dark circle) is seen over the full rotation.

and a flat detector. It is worth noting (and discussed in greater detail in a later section) that this prevalent approach applied to a circular source-detector orbit provides "exact" reconstruction only in the central axial plane, and CT number (i.e., voxel value) inaccuracies and artifacts occur with increased severity at greater distance from the central plane. Violation of "Tuy's condition" results in a "null cone" in the Fourier domain for which a circular orbit does not allow accurate reconstruction of the complete spatial frequency content of the object. The resulting and much discussed "cone-beam artifact" is presented in the following section.

Neglecting for the moment the particulars of projection image processing (e.g., offset-gain calibration) and geometric calibration (i.e., small excursions from a perfect circular orbit), the "voxel-driven" implementation of the FDK algorithm is summarized as follows, with a summary flowchart for 3D reconstruction given in Figure 5.5.

A simple step-by-step description of the basic FDK algorithm is provided below in the style of the excellent summary provided by (Hoppe et al., 2007). We begin simply with a projection image, $p(u,v)$, acquired at a given angle θ as given by the Beers-Lambert law

$$p(u,v;\theta) = p_0 e^{-\int_0^{\mathrm{SDD}} \mu(x,y,z)dy}, \qquad (5.9)$$

where p_0 indicates the bare-beam (unattenuated) detector signal, $\mu(x,y,z)$ is the object function of true attenuation coefficients to be reconstructed, the transform from (x,z) to (u,v) is implicit in the geometry of Figure 5.3, and we have neglected effects of a polyenergetic beam.

(i) Log weighting: We first normalize the projection by the bare-beam detector signal and rewrite as a "line integral" given simply by the natural logarithm

$$p_1(u,v;\theta) = \ln\left(\frac{p_0}{p(u,v;\theta)}\right) = \int_0^{\mathrm{SDD}} \mu(x,y,z)dy. \qquad (5.10)$$

(ii) Ray density (cosine) weighting: The projection data are weighted to account for variation in the density of rays intersecting a flat detector surface at nonorthogonal angles

$$p_2(u,v;\theta) = p_1(u,v;\theta)\left[\frac{\mathrm{SDD}}{\sqrt{\mathrm{SDD}^2+u^2+v^2}}\right], \qquad (5.11)$$

where $(u = 0, v = 0)$ is given by the piercing point. The weighting is distinct from an inverse-square correction for a flat detector in that it scales pixel values downward at locations distant from the piercing point.

(iii) Parker weights (data redundancy): Backprojection of data over precisely $(180° + \varphi_{\mathrm{fan}})$ or $360°$ naturally weights all projections equally, with uniform weighting of 1.0 or 0.5, respectively. However, orbits spanning any intermediate angular range require weighting to properly weight redundant data. We write

$$p_3(u,v;\theta) = p_2(u,v;\theta)w_3(u,v;\theta), \qquad (5.12)$$

where

$$w_3(u;\theta) = \begin{cases} \sin^2\left(\dfrac{\pi\theta}{4\left(\dfrac{1}{2}\phi_{\mathrm{fan}} - \tan^{-1}\left(\dfrac{u}{\mathrm{SDD}}\right)\right)}\right) & \text{for } 0 \leq \theta \leq \phi_{\mathrm{fan}} - 2\tan^{-1}\left(\dfrac{u}{\mathrm{SDD}}\right) \\ 1 & \text{for } \phi_{\mathrm{fan}} - 2\tan^{-1}\left(\dfrac{u}{\mathrm{SDD}}\right) \leq \theta \leq \pi - 2\tan^{-1}\left(\dfrac{u}{\mathrm{SDD}}\right) \\ \sin^2\left(\dfrac{\pi(\pi+\phi_{\mathrm{fan}}-\theta)}{4\left(\dfrac{1}{2}\phi_{\mathrm{fan}} + \tan^{-1}\left(\dfrac{u}{\mathrm{SDD}}\right)\right)}\right) & \text{for } \pi - 2\tan^{-1}\left(\dfrac{u}{\mathrm{SDD}}\right) \leq \theta \leq \pi + \phi_{\mathrm{fan}} \end{cases}$$

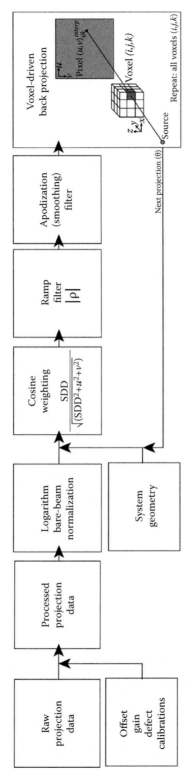

FIGURE 5.5 Flowchart illustration of basic steps intrinsic to voxel-driven 3D filtered backprojection as in the FDK algorithm for CBCT reconstruction.

(iv) Ramp filter: A ramp filter (so-called, because the frequency domain representation is simply a high-pass filter $|\rho|$) is applied to the projection data to account for the $1/r$ reduction in radial density of backprojected rays. The filter may be applied as a multiplication in the Fourier domain

$$p_4(u,v;\theta) = FT^{-1}\left[FT\left[p_3(u,v;\theta)\right]|\rho|\right], \qquad (5.14)$$

where ρ corresponds to the "lateral" spatial frequency domain (f_u). Alternatively, the ramp filter may be applied as a convolution in the spatial domain

$$p_4(u,v;\theta) = p_3(u,v;\theta) * \left(-\frac{1}{2\pi^2 u^2}\right), \qquad (5.15)$$

where the term in parentheses corresponds to the spatial domain "convolution kernel" associated with the ramp filter. Note that the ramp filter only affects the projection data in the lateral, u-direction.

(v) Apodization (smoothing) filter: A smoothing filter is often applied to reduce high-frequency noise amplified by the ramp filter. The choice of smoothing filter is optional, with common choices being the Shepp-Logan or Hann filters. A generic form for a cosine filter is as follows:

$$T_{win}(f) = h_{win} + (1 - h_{win})\cos(2\pi f \Delta), \qquad (5.16)$$

where h_{win} is an arbitrary, tuneable parameter in the range 0.5–1.0 (e.g., $h_{win} = 0.5$ for a smooth Hann filter or $h_{win} = 1.0$ for a sharp Ram-Lak filter), and Δ is the sampling step size of the detector elements. Note that the apodization filter is generally two-dimensional (affecting both the u and v directions of the projection data), whereas the ramp filter is only applied in the u-direction. The apodized projection data are therefore,

$$p_5(u,v;\theta) = FT^{-1}\left[FT\left[p_4(u,v;\theta)\right]T_{win}(f)\right], \qquad (5.17)$$

written as a multiplication in the Fourier domain, or alternatively

$$p_5(u,v;\theta) = p_4(u,v;\theta) * t_{win}(u,v), \qquad (5.18)$$

where $t_{win}(u,v)$ is the spatial domain convolution kernel corresponding to $T_{win}(f)$. The selection of smoothing filter depends on the imaging task, as it imparts a tradeoff between noise and spatial resolution in the 3D reconstruction. A smoother filter (lower h_{win}) reduces noise at the cost of spatial resolution, and a sharper filter (higher h_{win}) is associated with higher noise and higher spatial resolution. Reconstruction filters should therefore be chosen in a manner "optimal" to the imaging task.

(vi) Interpolation: For "voxel-driven reconstruction," a given voxel in the 3D reconstruction draws its value from a ray back-projected from a location (u,v) on the detector plane that contains the x-ray source and the center of that voxel, repeated for each projection view. Ideally, the projection data would be continuously described at any position in the detector plane. Since the projection data are discrete, however, and the positions of back-projected rays do not necessarily correspond to pixel centers, the projection data are "interpolated" or "up-sampled" to reduce error associated with discrete pixel sampling. Bilinear interpolation is a reasonable choice, such that the projection image signal at an arbitrary location (u,v) on the detector plane is given by 2D bilinear interpolation of adjacent pixel values. Alternatively, the projection data are "up-sampled"—for example, by a factor of 2 or 4—to effect a finer pixel size, drawing each back-projected ray from the nearest-neighbor pixel of the up-sampled projection data and avoiding a more computationally expensive continuous bilinear interpolation for each back-projected ray. We write for the interpolated projections

$$p_6(u,v;\theta) = \text{interp2}\left[p_5(u,v;\theta)\right], \qquad (5.19)$$

where the operator interp2 is left fairly generic for present purposes simply to designate that $p_6(u,v;\theta)$ can now be considered approximately continuous in the (u,v) domain. The interpolation step correspondingly limits the influence of high-frequency "aliased noise" in 3D reconstruction via the (low-pass) transfer function associated with the interpolation method—for example, a sinc^2 function for bilinear interpolation and a sinc function for nearest-neighbor. The choice of interpolation and up-sampling method has distinct effects on the noise and spatial resolution in CBCT reconstructions, as detailed in Tward and Siewersden (2009).

(vii) Reconstruction matrix: The 3D reconstruction matrix may be arbitrarily defined according to a given FOV in axial (x,y) and longitudinal (z) directions—a region of extent FOV_{xy} and FOV_z, respectively, recognizing the maximum FOV associated with the detector size and system geometry as described in the previous section. The reconstruction is typically centered about the central plane and axis of rotation (i.e., the center of reconstruction is the system isocenter), but such is not a strict requirement, and the reconstruction volume may be defined anywhere within the region of support associated with the detector size and system geometry. Similarly, the voxel size may be arbitrarily defined according to a given aperture in axial and longitudinal directions—a_{xy} and a_z, respectively, the former representing the axial voxel size and the latter the longitudinal voxel size or "slice thickness."

(viii) Voxel-driven reconstruction: As illustrated in Figure 5.5, voxel-driven reconstruction proceeds as follows. For a given projection $p_6(u,v)$ at a specified angle θ, the algorithm loops over all voxels (i,j,k) in the reconstruction matrix. For each voxel, one computes the point of intersection between the x-ray focal spot, the center of the voxel, and the detector plane at location $(u, v)_{ijk}^{\text{interp}}$. The pixel value at position $(u, v)_{ijk}^{\text{interp}}$ is then added to the current voxel value at (i,j,k). The process is repeated for all voxels (i,j,k) and subsequently for all projection views over the entire source-detector orbit.

There are numerous real, practical aspects of image processing and numerical computation that have been brushed aside in the above summary. For example, high-quality 3D reconstructions free of ring artifacts rely upon the quality of offset-gain corrections in the projection data, as mentioned below. Furthermore, we have set aside the important aspects of nonidealities in the system geometry—that is that the source and detector do not move through a perfect circular orbit, owing to mechanical flex of the imaging system as it rotates under gravity. These have been important areas of investigation, with solutions typically relying on an accurate calibration of system geometry—that is., specification of each degree of freedom in the imaging system for all projection angles—and the reproducibility of such during system acquisition. While this task may seem daunting, a number of calibration methods have been reported (Cho et al., 2005; Fahrig and Holdsworth, 2000; Hoppe et al., 2007; Navab et al., 1996; Noo et al., 2000; Rougee et al., 1993, 1988; Von Smekal et al., 2004), and CBCT systems developed for IGRT have been shown to provide a high degree of reproducibility in the nonidealities of each degree of freedom.

Finally, it is worth noting that while the FDK algorithm is the most commonly used CBCT reconstruction approach, a variety of other methods exist. For example, while FDK-based approaches have been extended to noncircular geometries (e.g., helical CBCT), the reconstruction is approximate. Exact reconstruction methods for helical geometries have been developed based on pi-line approaches (Noo et al., 2003; Yu and Wang, 2004) or more generalized exact methods based on the work of Katsevich (Katsevich, 2002; Ye et al, 2005; Zou and Pan, 2004) that also apply to more general geometries (Yu et al., 2005; Pack and Noo 2005). Numerous iterative reconstruction methods also exist based either on the algebraic solution of the forward model (Guan and Gordon, 1996; Nielsen et al., 2005) or more sophisticated techniques (e.g., maximum-likelihood methods (Lange and Carson, 1984, Manglos et al., 1995)) that also model the statistics of the detection process. Within the class of statistical reconstruction methods, there are also numerous regularization approaches (or objective function modifications) to control noise in the reconstructed images. Such techniques include penalized-likelihood approaches (Erdogan and Fessler, 1999; Fessler and Hero, 1995; Wang et al., 2009), which can also include polyenergetic forward models (De Man et al., 2001; Elbakri and Fessler, 2002) for more quantitative imaging, as well as methods based on modified norms like total variation or compressed sensing techniques (Sidky and Pan 2008a,b, Chen et al. 2008), which can provide excellent performance under conditions of limited (angularly undersampled) data. Such methods present a vibrant area of ongoing research, with advances in computing speed making such approaches more clinically practical.

5.1.5 CBCT Acquisition Orbits

Most of the discussion above relates to a circular source-detector orbit, and such is the basis for the basic FDK algorithm that is so prevalent in CBCT imaging for IGRT. Such circular trajectories can encompass a full 360° orbit or a "half-scan" encompassing $(180° + \varphi_{\text{fan}})$. Orbits intermediate to these are also possible and do provide complete, fully 3D reconstructions (with proper application of data redundancy weighting, as noted above). Orbits shorter than these are technically "incomplete" due to less-than-complete sampling and fall within the domain of "tomosynthesis," which is the use of limited sampling to compute tomographic images as detailed in Chapter 9. Such scans do not provide sufficient projection data to reconstruct a fully 3D image with isotropic spatial resolution. The main limitation of such reconstructions is a lack of depth resolution (the y-direction in Figure 5.3), causing superposition of structures from out-of-plane. Particularly for high-contrast structures, out-of-plane distortion can significantly limit the accuracy of 3D localization. The advantage of such incomplete orbits, of course, is the potential for faster scans over a shorter arc, lower dose, and faster computation times. Research aimed at more complete reconstruction from limited arcs is an active area of work—for example, using prior information and/or non-FDK reconstruction techniques. Finally, there is considerable interest in noncircular trajectories—for example, helical CBCT to cover longer volumes and avoid cone-beam artifacts.

5.1.6 Clinical Implementations

Following the feasibility studies demonstrating a CBCT scanner integrated with a linear accelerator producing images with soft-tissue contrast at acceptable dose levels (Jaffray et al., 2002), CBCT systems for radiotherapy guidance became commercially available from a variety of corporate vendors (Figure 5.6). First, Elekta (Elekta Oncology Systems, Crawley, West Sussex, UK) developed their Synergy system that received regulatory clearance in 2003. Subsequently, Varian (Varian Medical Systems, Palo Alto) received regulatory clearance in 2004 for their On-Board Imaging (OBI) system. Both CBCT scanners featured an x-ray tube and FPD mounted orthogonally to the central axis of the treatment beam and provided FDK-based reconstruction concurrent with image acquisition producing scans within two minutes. CBCT-to-planning CT image registration was used to demonstrate differences between patient positioning at planning and treatment and to calculate an optimal couch correction. At the time of writing, the majority of radiotherapy linear accelerators sold in the world feature an integrated CBCT option. More recently (Kamino, et al., 2006), Mitsubishi (Mitsubishi Heavy Industries, Tokyo, Japan) introduced the Vero TM2000 with regulatory clearance in 2008, which contains a dual kV-source

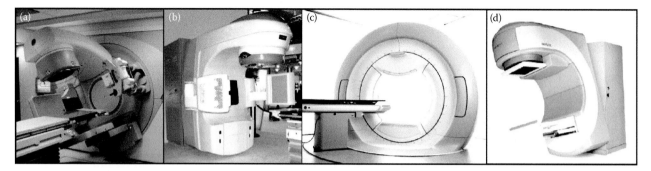

FIGURE 5.6   Illustration of various clinical implementations of kV CBCT for IGRT: (a) Synergy (From Elekta Oncology Systems), (b) OBI (From Varian Medical Systems), (c) Vero (From Mitsubishi), and (d) Artiste (From Siemens Healthcare).

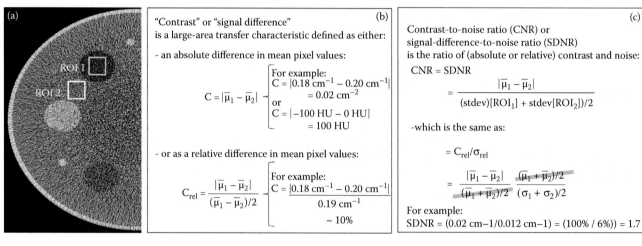

FIGURE 5.7   (a) Example axial slice of a soft-tissue simulating phantom in CBCT illustrating (b) contrast and (c) contrast-to-noise ratio.

imaging pair capable of CBCT imaging on an O-ring gantry structure. Finally, Siemens announced a kV CBCT design in 2005, complementing their MV CBCT approach (see Chapter 10) with the central axis of the imaging system in line with the central axis of the treatment beam. At the time of writing, however, this system is not commercially available, and experience has been limited to a prototype installed at the German Cancer Research Center (DKFZ, Heidelberg, Germany).

5.2 Image Quality Fundamentals

In this section, the essential metrics of imaging performance are briefly reviewed in terms relevant to CBCT, details of which can also be found in a variety of textbooks on the physics of medical imaging (Bushberg et al., 2002; Hendee and Ritenour, 2002). We touch on the basic metrics of contrast (signal difference), noise, signal-difference-to-noise ratio (SDNR), and basic measures of spatial resolution, as well as more sophisticated Fourier domain metrics, such as the MTF, noise-power spectrum (NPS), and noise-equivalent quanta (NEQ), each in the context of CBCT. A summary overview of CBCT artifacts and methods for artifact reduction is also reviewed, focusing on those most pertinent to CBCT. In general, these image-quality metrics can be formulated for any design of imaging device,

though particular source-detector geometries (fan beam, cone beam), sampling/acquisition schemes (orbits, helices, fixed/finite projections), x-ray beam energies (kV, MV), and reconstruction algorithms must be appropriately specified.

5.2.1 Contrast, Noise, and CNR (SDNR)

Among the simplest imaging performance metrics is the signal difference exhibited between two structures in the image relative to the magnitude of stochastic fluctuations in the image background. The signal difference ("contrast") refers to the difference in mean values between two "large" objects (i.e., objects with extent much greater than the voxel size or "correlation length")

$$C = \bar{\mu}_1 - \bar{\mu}_2, \qquad (5.20)$$

where $\bar{\mu}_1$ and $\bar{\mu}_2$ are the average voxel values over of interest as (ROI) illustrated in Figure 5.7. The term written this way may be considered the "absolute" contrast and carries units of the image—that is of the voxel value, such as attenuation coefficient (mm^{-1}) or Hounsfield units (HU). The "relative" contrast is alternatively

$$C_{rel} = 2\frac{\bar{\mu}_1 - \bar{\mu}_2}{\bar{\mu}_1 + \bar{\mu}_2}. \qquad (5.21)$$

For example, $\bar{\mu}_1$ and $\bar{\mu}_2$ could refer to the mean voxel value within a tumor and normal background, respectively. Ideally—for complete, accurate reconstruction in the absence of x-ray scatter, etc.—these voxel values are simply the linear attenuation coefficient of the materials. As discussed below, effects such as x-ray scatter tend to reduce the difference between voxel values to less than that of the actual, intrinsic linear attenuation coefficients.

For digital imaging modalities (including digital radiography, CT, and CBCT), the contrast in itself is important primarily in proportion to the magnitude of image fluctuations—that is the image noise—since the window and level can be simply adjusted to display arbitrarily low contrast. Under conditions of low-contrast between the two ROIs, the image noise is most simply characterized as the standard deviation in voxel values over one or both ("large") regions of support

$$\sigma = \langle \text{stdev}(\text{ROI}_1), \text{stdev}(\text{ROI}_2) \rangle, \qquad (5.22)$$

written as the "absolute" noise (which carries the same units as the image) or alternatively as the relative noise

$$\sigma_{\text{rel}} = \frac{\overline{\sigma_1} + \overline{\sigma_2}}{\overline{\mu_1} + \overline{\mu_2}}. \qquad (5.23)$$

The fundamental source of image noise is the Poisson-distributed x-ray quanta incident upon the detector in each projection, and the dependence of the 3D image noise upon radiation dose as well as various CT reconstruction parameters was first described in Barrett et al. (1976) with analysis extended to CBCT by Siewerdsen and Jaffray (2000a,b), Siewerdsen and Jaffray (2003), and Tward and Siewerdsen (2008)

$$\sigma^2 = \frac{\mu_e E}{D_o e^{-\mu d/2} \rho} \frac{1}{\eta} \frac{K_{xyz}^2}{a_{xy}^3 a_z}, \qquad (5.24)$$

where σ^2 is the "variance" (and σ is the "noise"). The term D_o refers to the dose delivered to the center of the (cylindrical) phantom, and ρ is the material density. The factor η is the detector efficiency [specifically, the zero-frequency detective quantum efficiency, DQE(0)]. Tradeoffs between noise and spatial resolution become evident in the dependence on a_{xy} (the voxel size in axial planes), a_z (the voxel size in the longitudinal direction—most commonly referred to as "slice thickness"), and K_{xyz} (a 3D "bandwidth integral" over transfer functions and applied filters in the detection and reconstruction process). Classic dependencies are evident, namely the inverse proportionality between noise and the square root of dose (e.g., number of quanta) and slice thickness.

The contrast-to-noise ratio (CNR) or more precisely the SDNR is therefore

$$\text{SDNR} = 2 \frac{\overline{\mu_1} - \overline{\mu_2}}{\sigma_1 + \sigma_2}, \qquad (5.25)$$

in its empirical form or in a more theoretical form

$$\text{SDNR}^2 = (\overline{\mu_1} - \overline{\mu_2})^2 \frac{D_o e^{-\mu d/2} \rho}{\mu_e E} \eta \frac{a_{xy}^3 a_z}{K_{xyz}^2}. \qquad (5.26)$$

The SDNR therefore improves with dose and detector DQE and is degraded at finer voxel size and elevated levels of x-ray scatter. Relation to the classic Rose criterion (i.e., threshold detectability of an object around CNR ~3–5) is tempting but should be carefully regarded in relation to the assumptions of both the Rose criterion and the noise characteristics of CBCT.

5.2.2 Spatial Resolution: Impulse Response Functions and MTF

The spatial resolution of a CBCT imaging system can be described in terms of simple spatial domain characteristics referring to the minimum resolvable feature size or in somewhat more quantitative, observer-independent terms in the Fourier domain. In the former case, for example, the spatial resolution can be characterized in terms of the full-width-at-half-maximum (FWHM) in the (axial) image of a thin wire oriented along the longitudinal axis, as in Figure 5.8. For a very thin wire (or deconvolving the wire function from the image), the axial image represents the point-spread function (PSF) of the imaging system, and the FWHM of the PSF provides a quantitative measure of spatial resolution that is intuitive and exhibits expected dependence, for example, on the choice of reconstruction filter. Alternatively and as mentioned below in relation to quality assurance tests, a phantom presenting patterns of line-pairs at increasing spatial frequency provides a measure of spatial resolution in terms of the minimum resolvable line-pair.

The MTF provides a Fourier-domain characterization of spatial resolution. Specifically, the MTF describes the factor by which change in image signal at a given spatial frequency (e.g., a set of line-pairs or a sinusoidally varying pattern in the image) is modulated in its mean signal at the output of the imaging system. For example, a slowly varying pattern (low-spatial frequency) may be transferred without loss of contrast—that is without signal modulation, implying the MTF at low spatial frequencies is ~1. Conversely, a rapidly varying pattern of fine detail (high spatial frequency) may suffer a loss of contrast in the signal pattern—that is modulated signal, with MTF at higher spatial frequencies <1. An MTF greater than one is also possible (e.g., by digital filtering) and implies, for example, an edge enhancement effect.

The relationship of the MTF to the PSF (e.g., the image of a thin wire) as well as the line-spread function (LSF) and edge-spread function (ESF) is illustrated in Figure 5.9. We see that the MTF is defined in terms of the Fourier transform of the LSF, which in turn is given by the Radon transform of the PSF or the derivative of the ESF. While a wire PSF gives the simplest practical measurement of MTF, it is somewhat limited in that such measurements usually consider only the wire oriented along the

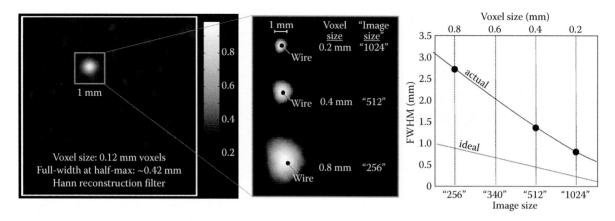

FIGURE 5.8 CBCT spatial resolution as illustrated in an axial slice image of a thin steel wire. The center panel shows wire images reconstructed at various voxel sizes, illustrating the degradation in underlying FWHM for coarser voxels. Voxel size (and image format) affects spatial resolution, but they are not in themselves meaningful metrics of spatial resolution. One should avoid characterizing system resolution by voxel size (e.g., saying the resolution is "0.4 mm" simply because that is the voxel size) or image size (e.g., a "512" reconstruction). As illustrated in the graph on the right, the "actual" resolution length is considerably larger than the "ideal" suggested by the voxel size. Instead, the underlying correlation length as described by the FWHM of the PSF or, better, a more complete description as given by modulation transfer function (MTF) is the more appropriate way to characterize system spatial resolution.

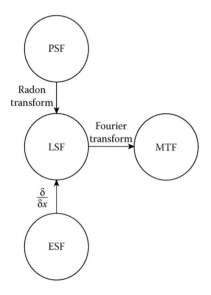

FIGURE 5.9 Basic relationship among the point-spread function (PSF), the line-spread function (LSF), the edge-spread function (ESF), and the modulation transfer function (MTF).

longitudinal axis and therefore describe only the axial MTF (and not the longitudinal or fully 3D MTF). Still, it is a useful, practical approach to MTF measurement, and Silverman et al. (2009) described a method whereby orienting the wire at a slight angle to the longitudinal axis allows the analysis of an "oversampled" PSF and LSF, yielding the "presampling" MTF analogous to the angled slit method of Fujita et al. (1992) that is common in 2D radiography. The method is illustrated graphically in Figure 5.10. Alternative methods for spread-function measurement include the direct LSF measurement of Boone (2001) based upon a thin metal sheet and the fully 3D ESF measurement based upon the image of a sphere, which gives an estimate of the fully 3D MTF.

The choice of reconstruction filter directly affects the spatial resolution and noise—for example, "smooth" or "sharp" filters as illustrated in Figure 5.11.

5.2.3 Fourier Metrics of Noise and Signal-to-Noise Ratio

Image noise can be similarly described in terms of Fourier-domain metrics that characterize not only the magnitude of image fluctuations (i.e., σ) but also the correlations ("texture") therein. Specifically, the NPS is defined in terms of the Fourier transform of "noise-only" image realizations

$$\mathrm{NPS}(f_x, f_y, f_z) = \frac{a_x a_y a_z}{N_x N_y N_z} \left\langle \left| FT_{3D} \{ \Delta\mu(x, y, z) \} \right|^2 \right\rangle, \quad (5.27)$$

where $\Delta\mu(x,y,z)$ denotes a "noise-only" image containing only the image fluctuations about the mean voxel values—for example, obtained by global mean subtraction, detrending, or double-image subtraction (accounting for a factor of two noise amplification in subtracting uncorrelated images). The operator FT_{3D} refers to the three-dimensional Fourier transform, the | | brackets denote the modulus, and the ⟨ ⟩ brackets refer to the ensemble average over all realizations. The scale factor includes a_x, a_y, and a_z (the voxel dimensions in the x, y, and z directions, respectively) and N_x, N_y, and N_z (the number of voxels in each direction in each realization, respectively). The process for experimental determination of the NPS is illustrated in Figure 5.12.

As common in spectral estimation, the voxel size determines the highest spatial frequency for which the NPS is measured (i.e., the Nyquist frequency $f_{x\text{-Nyq}} = f_{x\text{-max}} = 1/2a_x$), the size of the realization determines the lowest spatial frequency for which the NPS is measured ($f_{x\text{-min}} = 1/a_x N_x$), and the number of

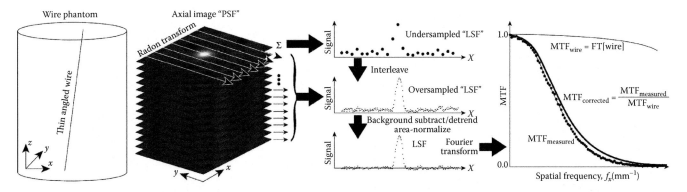

FIGURE 5.10 Illustration of MTF measurement from a thin-angled wire. Axial images present a "PSF," the Radon transform of which gives an (undersampled) "LSF." By interleaving undersampled LSFs according to the angle of the wire [analogous to the angled slit method of (Fujita et al., 1992)], an oversampled LSF is obtained, the Fourier transform of which gives the presampling MTF.

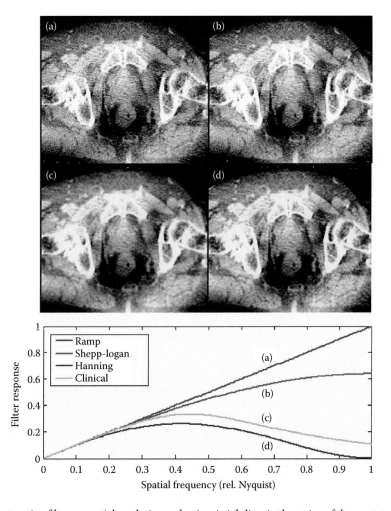

FIGURE 5.11 Effect of reconstruction filter on spatial resolution and noise. Axial slices in the region of the prostate reconstructed with different reconstruction filters: (a) Ramp filter, (b) Shepp-Logan filter, (c) Hann or Hanning filter, and (d) a Wiener filter. Each filter is shown in the frequency domain in the bottom figure, showing progressively smoother filters for (a)–(d). Correspondingly, while the spatial resolution degrades in images (a)–(d), the noise is reduced.

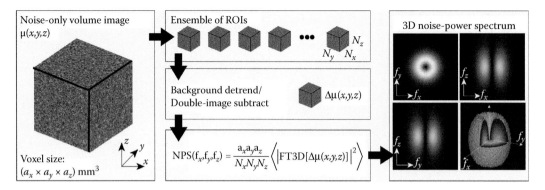

FIGURE 5.12 Illustration of the process by which the fully 3D NPS is estimated from CBCT images. Note that a fully 3D image is properly characterized by a fully 3D NPS analyzed, for example, by 3D Fourier transform of zero-mean, noise-only 3D ROIs. Such yields a 3D NPS with units of volume times signal-squared—for example, (mm³) (HU²). Such analysis should not be confused with a 2D Fourier transform of individual "slices" taken from the CBCT image, which is an erroneous representation of the NPS in that it ignores correlations orthogonal to the slice, does not carry proper units, and is not simply related to the 3D NEQ.

realizations determines the standard error in the NPS measurement (in inverse-square-root proportion, with $N_{\text{realizations}}$ typically in the range ~50–100 or more). For properly normalized CBCT reconstructions (i.e., images for which the mean voxel value in a uniform medium is independent of dose), the NPS is also normalized such that it is inversely proportional to dose. Note that the fully 3D NPS written in Equation 5.27 carries units of [signal²][mm³], which is either [HU²][mm³] for an image scaled to Hounsfield units, or for an image with voxel values of linear attenuation coefficient, [(1/mm)²][mm³], where terms could be cancelled to yield units of [mm], but are left as either [(1/mm)²][mm³] or symbolically [μ²mm³] to be explicit.

Note further that the fully 3D NPS described here (obtained by 3D Fourier transform of 3D realizations, etc.) is distinct from the power spectrum that might be obtained from individual 2D slices. Specifically, the latter is prone to error in ignoring correlations in the direction orthogonal to the analyzed slice. For example, a 2D power spectrum analyzed from an ensemble of 2D axial slices "extracted" from a fully 3D volume is *not* a slice of the 3D NPS; rather, it is equal to the 3D NPS convolved with the system MTF along the orthogonal direction. The 2D power spectrum (PS_{2D}) analyzed from axial planes is therefore related to the 3D NPS by

$$PS_{2D}(f_x, f_y) = \int NPS(f_x, f_y, f_z)MTF^2(f_z)df_z, \quad (5.28)$$

but it should *not* be confused with the image NPS, nor should it be used to obtain the NEQ, etc. Only in the case that noise is uncorrelated along the f_z direction is this simply related to a slice of the 3D NPS (differing by a factor of the slice thickness, a_z), and in general, the PS_{2D} underestimates the fully 3D NPS by a factor related to the bandwidth integral (blur) in the orthogonal direction. Furthermore, and more fundamentally, the units of the 2D power spectrum ([signal²][mm²]) are distinct from those of the 3D NPS ([signal²][mm³]), so it is important to appreciate

the full dimensionality of the data in the analysis of such Fourier metrics (Siewerdsen et al., 2002). Failure to do so will yield erroneous conclusions that fail to account for fully 3D correlations in the image data, or—worse—are meaningless in that they do not carry units appropriate to the dimensions of the data.

The NPS is a useful quantitative metric of image noise recognized in early work on CT image quality (Hanson, 1979; Wagner et al., 1979). It captures both the magnitude of image fluctuations through the relationship

$$\sigma^2 = \int_{-f_{\text{Nyquist}}}^{+f_{\text{Nyquist}}} NPS(f_x, f_y, f_z)df_x df_y df_z, \quad (5.29)$$

and the correlations (or "texture") of the noise therein.

The MTF and NPS metrics can be combined in a spatial-frequency-dependent description of the signal-to-noise ratio, usually denoted the noise-equivalent quanta (NEQ)

$$NEQ(f_x, f_y, f_z) = \theta_{\text{tot}} f \frac{MTF^2(f_x, f_y, f_z)}{NPS(f_x, f_y, f_z)}, \quad (5.30)$$

where θ_{tot} is the extent of the angular range (e.g., π or 2π). Note again the fully 3D dimensionality of the $NEQ(f_x, f_y, f_z)$, its units ([photons/mm²]), and the proportionality to dose (since the NPS is normalized and inversely proportional to dose). An intuitive interpretation of the NEQ is the total fluence of x-ray quanta "used" in forming the 3D image. Similarly, the fraction of x-ray quanta contributing to the 3D image is given by the detective quantum efficiency (DQE)

$$DQE(f_x, f_y, f_z) = \frac{\theta_{\text{tot}} f}{N_{\text{proj}} \overline{q_0}} \frac{MTF^2(f_x, f_y, f_z)}{NPS(f_x, f_y, f_z)}. \quad (5.31)$$

The NEQ and DQE written this way have similar utility as prevalently applied in 2D radiographic imaging applications. At low spatial frequencies, the 3D DQE is typically close to that of the 2D DQE of the FPD, but the process of 3D CBCT reconstruction—although mathematically deterministic—is irreversible and can degrade the DQE below that of the projection data. Specifically, the choice of CBCT reconstruction filter, voxel size, and voxel sampling all impart nontrivial, non-negligible effects on the 3D DQE—for example, via 3D "aliased noise" (Siewerdsen and Jaffray, 2000a; Tward and Siewerdsen, 2008). Because of the asymmetric processing imparted in 3D reconstruction (e.g., the ramp filter and/or asymmetric voxels in a_{xy} and a_z), the NEQ and DQE are correspondingly asymmetric in axial and longitudinal directions: the axial (f_x,f_y) domain is governed by the application of the ramp filter in the u-direction only, whereas the longitudinal (f_z) direction is governed primarily by the transfer characteristics of the detector and, possibly, other applied filters (but not the ramp).

Finally, the NEQ and DQE can be extended to models of observer performance in a manner that provides a guide for system optimization. For example, a simple ideal observer model computes a detectability index (d') as the integral of the NEQ weighted by the spatial frequencies of interest (characterized by a model task function, W_{task})

$$d'^2 = \iiint \mathrm{NEQ}\left(f_x,f_y,f_z\right) W_{task}^2\left(f_x,f_y,f_z\right) df_x df_y df_z. \quad (5.32)$$

Such analysis has shown to be useful in the design and optimization of kV CBCT imaging systems for IGRT—for example, in analyzing the optimal system geometry in a manner that balances tradeoffs of focal spot blur, x-ray scatter, and detector response (Siewerdsen and Jaffray, 2000b).

5.2.4 Image Artifacts

Consider an object defined by a 3D distribution of linear attenuation coefficient $\mu_{object}(x,y,z)$ [or a linearly transformed version of μ_{obj}, such as conversion to Hounsfield units, $\mathrm{HU}_{object}(x,y,z)$], and a reconstructed 3D image $\mu_{image}(x,y,z)$ [similarly $\mathrm{HU}_{image}(x,y,z)$ etc.]. Ideally, the image represents a "true" reconstruction, such that

$$\mu_{image}(x,y,z) = \mu_{object}(x,y,z). \quad (5.33)$$

In practice, the reconstructed image differs from the object function due to numerous sources of image degradation. The most common source of degradation is stochastic noise, such that

$$\mu_{image}(x,y,z) = \mu_{object}(x,y,z) + \Delta_{random}(x,y,z), \quad (5.34)$$

where $\Delta_{random}(x,y,z)$ represents a zero-mean random process associated with purely stochastic noise—for example, quantum noise, as discussed in previous sections. The component of the image associated with purely stochastic noise, $\Delta_{random}(x,y,z)$ is independent from one image to the next and is described statistically—for example, in terms of the voxel noise, σ_{vox}, and NPS, as mentioned above.

Image "artifacts" refer to nonstochastic deviations from the true image. The nonstochastic nature of such image degradation is usually associated with errors or view-to-view inconsistency in the measured projection data and/or errors in the algorithmic handling of data during 3D reconstruction. Analogous to the above, we write

$$\mu_{image}(x,y,z) = \mu_{object}(x,y,z) + \Delta_{random}(x,y,z) + \Delta_{artifact}(x,y,z). \quad (5.35)$$

Common presentations of $\Delta_{artifact}(x,y,z)$ include shading, streaks, and distortion. They depend intrinsically on the specific imager configuration (detector type, geometry, etc.), imaging technique (kVp, mAs, number of views, etc.), reconstruction technique (projection normalization, sampling, etc.), and upon the object itself (the subject being imaged). In this way, artifacts are often deterministic (i.e., not stochastic), and the $\Delta_{artifact}(x,y,z)$ component of the image is reproducible for repeated scans.

The sections below briefly review a number of the most common and significant image artifacts in kV CBCT. The topic of image artifacts has represented a significant area of research, development, and continuous improvement since the inception of x-ray CT, and it is the subject of numerous articles and general textbooks. Essentially every artifact of significance in kV CT is relevant in the context of kV CBCT as well, and often of greater consequence in the latter due to various limitations in this comparatively new modality. For example, artifacts arising from x-ray scatter, defective detector elements, and object truncation are typically stronger in CBCT than in CT due to, respectively, a larger x-ray scatter fraction, less highly optimized detectors, and smaller detector FOV. Furthermore, conventional CBCT introduces artifacts of its own—most notably the "cone-beam" artifact associated with a circular source-detector orbit and divergent beam in filtered backprojection. A brief list of artifacts is summarized below, and the reader is referred to other general texts discussing image artifacts and correction techniques in CT.

5.2.4.1 CT Number Accuracy

As implied by Equation 5.27, all image artifacts impart some form of inaccuracy in the reconstructed voxel value ("CT number"). These include shading artifacts (a reduction in voxel value), streak artifacts (light or dark variations in voxel values with strong directional dependence), and so-called distortions (e.g., out-of-plane blur due to an incomplete orbit). For some applications (e.g., radiation therapy planning or calculation of accurate DRRs), the accuracy of voxel values is critical, so we address the point separately here. We limit discussion in this section specifically to global inaccuracy in the mean CT number in an otherwise uniform object—for example, a water cylinder for which the true CT number is 0 HU, but artifacts may impart an erroneous mean value and/or slowly varying (shading) artifacts.

Aside from the physical sources of CT number inaccuracy (e.g., x-ray scatter, beam hardening, etc. discussed below), several purely algorithmic sources of inaccuracy exist as well. For example, accurate normalization of projection data by the "bare-beam" signal (I_0) is required in basic filtered backprojection

$$\ln(I_0/I) = \mu d, \tag{5.36}$$

where all terms are recognized from the basic Beers-Lambert law of attenuation. Determination of I_0 can be gained from the projection data directly (e.g., at the edge of the projection) if the object is entirely within the FOV and a region of bare (unattenuated) beam exists for all projections. Alternatively (perhaps more commonly), the bare-beam signal can be measured in calibration procedures ("air scans"). In either case, errors in I_0 will impart errors in the reconstructed μ values. Similarly, improperly normalized filters employed in the reconstruction process can erroneously shift voxel values.

A second potential source of error is the basic scaling of reconstructed images and conversion to Hounsfield units. The proper conversion is given by

$$HU(x, y, z) = 1{,}000\frac{\mu(x, y, z) - \mu_{water}}{\mu_{water}}, \tag{5.37}$$

(with some systems adding an extra 1,000 units to the result such that the voxel values are non-negative). Accurate conversion to HU requires an accurate value of μ_{water}, which of course is energy-dependent. Errors in $\mu(x,y,z)$ and μ_{water} for the particular imaging configuration will impart errors in $HU(x,y,z)$. Similarly, some reconstruction algorithms may disregard accuracy in the computed voxel values altogether—for example, scaling results arbitrarily across a 12-bit scale for purposes of display.

Developers and users of kV CBCT should be aware of such basic inaccuracies and can measure the accuracy (or "CT linearity") of a system using standard CT quality assurance phantoms. For example, specially engineered plastics representing specific electron densities and simulating a broad range of tissue types are commonly available. A common CT number accuracy and linearity test involves measuring the mean value reconstructed within an assortment of such materials and comparing to the value specified by the manufacturer and/or measured on an independently validated/calibrated CT scanner. This test is a common step for the commissioning of a CT simulator and radiation treatment planning system, to enable the proper computation of dose for nonhomogeneous conditions, and an example CT linearity measurement is shown in Figure 5.13.

As some applications such as dose calculation, radiation therapy planning, and adaptive plan modifications rely on accurate determination of CT number, various means of calibrating and correcting measured CBCT voxel values have been an area of considerable interest. Such corrections are nontrivial, since inaccuracies can be imparted by numerous sources

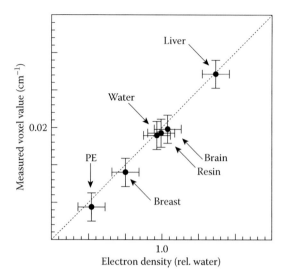

FIGURE 5.13 Example CT linearity measurement. The vertical axis represents mean values measured on a kV CBCT scanner, and the horizontal axis is the expected CT number as measured on a calibrated CT scanner.

of error—with x-ray scatter and object truncation (each discussed below)—being perhaps the greatest sources of bias. As these sources are patient-specific, straightforward machine calibration will not suffice (Hatton et al., 2009) in the absence of accurate scatter and truncation corrections. Two types of correction methods can be distinguished: (i) methods assigning a constant density value to different regions of the image (bulk density replacements) and (ii) methods that apply a continuous correction to the projection images or reconstruction. Examples of the first category are (Chi et al., 2007) who applied a stepwise density table to the CBCT data and (Boggula et al., 2009) who replaced regions in the CBCT scan identified as air, soft tissue, and bone with the mean value from the corresponding regions in the planning CT image. An example of the second category is found in Létourneau et al. (2007) who optimized a sixth-order polynomial correction to the pixel values of the projection images to convert measured attenuation to equivalent thickness of water prior to CBCT reconstruction. Marchant et al. (2008), on the other hand, derived a scan-specific shading correction by calculating a low spatial-frequency ratio field between CBCT and the corresponding planning CT from a calibrated scanner. Finally, Yang et al. (2010) utilized deformable planning CT-to-CBCT registration to propagate CT# from a calibrated scanner to the CBCT scan. Note that corrections from the first category reduce the image quality while methods of the second category have the potential to improve image quality.

In the absence of CT number corrections, deviations up to 200–300 HU are not uncommon, especially for high-density materials, corresponding to 20% errors in dose calculation in extreme cases (Hatton et al., 2009). After corrections, dose calculation accuracy is typically within 3%.

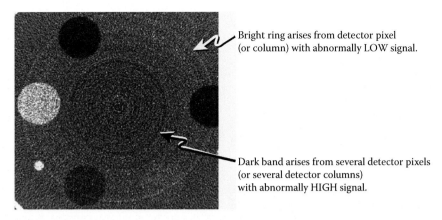

Bright ring arises from detector pixel (or column) with abnormally LOW signal.

Dark band arises from several detector pixels (or several detector columns) with abnormally HIGH signal.

FIGURE 5.14 Example images illustrating CBCT ring artifacts. Rings in the axial plane (as shown) appear as vertical streaks in coronal or sagittal planes.

5.2.4.2 Ring Artifacts

Ring artifacts—as their name implies—appear as (light or dark) circular bands in axial slices concentric about the axis of rotation. An example is shown in Figure 5.14. A ring artifact arises from a measurement that is fixed in the projection domain from view-to-view—for example, a measurement arising from a dead or defective pixel on the detector. A defective detector line (parallel to the axis of rotation) would similarly produce a ring artifact in every axial slice of the 3D reconstruction. Likewise, a scratch or impurity on the x-ray tube collimator window or added filter can produce a signal that is stationary from view-to-view in the projection data and, therefore, create a ring artifact in the reconstruction.

The most common source of ring artifacts in FPD-based CBCT is insufficient offset-gain-defect detector calibration. Offset corrections (also called "dark" corrections) are intended to correct for spatial variations in detector dark current. Similarly, gain corrections (also called "flood-field" corrections) are intended to correct for variations in the detector response under otherwise uniform x-ray irradiation. In practice, the gain correction may be combined with the bare-beam (I_0) calibration implied by Equations 5.10 and 5.36. Defect calibrations are intended to identify and filter detector pixels that show erroneous offset or gain characteristics, including aberrant dark signal, dark noise, flood-field signal, flood-field noise, and linearity—for example, dead or noisy pixels. Once identified, pixel defects are typically filtered (e.g., median filtration) prior to filtered backprojection.

The best means of correcting ring artifacts is therefore good offset-gain-defect calibration—particularly for pixels near the center of the detector, where the visibility of ring artifacts is likely to be most pronounced. In practice, FPD dark fields tend to be variable with time and temperature and are calibrated frequently (or even prior to each scan). Flood-field response and defect pixel behavior are more stable and are typically calibrated on a monthly (or even biannually) basis. Dark-field corrections typically involve pixelwise subtraction of the mean dark image determined from ~50 dark images acquired at the same frame rate as the projection data. Flood-field corrections

similarly involve pixelwise division by the (dark-subtracted) mean flood-field (gain) image determined from ~50 flood-field images acquired at the same technique as the projection data (and with all added filtration, bowtie filter, and antiscatter grid in place). The basic offset-gain-corrected projection is therefore given by

$$I_{\text{proc}}(u,v) = K \frac{I_{\text{raw}}(u,v) - \overline{I_{\text{offset}}(u,v)}}{I_{\text{gain}}(u,v) - I_{\text{offset}}(u,v)}, \tag{5.38}$$

where I_{proc} is the corrected image, I_{raw} is the uncorrected projection, I_{offset} is the (mean) offset image, I_{gain} is the (mean) flood-field image, and K is a scale value that gives the correct mean signal in I_{proc}. An improved version of such is given by exposure-dependent mean flood images acquired at various levels (~3–10 exposure levels) within the detector latitude. Other techniques for ring artifact correction have been reported that operate on the reconstructed data—for example, transforming the rectilinear axial slice to polar coordinates, median filtering in the polar domain.

5.2.4.3 Geometric Calibration Artifacts

As mentioned in the previous section on 3D reconstruction from a circular orbit, real implementations of CBCT exhibit geometric nonidealities resulting, for example, from mechanical flex of gantry components as the system rotates within a gravitational field. Uncorrected, such excursions from a perfect circular orbit induce deviations from the system geometry used in the reconstruction algorithm and result in image artifacts as illustrated in Figure 5.15. The departure from a circular orbit does not in itself degrade image quality; it is the failure to correct for such excursions that result in such artifacts, and if motion of the source and detector is reproducible, then geometric nonidealities can be accommodated by way of a calibration. As mentioned above, numerous methods for geometric calibration have been reported, typically involving a phantom of known geometry (e.g., an array of BBs) projected in the detector domain and analyzed in a manner to deduce the system pose at each projection angle (Cho et al., 2005;

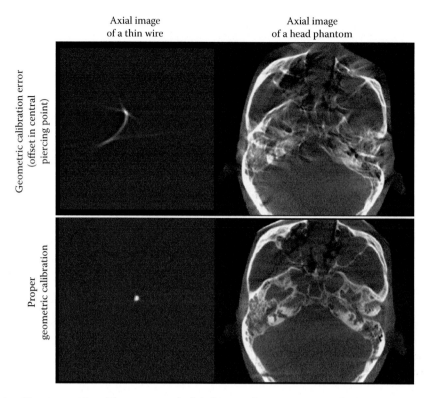

FIGURE 5.15 Geometric calibration artifacts. The images on the left show axial reconstructions of a thin wire, and those on the right show an anthropomorphic head phantom—each imaged using a half-scan rotation of the source and detector. Failure to correct geometric nonidealities (e.g., deviations from a circular orbit) can impart significant artifacts, as in the top row of images, where an uncorrected offset in the piercing point causes the entire image to be convolved with a crescent-shaped (half-scan) distortion. Proper geometric calibration (bottom row) allows accurate image reconstruction even under large geometric nonidealities in source-detector orbit, provided such motion is reproducible between the calibration and image acquisition.

Fahrig and Holdsworth, 2000; Hoppe et al,. 2007; Navab et al., 1996; Noo et al., 2000; Rougee et al., 1993, 1998; Von Smekal et al., 2004). The simplest method (and one still encountered in practice) involves a single BB placed at isocenter to estimate the position of the piercing point in each projection angle (Jaffray et al., 2002). Navab et al. (1996) used a helical pattern of BBs combined with an iterative solution to the system pose. Noo et al. (2000) used a line of BBs and analyzed the ellipses projected in the detector domain. Cho et al. used two rings of BBs and derived a direct analytical solution to all 9 degrees of freedom [$(x,y,z)_{source}$, $(x,y,z)_{detector}$, $(\eta,\theta,\varphi)_{detector}$] from each individual projection view. Provided the motion of the source and detector is reproducible, geometric calibration has been shown to restore image quality to a high degree, as illustrated in Figure 5.15 (Daly et al., 2008).

5.2.4.4 X-Ray Scatter

(i) The nature of x-ray scatter and its effect on CBCT image quality.

X-ray scatter has been identified as one of the main physical factors of image quality degradation in CBCT. The basic reason for high x-ray scatter fractions is the large volumetric FOV with a correspondingly large volume of irradiated tissue. X-ray scatter degrades CBCT images in at least three ways: (1) it causes inaccuracy (underestimation) in reconstructed voxel values; (2) it

imparts an intrinsic reduction in the contrast (signal difference) between reconstructed tissues; and (3) it affects the noise characteristics and can be considered to degrade system DQE.

The scatter fluence presented to the detector represents an overestimation of transmission in the projection measurements and a corresponding underestimation of $\mu(x,y,z)$ in the reconstruction. In situations for which the x-ray scatter fluence is slowly varying in the projection domain, the resulting artifacts tend to be slowly varying (low-frequency) in the reconstruction as well—for example, the classic "cupping" or shading artifact as illustrated in Figure 5.16. However, such is not always the case, and relatively sharp fluctuations in scatter-to-primary at the detector (for example., behind a strongly attenuating bone) can result in sharply varying artifacts as well—e.g., the "streak" artifact as illustrated in Figure 5.16. An intuitive description of these effects—as well as the fact that x-ray scatter artifacts always underestimate the true voxel value—can be found among the earliest work on CT image quality (Glover, 1982).

The second form of image degradation associated with x-ray scatter is an intrinsic reduction in reconstructed attenuation coefficients, related to the underestimation noted above. As shown in Johns and Yaffe (1982) as well as in Siewerdsen and Jaffray (2001), the measured contrast (signal difference, $\Delta\mu_{measured}$) in soft tissues reconstructed in the presence of scatter

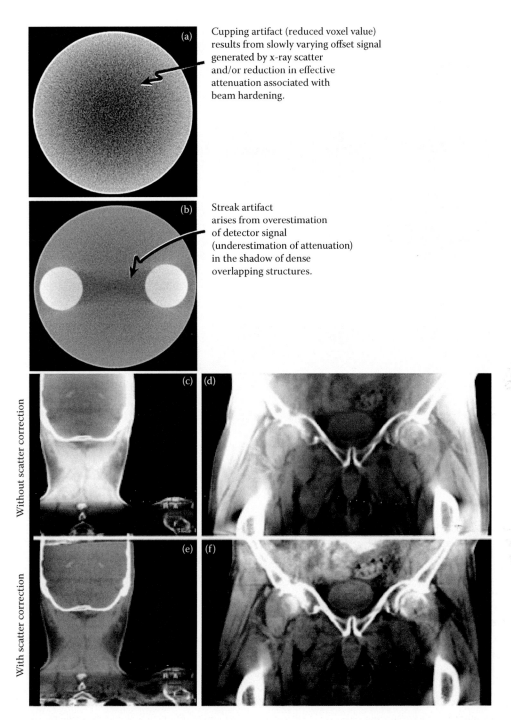

Cupping artifact (reduced voxel value) results from slowly varying offset signal generated by x-ray scatter and/or reduction in effective attenuation associated with beam hardening.

Streak artifact arises from overestimation of detector signal (underestimation of attenuation) in the shadow of dense overlapping structures.

FIGURE 5.16 Example images illustrating x-ray scatter artifacts. (a) Shading artifact within a uniform water phantom. (b) Streak artifact between two highly attenuating objects (simulated cortical bone). Note that x-ray scatter artifacts and beam-hardening artifacts (discussed below) can be difficult to distinguish. For example, the streak artifact in (b) could be equally attributed to beam hardening in views associated with attenuation by the two overlapping bone structures. (c,d) Coronal CBCT images of the head-and-neck and pelvis without scatter correction. (e,f) The same images reconstructed with the simple scatter correction method adapted from the work of (Boellaard, R. et al., *Radiother Oncol.*, 44: 149–157, 1997.)

is degraded in proportion to the scatter-to-primary ratio (SPR) at the detector

$$\Delta\mu_{\text{measured}} = \Delta\mu_{\text{true}} + \left(\frac{1}{d}\right)\ln\left[\frac{1+\text{SPR}\,e^{\Delta\mu_{\text{true}}d}}{1+\text{SPR}}\right], \quad (5.39)$$

where $\Delta\mu_{\text{true}}$ is the true difference in soft-tissue attenuation coefficients, and d is the size of the soft-tissue target. Whether the target exhibits positive or negative contrast relative to surrounding tissue, the result is that scatter (i.e., SPR > 0) always causes $\Delta\mu_{\text{measured}}$ to be less than $\Delta\mu_{\text{true}}$. Over a range in SPR varying from ~5% to ~150% (corresponding to the range from fan-beam

CT to volumetric CBCT), soft-tissue contrast can be degraded by a factor of ~2 or more due to x-ray scatter.

X-ray scatter contributes uncorrelated quanta to detector signal, thereby adding signal that carries no (or little) actual imaging information. The expected increase in noise (per unit dose to the detector) can be measured as a function of SPR, recognizing that absolute noise (per unit dose to the patient) in a uniform phantom can actually decrease with SPR, since scattered quanta still contribute detector signal (Siewerdsen and Jaffray, 2001). Still, the SDNR degrades with SPR. The effect of x-ray scatter on image noise is best appreciated in terms of its effect upon the detective quantum efficiency (DQE), sometimes referred to as the "system" DQE when scatter is included. Considering the simple case in which x-ray scatter is presumed to contribute uncorrelated noise in the projection data (and that the x-ray scatter spectrum is shifted negligibly from that of the primary spectrum), the DQE is degraded from the scatter-free case by a factor related to SPR

$$DQE_{sys} = \frac{1}{1+SPR} DQE. \qquad (5.40)$$

Siewerdsen and Jaffray (2000b) showed that scatter can be included in a model for CBCT signal and noise propagation as "additive quantum noise," yielding Equation 5.40 under conditions for which the detector is input-quantum-limited. The general form for the effect of scatter on system DQE is given in Siewerdsen and Jaffray (2000b).

(ii) Methods to physically reject x-ray scatter.

The question immediately arises as to how the magnitude of x-ray scatter reaching the detector can be minimized in order to mitigate such degradation in CT number accuracy (artifacts), contrast, and noise. Numerous basic methods for physically minimizing the amount of x-ray scatter may be briefly summarized.

- First, the FOV (i.e., volume of tissue irradiated) should be minimized by restricting the collimation to an extent consistent with the imaging task. For example, the longitudinal (z-direction) FOV should be restricted to cover the extent of anatomical structures of interest, for example, ~8 cm to cover the prostate. The lateral (x–y) FOV can be similarly restricted, recognizing that such will increase the presence of truncation artifacts.

- Second, a bowtie filter or region-of-interest (ROI) filter, placed in the x-ray beam during image acquisition, is a simple, common means of reducing the scatter fluence (and patient dose) by irradiating a smaller tissue volume. Such can also alleviate dynamic range requirements of the detector by "flattening" the x-ray beam transmitted to the detector.

- Third is the selection of system geometry with a large air gap (distance between the patient exit surface (or isocenter) and the detector), thereby increasing the distance between the detector and the "effective scatter source" and reducing the scatter fluence in a manner similar to the

inverse square law (under the assumption of a scatter point source). Neitzel (1992) showed that reduction in x-ray scatter is a strong function of the air gap distance and that applications allowing a large gap benefit more from the air gap than from an antiscatter grid. Such modeling was applied in the design of early CBCT-guided radiotherapy systems (Siewerdsen and Jaffray, 2000b, 2001) and showed that the extended geometries typical of IGRT benefited significantly from an optimally selected air gap.

- Finally, antiscatter grids may be incorporated in CBCT systems to physically reject x-ray scatter from reaching the detector. Such rejection comes at the cost of some attenuation of primary x-rays, with typical primary transmission factors of ~0.6–0.8. Grids therefore may carry a necessary increase in patient dose to maintain a given exposure to the detector and image noise level, the so-called Bucky factor, which may or may not be important to maintaining input-quantum-limited performance in modern FPDs. For the extended geometries of IGRT, antiscatter grids have been found to improve image uniformity (i.e., reduce cupping artifacts) but impart tradeoffs in contrast-to-noise ratio (Siewerdsen et al., 2004). For other applications and scanner geometries for which a large air gap is not feasible, the selection of an optimal antiscatter grid is likely to be significantly more important.

(iii) Methods to algorithmically correct x-ray scatter.

Even with the various physical methods outlined above, x-ray scatter can still be a significant source of image quality degradation, and methods to correct scatter artifacts have been a topic of significant activity in the scientific and patent literature since the early days of CT. The usual means of scatter correction is to estimate the scatter fluence contributing to the projection data, subtract this fluence from the projections, and reconstruct the estimated primary-only data. This clearly relies upon a means of accurately estimating the scatter fluence, for which one can consider two broad classes of scatter estimation—measurement and modeling.

Numerous methods for measuring the scatter fluence have been reported, ranging from simple calibrations (in which the scatter fluence is measured, for example, in a variety of water cylinders, and the scatter fluence in real patient data is estimated directly from the detector signal) to more innovative methods that extract the scatter fluence directly from the measured projections or Monte Carlo simulations (Bani-Hashemi et al., 2005; Bertram et al., 2005; Jarry et al., 2006; Liu et al., 2005; Ning et al., 2004; Siewerdsen et al., 2006; Spies et al., 2001, Zhu et al., 2005). Many of these involve the introduction of an object within the FOV (between the x-ray source and patient) to either completely or partially attenuate the primary + scatter fluence reaching the detector. For example, an array of highly attenuating "blockers" in the projections offers a fairly straightforward means of estimating scatter fluence derived from the detector signal behind the blockers. Such methods introduce the challenge of either ignoring or interpolating over the blockers prior to reconstruction or performing a second scan with the blocker pattern removed. A more elegant method involves a weakly attenuating pattern introduced in the projections—for example, a checkerboard of aluminum or other partially attenuating material—from which the pattern and low-frequency characteristics of x-ray scatter may be decomposed in the spatial frequency domain. Alternatively, a simple estimate of the scatter fluence can be obtained from the detector signal behind the *z* collimator blades, which are often present in the projection data (per the recommendation above that longitudinal FOV be minimized). Under the assumption that the signal in collimator shadows is scatter-only, the scatter fluence in each projection can be estimated by interpolating over the scatter + primary field—a reasonable assumption for cylindrically symmetric objects, but subject to possible over- or underestimation for complex objects with internal or external surface shapes that vary strongly in the *z* direction.

Several such methods involve modeling the x-ray scatter fluence, including analytical and Monte Carlo methods for deriving the scatter fluence from a given source and object model. For example, "two-pass" model-based scatter correction involves: an initial CBCT reconstruction based on the uncorrected primary + scatter fluence; an estimate of the scatter fluence in each projection computed from the object model yielded in the previous step—either analytically (with a simplified object model) or by Monte Carlo (on the initial reconstruction directly); subtraction of the scatter fluence estimate; a second-pass reconstruction based on the corrected primary-only estimate; and possible iteration on this approach through multiple passes. The increasing speed and sophistication of Monte Carlo and multiple-pass 3D reconstruction makes this a potentially promising area of future research, development, and clinical application.

In practice, none of the physical or algorithmic methods summarized above provide a perfect solution to the significant effects of x-ray scatter in CBCT. As a result, system design and good practice often represent a combination of numerous approaches—for example, minimizing collimator FOV, knowledgeable selection of gap and/or grid, subtraction of scatter estimates from measured projections, and model-based scatter correction.

5.2.4.5 Beam Hardening

As a polyenergetic x-ray beam passes through material, low-energy ("soft") x-rays are more likely to be absorbed than high energy ("hard") x-rays in accordance with the Beers-Lambert law and (apart from K-edge effects) monotonically decreasing attenuation coefficient, $\mu(E)$. The shift in the polyenergetic spectrum to higher energies is referred to as "beam hardening." As a result, the effective attenuation coefficient within a material changes (reduces) as the beam hardens. The effect on 3D reconstruction is an underestimation in attenuation coefficient due to the hardening of the beam and/or over-response of the detector to higher-energy x-rays (Brooks and DiChiro, 1976). The resulting artifacts are similar in form to the "shading" and "streak" artifacts discussed above in relation to x-ray scatter, see Figure 5.16.

Beam hardening artifacts may be reduced through physical and algorithmic techniques. The physical methods are analogous to the bowtie filter employed to "flatten" the x-ray fluence transmitted to the detector. One such method employs added beam filtration to pre- or postharden the beam; however, this method can degrade the detector signal, resulting in increased noise. Another method employs a wedge calibration relative to a cylindrical object (e.g., water). However, this method requires scanning objects with cylindrical geometry and has limited clinical applicability.

Algorithmic corrections can be similarly (and perhaps more successfully) applied to reduce the effects of beam hardening on image quality. In images containing only soft tissues, where the attenuation coefficients possess energy dependence similar to water, a nonlinear correction algorithm based on a previously acquired water calibration can greatly reduce beam hardening effects (Joseph and Spital, 1978). In images where bone is present, an additional correction factor related to the energy dependence of the attenuation coefficient of bone must be applied. Alternatively, an iterative correction algorithm can significantly reduce the effects of beam hardening on image quality (Hsieh et al., 2000) with the advantage of correcting artifacts associated with multiple high-density materials. Overall, artifacts associated with beam hardening tend to be similar in appearance to those arising from x-ray scatter, but tend to be lesser in magnitude and more easily corrected using the algorithmic methods mentioned above.

5.2.4.6 Metal, "Zero-Data," and Photon Starvation Artifacts

The term "metal artifact" somewhat broadly refers to several potential sources of image degradation in regions about strongly attenuating metal structures within the patient, for example, dental fillings and metallic implants. These include beam-hardening effects (i.e., strong shifts in the x-ray spectrum associated with absorption in high-Z materials) and photon starvation effects (i.e., low detector signal in the shadow of metal objects) as described above. In the extreme case of total or near-total x-ray attenuation within a metal structure, a distinct artifact arises—referred to as a zero-data artifact—in which the detector signal is approximately zero (including only x-ray scatter and electronics noise). Depending on the exact implementation of the 3D reconstruction algorithm, the presence of zero-data may completely confound backprojection along views for which detector signal is zero. The effect on the reconstruction is typically bright streaks (corresponding to very high attenuation) along the corresponding zero-data views. Correction of metal artifacts include beam-hardening corrections (mentioned earlier) as well as a variety of projection-based and multipass reconstruction-based algorithms that seek to restore the projection data to reasonable detector signal values (Figure 5.17).

The term "photon starvation" refers to noise in 3D reconstructions arising from projections for which the exposure to the detector is low, and the detector signal-to-noise ratio is correspondingly poor. For example, projections through the lateral

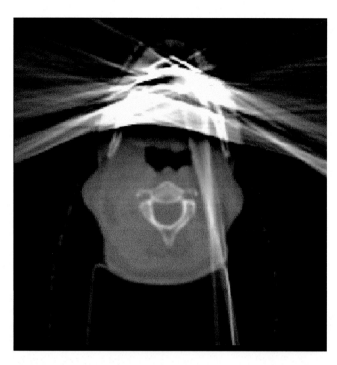

FIGURE 5.17 Example images illustrating zero-data artifacts arising from near complete x-ray attenuation in metal (dental fillings).

direction of a large pelvis suffer very strong x-ray attenuation through the thickest regions of the body, resulting in noisy projections and correspondingly high noise along the direction associated with those projection views. Therefore, photon starvation is not really an artifact in the terms defined above, since it is not a deterministic effect. Rather, it is a stochastic effect associated with increased quantum noise along strongly attenuated views. It often gives the appearance of a deterministic artifact—specifically, streakiness along specific directions in the object or between strongly attenuating structures—but, strictly speaking, it is simply strongly correlated noise (and not artifact). Its implications can be fairly significant in certain imaging tasks where strong asymmetry in the noise characteristic can confound detectability of subtle soft tissues or the delineation of tissue boundaries in regions dominated by photon starvation streaks. Methods for managing or correcting the effect range from algorithmic corrections in the reconstruction (e.g., penalized reconstruction methods that weight noisy projection data) to physical methods that boost x-ray intensity in projections that would otherwise yield very low detector signal (e.g., mA modulation in which the x-ray tube current is increased for lateral projections).

5.2.4.7 Image Lag

FPDs typically incorporate amorphous semiconductor components (such as a-Si:H) with material characteristics that (while quite advantageous in terms of large-area fabrication, radiation damage resistance, etc.) exhibit lower mobility and increased charge trapping effects in comparison to crystalline semiconductors. One result of such material characteristics is a relatively high level of "image lag" in the projection data, that is signal generated within a projection acquired at time t_0, "trapped" in long-lifetime metastable states, and subsequently released and read out in a projection at time t_1. There are other potential sources of image lag as well—including the x-ray converter (scintillator) and readout electronics—but the main source in the current generation of FPDs is typically the amorphous semiconductor within the pixel components (e.g., photodiode and/or TFT). Such has been the subject of considerable investigation since the early development of FPDs, with typical image lag magnitude on the order of ~1–5% (that is, 1–5% of signal read in a given projection was actually generated in the previous projection—the so-called "first-frame" lag—decreasing with each frame such that "tenth-frame" lag is typically on the order ~0.1%).

A separate effect is image "ghosting," which refers to a change in detector gain dependent on previous exposures. Such may arise from a change in sensitivity of the scintillator and/or FPD electronics. Although the terms "lag" and "ghosting" are sometimes interchanged or confused, they are distinct—the former referring to residual signal carried over from previous frames, and the latter referring to variation in detector sensitivity arising from previous exposures.

Image lag introduces a variety of artifacts in CBCT reconstructions. The one usually discussed is a so-called "comet" artifact evident as an azimuthal "tail" behind high-contrast structures, for example, the bright signal extending from the wire in the axial image of Figure 5.18. The origin of the comet tail is the residual signal (lag) at pixel locations no longer associated with the projected location of the wire (Siewerdsen and Jaffray, 1999). Note that the brightness and extent of the comet depend on the magnitude of image lag as well as the distance of the object from the center of reconstruction (more severe for objects at greater distance, since such objects involve a greater angular "velocity" from frame to frame, and residual signal therefore arises at distances farther removed from the actual projected location). The overall effect can be considered a radial convolution of a "blur" function related to the temporal MTF of the imaging system, applied in a manner that is spatially dependent in the reconstruction domain (stronger at greater distances from the center of reconstruction). Artifacts related to lag (and ghosting) can also be observed in particular near the skin line of large asymmetric objects, where the exposure level to the detector changes rapidly from frame to frame (e.g., at the lateral edge of the pelvis), creating a so-called "radar" artifact owing to inconsistencies in detector signal and/or gain—that is image lag (an increase in signal owing to previous exposures) and/or ghosting (an increase or decrease in detector gain owing to previous exposures). A variety of correction methods can be envisioned—for example, an empirically based correction based upon measured lag characteristics to give a weighted subtraction of previous projections from the current projection (Mail et al., 2008).

5.2.4.8 Lateral Truncation

While large-area FPDs were a critical advance in the practical application of CBCT in IGRT, the dimensions of the detector

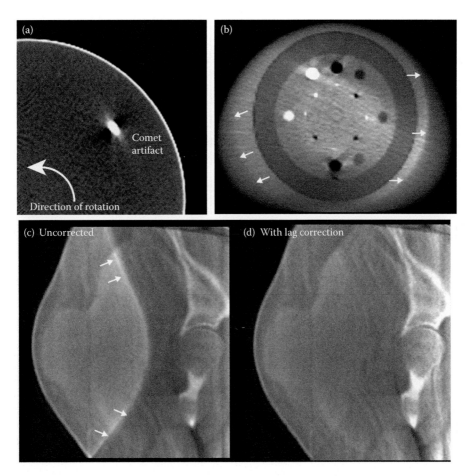

FIGURE 5.18 Example images illustrating image lag and/or ghosting artifacts. (a) A comet artifact associated with residual signal from projection-to-projection. (b) A radar artifact associated with lag and/or ghosting in regions of projections receiving high bare-beam exposure, followed by strong attenuation. The arrows mark the boundary of a circular "radar" shading artifact. (c) Sagittal view in CBCT of a sarcoma patient reconstructed without correction for lag. (d) The same as (c) with lag correction.

are often insufficient to completely cover the lateral extent of the patient and/or patient support. Thus, lateral truncation is somewhat the norm in CBCT, and truncation artifacts can arise as a result of the incomplete projection data. Such artifacts are evident as a combination of CT number inaccuracy (typically a reduction in CT# near the center of reconstruction, shading artifacts (a bright ring in the axial image about the periphery of the reconstruction), and streaks (for example, bright streaks arising from a highly attenuating object that is within the FOV for some, but not all, projections). Example images illustrating such effects are shown in Figure 5.19.

A variety of truncation artifact correction methods have been reported. The simplest involves lateral extrapolation of the projection data at the "left and right" edges of the projection data—for example, a smooth extrapolation from the measured pixel values at the edge of the detector to zero attenuation at some distance imagined to encompass the actual lateral extent of the object. While directly "padding" the projections with such extrapolated data is possible, doing so unnecessarily increases the image reconstruction time (due to larger format input projection). Since the extrapolated data are deterministic (e.g., an analytical linear or exponential extrapolation to zero), they can

be incorporated in the filtered backprojection process without explicit padding. Other approaches utilize prior information (e.g., the prior CT scan) to give a better estimate of the missing data, for example, expanding the measured CBCT sonogram to include data from the prior image at the lateral edges. Such methods are promising in applications such as IGRT, where prior information abounds, but requires careful implementation to ensure proper registration of current and prior datasets.

5.2.4.9 The "Cone-Beam" Artifact

Perhaps the most notorious artifact in CBCT (and one might argue, undeservedly so) is the so-called "cone-beam" artifact associated with a simple circular source-detector geometry. This typical CBCT imaging arrangement violates Tuy's condition for exact reconstruction, which requires that every plane passing through a voxel in the reconstruction intersects the source-detector plane. For a simple circular source-detector geometry, the only voxels in a CBCT image that obey Tuy's condition are those on the central axial slice. All other voxels suffer incompleteness in projection data. For example, a voxel at a given height (z) above the central plane contains at least one plane that does not intersect the source-detector orbit, for example, a plane parallel

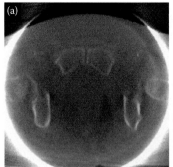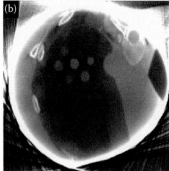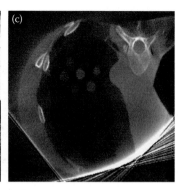

FIGURE 5.19 Example images illustrating lateral truncation artifacts. Uncorrected lateral truncation in (a) a prostate image and (b) a chest phantom is evident as a bright ring about the circle of reconstruction and a reduction of attenuation coefficients therein. (c) The same image as (b) corrected using a simple extrapolation of the projection data edges.

to the orbit, and is therefore not reconstructed accurately. Note that violation of Tuy's condition (and the associated "cone-beam artifact") is not a shortfall of the FDK algorithm in itself; rather, it is a result of the circular source-detector geometry.

Similarly, the effect can be considered in terms of the portion of the 3D Fourier domain that is sampled in 3D filtered back-projection from a circular orbit. A "null cone" about the z-frequency axis corresponds to the inability to reconstruct the f_z-component of structures in the image. The angle of the null cone is determined by the system geometry—the "cone angle" corresponding to a given voxel at some height above the central plane. The effect is typically manifest as a reduction in CT number and a loss of z-frequency content in the image—each referred to generically as "cone-beam" artifact.

The degree of incompleteness depends on the location within the 3D reconstruction (more severe for greater distances from the central axial plane) and is illustrated well in the Fourier domain. For voxels in the central axial plane, the Fourier domain is fully sampled, and all frequency components of the object are faithfully reconstructed. (In fact, this is a simplification as well, and the divergent beam and finite sampling impart completeness conditions of their own.) For voxels off the axial plane by a distance z (i.e., by some angle φ), sampling is incomplete as characterized by a cone about the f_z axis of extent φ, and spatial frequency components of the object residing within this "null cone" are not reconstructed. The effect is therefore spatially dependent—increasing for greater distances from the central axial plane, with the null cone "precessing" in a manner associated with the distance from the longitudinal axis (Bartolac et al., 2009).

A CBCT reconstruction of an object is therefore inaccurate in a manner related to the spatial frequency content of the object and the location within the 3D image. In general, the reconstructed image is lacking spatial frequency components associated with the spatially dependent "null cone" described above. The most egregious example of such is the image of a disk (or stack of disks) oriented parallel to the axial plane: while the disk (with spatial frequency content located entirely along the f_z axis) may be faithfully reconstructed at the axial plane, for the disk located at some distance from the central axial plane the image

is grossly inaccurate, since the object spatial frequency content is almost entirely within the null cone. While this effect presents a clear analytical shortfall of CBCT reconstruction from data collected on a simple circular trajectory (which is that assumed in the usual FDK algorithm), the spatial frequency content of natural anatomy is sufficiently rich (i.e., filling the Fourier domain) that the missing frequencies associated with the null cone may have a fairly small effect on image quality, depending on the imaging task—for example in reconstructing a spherical object for determination of its centroid, localizing a soft-tissue tumor in IGRT, or visualizing trabecular detail in bone—as illustrated in Figure 5.20.

5.2.4.10 Patient Motion

All of the artifacts mentioned above arise in some way from projection data inconsistency, for example, inconsistencies in the x-ray fluence (e.g., beam hardening), the detector signal (e.g., image lag), and/or the object itself. A moving object, for example, presents obvious projection data inconsistencies that will result in image artifacts—typically "streaks"—with the most common examples in IGRT being cardiac and/or respiratory motion.

As summarized early in the chapter, the basis for (cone-beam) CT is a series of projection views of an object acquired from different angles. In the event that (parts of) the object moves during acquisition, however, these views (a) are no longer from exactly the same object and/or (b) are from incomplete sets of views that are uncorrelated. Such motion therefore induces artifacts in the reconstructed images. The form and magnitude of such motion artifacts are related to a multitude of factors, such as the acquisition period relative to the direction and magnitude of object motion. While conventional diagnostic CT scanners offer fast gantry rotation time of typically ~0.3 ms, the various CBCT scanners mentioned above for IGRT have typical rotation times of ~60–120 s, limited in part by IEC requirements (IEC 1998). Such long acquisition times clearly present significant challenges with respect to patient motion. Moreover, in a fully 3D CBCT, inconsistent projection data can pollute the entire volume, whereas for axial CT it mainly impacts the spatial consistency of subsequent slices.

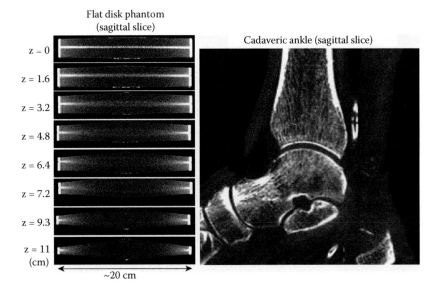

Flat disk phantom
(sagittal slice)

z = 0
z = 1.6
z = 3.2
z = 4.8
z = 6.4
z = 7.2
z = 9.3
z = 11
(cm)

~20 cm

Cadaveric ankle (sagittal slice)

FIGURE 5.20 Example images illustrating the "cone-beam" artifact in sagittal images. (a) A disk phantom highlights the effect as a loss of horizontal edge resolution at increasing distances from the central plane. (b) A cadaver specimen exhibits little such effect over a similar range in *z* (~11 cm range from the central axial slice), given the rich spatial frequency content of natural anatomy.

It is worthwhile to distinguish patient motion artifacts from possible artifacts associated with the normal motion of the x-ray source and detector. For pulsed x-ray exposures (the usual approach in systems mentioned above), the exposure time per projection image is typically too short (10–30 ms) to induce appreciable motion artifacts directly in the individual projections. For continuous x-ray exposure (e.g., CW fluoroscopy) during acquisition, there is the potential for projection motion blur over the finite frame time of individual projections, resulting in a so-called "azimuthal blur" in reconstructions. (Kwan et al., 2007). For current IGRT CBCT systems, artifacts arising from these sources of projection blur over ~0.01–0.5 s time scales are typically minor in comparison to those associated with gross patient motion occurring over the ~60–120 s acquisition period.

Two types of organ motion can be distinguished: periodic motion, such as respiration (discussed in the following section), and random/erratic motion, such as peristalsis. An example of such erratic motion is shown in Figure 5.21. Projection images (top row) show a large, moving gas pocket (bright structure) emerging in the rectum over a period of ~17 s at a position coinciding with projections of the prostate. Strong streak artifacts induced by such a moving gas pocket are shown in a CBCT axial slice in Figure 5.21, clearly reducing the visibility of the prostate due to strong black streak artifacts about the rectum.

Motion artifacts can be reduced by preventative measures or algorithmic techniques. Smitsmans et al. (2008) observed a significant decrease of moving gas and a corresponding improved image quality following the introduction of a dietary protocol for prostate cancer patients. Alternatively, in case of data redundancy, projection-images containing moving structures can be discarded to obtain a consistent subset of projection-images (Voogt et al., 2007).

5.3 Four-Dimensional Cone-Beam CT

Motion during CBCT acquisition violates the principles of computer tomography inducing motion artifacts as described above. For (semi) periodic motion that is fast relative to the CBCT acquisition time, these artifacts are mainly a blurring of the moving structures over their trajectory of motion (Sonke et al., 2005). As summarized below, several strategies have been proposed to mitigate these artifacts, and the topic remains an important area of research and development in IGRT.

5.3.1 Breath-Hold CBCT Acquisition

A straightforward approach to reduce respiratory motion artifacts is to acquire scans under breath-hold conditions. Borst et al. (2007) described a voluntary deep inspiration breath-hold protocol acquiring projection images over 200° in about 35 s for a short-scan protocol. For a full-scan protocol, Dawson et al. (Case et al., 2009; Hawkins et al., 2006) developed a "stop-and-go" protocol acquiring projection images over a full 360° rotation in three breath-holds (20 s each) using an active breathing control (ABC, Elekta Oncology Systems Ltd., Crawley, West Sussex, UK). To limit artifacts associated with breath-hold variability, only patients with diaphragm position reproducibility better or equal than 2 mm was permitted. Note, however, that the primary purpose of breath-hold CBCT scanning in these studies was to image the patients in treatment position rather than mitigating motion artifacts.

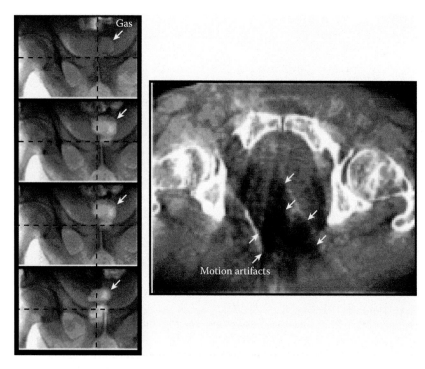

FIGURE 5.21 The impact of a large, moving gas pocket during image acquisition on the CBCT reconstruction. Projection images (left) show a large, moving gas pocket (bright structure) emerging in the rectum in a time span of 17 s at a position where the prostate would be projected. The reconstruction result, showing the streak artifacts in an axial slice of the CBCT scan. (Modified from Smitsmans et al., *Int J Radiat Oncol Biol Phys.* 63(4): 975–984, 2005.)

5.3.2 Respiratory-Correlated CBCT

In situations where patients are treated under free-breathing conditions, breath-hold CBCT scanning techniques are undesirable for image guidance. To reduce motion artifacts, time-resolved CBCT imaging was developed to correlate respiratory motion with image acquisition (Dietrich et al., 2006). As respiratory motion induces blurring of mobile structures, a slice selecting procedure to obtain a four-dimensional (4D) data set, as employed in respiratory correlated CT imaging, does not work. Therefore, respiratory correlation needs to be applied in projection space (Sonke et al., 2005). That is, cone-beam projections are snapshots representing a certain phase of the respiratory cycle, while different projections represent different respiratory phases. By sorting the projections into bins depending on their respective respiratory phase and subsequently reconstructing each bin separately into a 3D CBCT image or frame representing one phase of the respiratory cycle, a 4D CBCT image of the respiratory cycle is generated.

5.3.2.1 Breathing Signal Extraction

To correlate the projection images to the respiratory motion, a breathing signal is required (see Chapters 13 and 14). Such a signal can be determined by measurement of temperature differences between inhaled and exhaled air near the patient's nose (Rit et al., 2009; Sonke et al., 2009), by measuring changes in the circumference of the thorax using stretch/pressure sensors, or using reflective markers on the patient's chest. These types of measurements need to be synchronized with the exact

time at which cone-beam projection images are acquired. Alternatively, a breathing signal can be extracted directly from motion captured in the series of projection images. Zijp et al. (Zijp et al., 2004) developed an algorithm where each 2D projection is processed with a derivative filter in the craniocaudal direction to enhance diaphragmatic structures and projected on the craniocaudal axis in a 1D image. The concatenation of these 1D images for a few projections (>1 respiratory cycle) gives a 2D image representation loosely referred to as the "Amsterdam Shroud" (illustrated in Figure 5.22) from which the respiratory signal is extracted with a linear correlation of adjacent columns. Nguyen et al. (2009) described the use of a navigator channel placed on a projected dome of the diaphragm to measure intensity variations. The breathing signal thus obtained is synchronized by definition and eliminates the need for additional equipment.

5.3.2.2 4D CBCT Reconstruction

In 4D CBCT scans, the number of projections for each respiratory phase is significantly reduced compared to conventional (non-4D) CBCT scans. Considerable view aliasing artifacts are therefore present in the reconstructed images, and the contrast-to-noise ratio is also compromised in accordance with a reduced dose per 3D reconstruction in the 4D sequence. Increasing the frame rate of the detector will not significantly improve the image quality. Although the number of images per bin will proportionally increase, these will be grouped in bursts of images

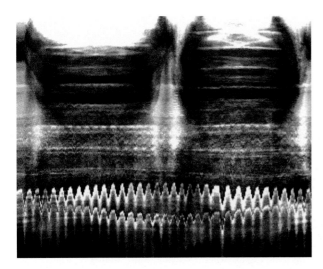

FIGURE 5.22 Illustration of the "Amsterdam Shroud" representation of motion inferred directly from the projection data of a CBCT acquisition series. The vertical axis in this representation is the v coordinate on the detector, while each column corresponds to a single projection image such that the horizontal axis represents projection angle (or time).

corresponding to the same phase of the same respiratory cycle separated by considerable angular gaps between corresponding phases of adjacent respiratory cycles and resulting in view aliasing (undersampling) effects in the reconstruction. Alternatively, slowing down the gantry rotation speed increases the number of respiratory cycles captured during the acquisition and thus reduces the angular gap between corresponding phases of adjacent respiratory cycles. Note that the imaging dose can be kept constant by decreasing the dose per projection in proportion to the gantry rotation speed. Similarly, acquiring multiple arcs also increases the captured number of respiratory cycles but provides less control on the angular gap.

The effect of gantry rotation speed on 4D CBCT image quality is illustrated in Figure 5.23 for the exhale phase of a dynamic thorax phantom, CIRC, Norfolk, Virginia. Scans were acquired over an arc of 200° for a motion period of 3 s and gantry rotation speeds of 0.5, 1, 2, and 4 rpm capturing 10, 20, 40, and 80 motion periods, respectively. It can be seen that clinically acceptable image quality can be obtained with 40–80 captured breathing cycles. In Figure 5.24, sagittal, coronal, and transverse slices of a 3D CBCT scan as well as for the respiratory phases peak-exhale, mid-inhale, peak-inhale, and mid-exhale of a 4D CBCT scan for lung cancer patient. Visual examination shows that the blurring of the moving objects is reduced considerably in the 4D data such that the shape of the moving structures can be identified more easily and accurately. Furthermore, the 4D data set provides information on the trajectory of these structures, absent in the 3D data.

Note that 4D CBCT imaging, similar to 4D CT imaging, relies on a regular breathing pattern, while irregular breathing induces artifacts in 4D reconstructions. Weighting of the projection data with the angular spacing between adjacent images within each phase-bin helps to mitigate the effect of changes in respiratory

frequency. Because of the slow gantry rotation speed relative to the respiratory frequency, irregularities in respiratory amplitude and baseline typically induce blurring over the residual motion within each subset of projection images.

As view aliasing artifacts limit 4D CBCT image quality, and slower gantry rotation speed have a negative impact on patient throughput, advanced CBCT reconstruction algorithms have been studied to produce streak artifact free images. Bergner et al. (2009) described an autoadaptive phase correlation (AAPC) reconstruction algorithm that estimates motion from the projections and areas that are unaffected by motion are then used for image reconstruction regardless of the motion phase. Leng et al. (2008a,b) described a McKinnon-Bates (MKB) based algorithm where a prior image is first reconstructed using all available projections without sorting, in which static structures are well reconstructed while moving objects are blurred. The view aliasing artifacts from static structures are estimated from this prior image volume and subsequently suppressed from the 4D CBCT. Iterative reconstruction algorithms like the algebraic reconstruction algorithm (ART) or the simultaneous algebraic reconstruction algorithm (SART) have the potential to reconstruct images with fewer artifacts and less image noise (Desbat et al., 2007). Similarly, compressed sensing (CS) based reconstruction algorithms such as prior image constrained compressed sensing (PICCS) (Leng et al., 2008a,b) and constrained total-variation minimization (Jia et al., 2010; Sidky and Pan 2008a, b) have the ability to reconstruct images based on a limited number of projection images. Although such algorithms show promising results, their value still needs to proven on a range of clinical data. Moreover, they are computationally complex and their implementation will require significant advances in computing power and speed to find real utility in clinical practice.

5.3.3 Motion-Compensated 4D CBCT Reconstruction

An alternative solution to reduce respiratory motion-induced artifacts in CBCT is motion-compensated reconstruction (Li et al., 2006a,b, 2007). In motion compensated CBCT reconstruction, the motion is estimated during the acquisition, producing deformation vector fields (DVF) for every motion state, which are then accounted for in the reconstruction algorithm. Thus, a 3D CBCT image at a reference position is reconstructed from all the projections, thus minimizing view aliasing artifacts and noise. If accurate motion information can be obtained, this approach can potentially compensate motion artifacts completely in the reconstruction algorithm. Estimating the motion, however, is computationally complex and challenging in real cone-beam projections (Zeng et al., 2007). Also, the incorporation of the motion compensation in the reconstruction is computationally complex, even for the "simple" FDK algorithm. To reduce the computational complexity (Rit et al., 2009) developed a method using an *a priori* model of the patient respiratory motion derived from the 4D planning CT. During CBCT

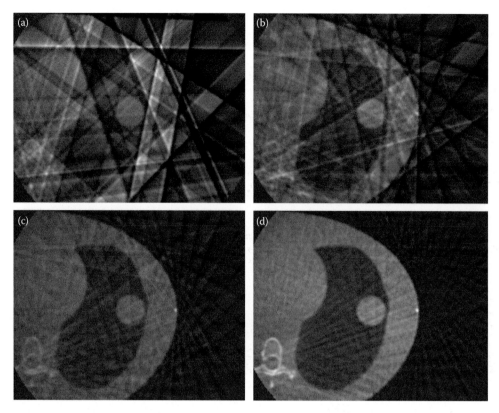

FIGURE 5.23 Transverse slice of the exhale phase of 4D CBCT scans of a dynamic thorax phantom, CIRC, Norfolk, Virginia with a 3 cm water-equivalent density spherical object in lung equivalent material moving with a 6 s motion period for various gantry rotation speeds: (a) 1 rpm/30 s acquisition, (b) 0.5 rpm/60 s acquisition, (c) 0.25 rpm/120 s acquisition, and (d) 0.125 rpm/240 s acquisition. Clearly, slowing down the gantry rotation speed reduces view aliasing artifacts.

acquisition, the model is correlated with the respiration using a respiratory signal extracted from the projections similar to the 4D CBCT approach. The estimated motion is next compensated in an efficient implementation of the FDK algorithm providing on-the-fly motion-compensated reconstruction, that is reconstruction that keeps up with the acquisition process. An example of the image quality that can be achieved with motion-compensated reconstruction is shown in Figure 5.25. Images free of streak artifact can be obtained even with fast gantry rotation speeds.

It is important to be aware what reference position is chosen for the motion-compensated reconstruction as potential biases are introduced in an image-guided correction procedure. In Rit et al. (2009), the motion compensated for is forced to be null on average over the acquisition time to ensure that the compensation results in a CBCT image that describes the mean position of each organ, even if the *a priori* motion model is inaccurate.

5.4 Radiation Dose for Volumetric CT

The measurement of radiation dose in conditions appropriate to CBCT requires modification to dosimetry standards that have evolved in the context of conventional axial CT. Specifically, the pencil chamber and CT dose index (CTDI)

concepts arising from AAPM Task Group Report #1 (Judy et al., 1977) are currently undergoing revision to better describe dose metrics for volumetric beams as in CBCT. A summary of conceptual underpinnings and basis for a new set of dosimetric standards appropriate to volumetric CT dosimetry is provided in AAPM Task Group Report #111 (Dixon, 2003; Dixon et al., 2010).

The conventional CT dosimetry standards called for the adoption of standard "head" (16 cm diameter) and "body" (32 cm diameter) acrylic cylinders typically ~15 cm length within which a 10-cm length pencil ionization chamber is placed (at the center and periphery). With the pencil chamber oriented along the longitudinal axis and centered on a scan of length L, comprising n discrete, contiguous axial slices of thickness T, the CTDI in its basic form is

$$\text{CTDI} = f\left(\frac{X}{T}\right)L, \tag{5.41}$$

where X is the exposure measured in the air ionization chamber, and f is a conversion factor based on the pencil chamber calibration. The conventional CTDI represents an integral of the longitudinal (z-direction) dose profile, normalized by the beam collimation (length nT)

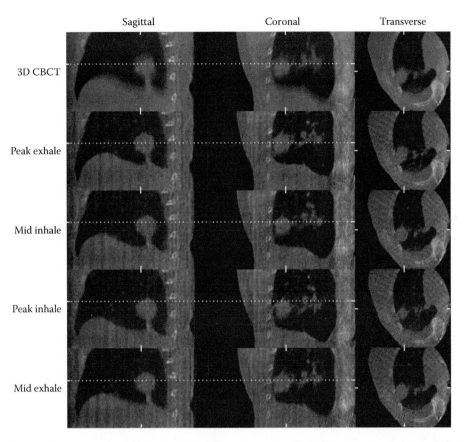

FIGURE 5.24 Sagittal, coronal, and transverse slices of a 3D CBCT scan as well as for the respiratory phases peak-exhale, mid-inhale, peak-inhale, and mid-exhale of a 4D CBCT scan for a lung cancer patient. The white dashes in each view identify the displayed slices in the corresponding views. The dashed lines in the coronal and sagittal views are drawn as a reference to appreciate the motion of the tumor in the 4D scan.

$$\text{CTDI} = \frac{1}{nT} \int_{-\infty}^{+\infty} D(z)\,dz. \qquad (5.42)$$

In practice for axial CT, the integral could be obtained from measurement using a 10-cm length pencil chamber. For volumetric beams in CBCT, the extent of the primary beam almost always exceeds 10 cm. Therefore, the conventional approach is not particularly well suited to CBCT, for which a 15-cm length phantom and 10-cm length pencil chamber are likely insufficient to capture the primary beam as well as potentially long tails associated with x-ray scatter.

An updated approach addresses the phantom length issue (i.e., properly measures the dose associated with broad volumetric beams and long scatter tails) either through the use of longer phantoms or extrapolation techniques based on previous measurements (Dixon, 2003; Dixon et al., 2010). In the former, for example, three conventional CTDI cylindrical phantoms could be "stacked" to facilitate a phantom ~45–50 cm in length. Such an approach captures the long scatter tails, although it triples the cost of the phantom and can be a bit cumbersome to transport and set up. A potential alternative is to use a shorter (~15 cm phantom) and extrapolate to the presumed "equilibrium" values associated with a phantom of sufficient length determined be previous measurements.

Approaches are furthermore under development to address the insufficiency of a 10-cm pencil ionization chamber, which is a poor choice for dose measurement in beams that typically cover ~20 cm length and exhibit long scatter tails. A brute force solution could entail the use of a very long pencil ionization chamber, although such introduces obvious factors of inconvenience and cost. Alternatively, and perhaps more natural to IGRT physicists well acquainted with the measurement of dose in broad volumetric beams (e.g., the MV treatment beam), is to use a small dosimeter—for example, a 0.6 cm³ Farmer chamber—for assessment of the "point" dose at the center of the volumetric beam within a long cylindrical phantom. The "Long-Phantom/Small-Dosimeter" approach illustrated in Figure 5.26 has been applied successfully in dose characterization for a variety of early CBCT imaging applications (Daly et al., 2006; Fahrig et al., 2006; Silverman et al., 2009).

5.5 Quality Assurance

Currently, there are no established quality assurance guidelines for kV CBCT systems. At the time of writing, AAPM Task Group Report 179 on "Quality assurance for image-guided radiation therapy utilizing CT-based technologies" is still in progress. Nevertheless, several groups have published on their quality

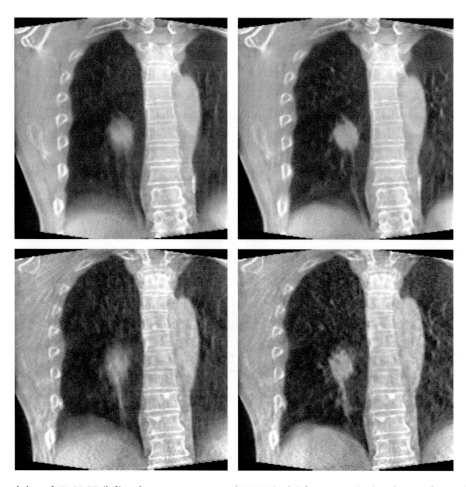

FIGURE 5.25   Coronal slice of 3D CBCT (left) and motion compensated CBCT (right) for a 4 min (top) and 1 min (bottom) acquisition time.

assurance programs (Bissonnette et al., 2008a,b; Lehmann et al., 2007; Saw et al., 2007; Schreibmann et al., 2009; Stock et al., 2009; Yoo et al., 2006). Basic quality assurance program components include assessments of geometric accuracy, image quality, and imaging dose, as now reviewed.

5.5.1 Geometric Accuracy

Traditionally, patient treatment setup errors were measured using MV portal imaging systems that determined the position of bony anatomy relative to the field edge. In such an approach, the imaging system is intrinsically calibrated to the treatment isocenter and thus required very little QA. A kV CBCT system integrated with a linear accelerator, on the other hand, has a separate imaging isocenter that needs to be calibrated to the treatment isocenter. Additionally, a geometric calibration correction has to be applied for gantry motion nonidealities for purposes of 3D image reconstruction, as described above. Note that calibration of imaging-to-treatment isocenter and gantry motion nonidealities are not specific for kV-CBCT guided systems and are also required for kV-planar and MV CBCT imaging.

The long-term stability of the geometric calibration (flex movements) of linac-integrated CBCT scanners is reported to be high (Bissonette et al., 2008; Sharpe et al., 2006; Yoo et al., 2006). For

example, Bissonette et al. reported reproducibility within ±0.5 mm (95% confidence interval). Ali and Ahmad (2009) on the other hand reported 1–2 mm discrepancies in flex and recommended regular quality assurance. While repeated flex measurements and/or trending of spatial resolution can identify subtle changes in the system geometry characteristics, for regular verification of accurate alignment of the kV and treatment coordinate systems, a simpler QA program is recommended (Bissonette et al., 2008b; De Jong et al., 2004). Based on a reference CT scan of an anthropomorphic phantom, a simple plan is created with two orthogonal beams and reference digitally reconstructed radiographs (DRRs) are generated. After alignment of the phantom to the room lasers, a CBCT scan and portal images are acquired. By both CBCT-to-planning CT registration and portal images-to-DRR registration, the position of the phantom is measured. Differences indicate discrepancies between the CBCT and treatment geometry. Typically, a tolerance of 2 mm for manual registration and 1 mm for automatic registration is applied. Two commercially available phantoms have been designed for this purpose: the Quasar Penta-Guide phantom (Modus Medical Devices Inc., London, ON, Canada) and the Mimi phantom (Standard Imaging Inc., Middleton, WI). Any other anthropomorphic phantom that has sufficient contrast on portal images and can be accurately positioned will be suitable for such a protocol.

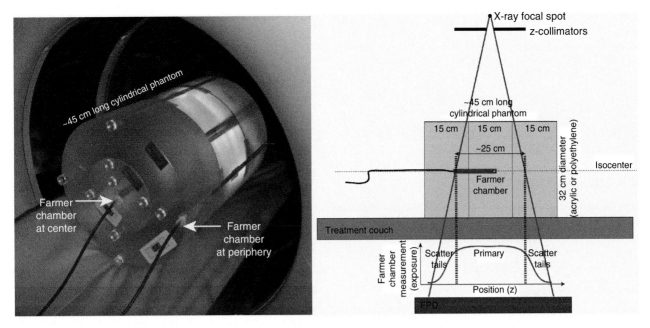

FIGURE 5.26 Illustration of dosimetry setup for volumetric CBCT. The photograph shows three conventional CTDI phantoms attached end-to-end to provide sufficient length to capture long x-ray scatter tails. The schematic at right shows such an arrangement to better cover the volumetric beam, with a small (0.6 cc) Farmer chamber placed at the center of the beam providing the most direct measurement of dose.

The frequency of geometric QA depends on the IGRT protocols implemented. In cases for which IGRT is limited to offline protocols or weekly imaging of conventional fractionated RT, weekly QA of geometric accuracy is probably sufficient. In cases for which online guidance is used for hypofractionated RT, daily QA is recommended. Note that different gantry rotation directions and imager positions are generally calibrated separately, since geometric deviations may differ based on mechanical variations in each direction of rotation. Full geometric QA, therefore, should check all such options. Note, however, that important sources of geometrical deviations such as changes in the source positions or panel position read-out electronics will affect all acquisition geometries, such that regular QA is often limited by one or a few panel positions/gantry rotations leaving the other options for (bi) annual QA.

5.5.2 Image Quality

Image quality control of conventional CT systems has been described in AAPM Report 74 "Quality control in diagnostic radiology" (Shepard et al., 2002). Recommendations of this report serve as a good starting point for image quality QA of kV CBCT systems for IGRT. Most image quality control tests can be performed using commercially available phantoms containing multiple inserts tailored to various aspects of image quality such as the Catphan 600 (The Phantom Laboratory, New York, USA), CIRS Model 610 AAPM CT (CIRS Inc., Norfolk, Virginia, USA) or GAMMEX 132 (Gammex Inc., Middleton, WI). Note, however, that most of such phantoms are designed for the conventional scanner geometry where the image performance is invariant along the axis of rotation, while in the

cone-beam geometry this is no longer true. Moreover, such phantoms tend to have a relatively small radius (e.g., ~16 cm) such that x-ray scatter effects tend to be lower than in practice with real patients.

The QA program of a CT-based IGRT system should be tailored to its utilization. The primary goal of an IGRT system is often to localize target and organs at risk in the treatment room and drive correction strategies to minimize geometrical uncertainties. Soft-tissue detectability is thus an important aspect. If the acquired CT scans are also used for dose calculations in, for example, an adaptive radiotherapy program, the CT number scale accuracy becomes important. Most CBCT guidance systems clinically operate at a spatial resolution that is substantially lower than their best possible (ideal) performance. As mentioned above, there is an intrinsic relationship and tradeoff in CT imaging between spatial resolution and noise in relation to low-contrast detectability. As low-contrast detectability can be critical to localizing organs at risk in IGRT, spatial resolution is sometimes traded off in favor of low-noise (higher CNR) images, for example, through the use of coarser voxels and smoother reconstruction filters. QA of the spatial resolution properties is nevertheless useful because a reduction in spatial resolution points to possible changes in scanner geometry, as described below.

Most studies report stable performance of linac-mounted CBCT scanners regarding the common image quality parameters described in Section 2, including image uniformity, low-contrast detectability, CT number accuracy, image scale accuracy, and spatial resolution. Despite the fact that kV CBCT guidance systems for radiation therapy operate in an aggressive environment of high energy (MV) x-rays, radiation damage to the kV FPDs has been uncommon. Nevertheless, regular image quality QA is recommended to prevent possible image quality degradation from interfering with the clinical process. Bissonette et al. (2008a,b) have recommended a six-month (semiannual) frequency or after machine service. During commissioning, baseline parameters should be established following vendor-recommended acceptance testing that can thereafter be compared to results acquired for quality assurance purposes. Tolerances relative to baseline should be aligned with the intended use of the images.

5.5.3 Imaging Dose

The imaging dose associated with kV CBCT guidance is commonly only a fraction of the therapeutic dose (Islam et al., 2006). Moreover, in case the guidance process justifies margin reduction, the reduced integral therapeutic dose often outweighs the integrated imaging dose. Nevertheless, quality assurance of imaging dose is recommended. For QA purposes, one can either check the actual imaging dose as described in Section 4 and/or check the x-ray tube output per projection using x-ray test instruments, such as the TNT 12000 X-Ray Test Device (Fluke Electronics Corporation, Everett, WA) or Diavolt Multi (PTW, Freiburg, Germany). The latter method is more straightforward and less time consuming, and is recommended for regular QA. Full dosimetric measurements (CTDI or similar metric) can be performed as a part of annual quality assurance procedures.

5.6 Clinical Applications

Numerous clinical applications of kV CBCT for IGRT have been published over the last few years, and a complete overview therefore falls outside the scope of this chapter. A brief description of important developments is given.

Initial studies focused on retrospective analysis of CBCT scans assessing the abilities of CBCT for IGRT and benchmarking the accuracy of CBCT to localize bony anatomy or fiducial markers against portal image analysis (Guckenberger et al., 2006; Létourneau et al., 2005; McBain et al., 200; van Herk et al., 2004). For example, potentially large discrepancies in target localization are observed due to registration by bony anatomy in comparison to registration on the soft-tissue target itself, as illustrated in cases of prostate treatment (Figure 5.27) and lung treatment (Figure 5.28). For several disease sites such as lung and breast, it was found that MV portal image analysis tends to underestimate bony anatomy setup error (Borst et al. 2007, Fatunase et al. 2008). Although kV CBCT was initially not developed for bony anatomy localization, it proved to be enabling technology for frameless stereotactic brain irradiation (Boda-Heggemann et al., 2006; Guckenberger et al., 200; Masi et al., 2008; Remeijer et al., 2007). That is, with a time interval of approximately 1 week between planning and treatment, the bony anatomy of the skull proved to be an excellent surrogate for the target position in image-guided SRT with a thermoplastic mask sufficiently limiting intrafraction motion.

For other treatment sites such a lung (Sonke et al., 2008; Wang Z et al., 2009), prostate (Létourneau et al., 2005; Moseley et al., 2007), rectum (Nijkamp et al., 2008), bladder (Yee et al., 2010), and breast (White et al., 2007), repetitive CBCT imaging over the course of radiotherapy has quantified considerable interfraction variability of the tumor relative to the skinmarks and bony anatomy. Repetitive 4D-CBCT additionally has provided information on respiratory amplitude variability for lung and liver (Case et al., 2009; Purdie et al., 2006; Sonke et al., 2008). Thus, these investigations have provided a rationale for the development and clinical implementation of protocols aimed at localization of soft-tissue targets.

CBCT guidance has been successful in the management of inter-fraction baseline variation for stereotactic body radiation treatment (SBRT) of pulmonary lesions (Grills et al., 2008; Guckenberger et al., 2007; Sonke et al., 2009), enabling considerable margin reduction of 5 mm and more. Possible differential motion between the primary tumor and involved lymph nodes, however, prevents large scale application for conventional fractionated therapy of higher stage patients. Soft-tissue guidance for prostate IGRT has also been described (Moseley et al., 2007; Smitsmans et al., 2005) but is more challenging due to lower contrast and peristaltic-induced motion artifacts. Here, similar accuracy can be achieved compared to fiducial-based corrections without using implanted markers. For other treatment sites such as liver cancer and bladder cancer, actual tumor visualization is challenging with the current level of CBCT image quality and correction protocols to infer tumor position rely on surrogates such as the locations of the diaphragm or organ contour (liver cancers) (Case et al., 2009; Hawkins et al., 2006) or injected lipiodol as a contrast agent (bladder cancer) (Pos et al. 2009).

Online coregistration of the CBCT and planning CT images presents a number of challenges. Aside from differences in image quality and image intensity (voxel value), variations in motion, patient posture, and target and normal tissue morphology can complicate accurate registration. For example, as illustrated in Figure 5.29, interfraction changes in neck flexion impart complex deformations throughout the head and neck. Because of the deformable (or piecewise rigid) nature of head and neck anatomy, a single rigid registration does not account for displacements throughout the entire FOV. Rigid registration constrained or bounded on specific regions of the anatomy (e.g., the upper cervical vertebrae versus the upper thoracic vertebrae) can resolve geometric discrepancies locally. Resolving such errors globally requires robust deformable registration methods, which are areas of active ongoing research.

Current clinically available CBCT guided systems facilitate online correction strategies through automatic couch shifts (Li et al., 2009). Day-to-day organ and target shape variability as well as differential motion, however, cannot be managed through such relatively simple correction strategies. As an alternative correction strategy to manage more complex variabilities, Yan et al. (1997) developed adaptive radiotherapy: a closed-loop radiation treatment process where the treatment plan can be modified using the systematic feedback of measurements.

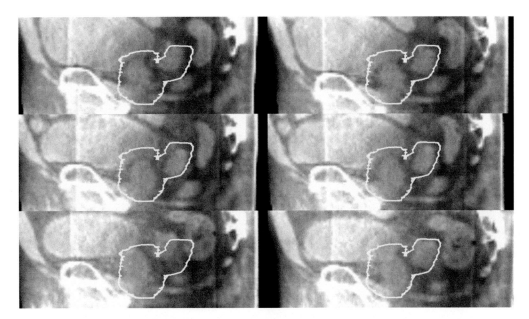

FIGURE 5.27 Example CBCT scans of a prostate cancer patient registered on bony anatomy (left) and registered on the prostate itself (right).

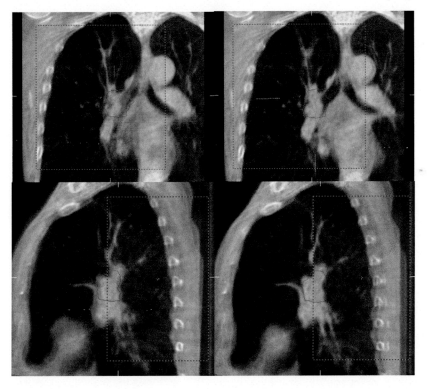

FIGURE 5.28 (See color insert) Illustration of the difference in bony anatomy alignment (left) and tumor alignment (right) for a lung cancer patient.

Several of such protocols are being developed or clinically implemented for head-and-neck posture and anatomy changes (Wu et al., 2009), prostate cancer (Nijkamp et al., 2008), esophageal cancer (Hawkins et al., 2010), bladder cancer (Foroudi et al., 2009), and lung cancer (Harsolia et al., 2008).

Despite the large-scale clinical implementation of kV CBCT guided radiation therapy, further improvements are still desirable.

As illustrated in Figure 5.30 (and other figures throughout this chapter) soft-tissue visualization in CBCT imaging typically does not match that of diagnostic quality CT images. The primary reasons for the reduced image quality are noise, contrast-to-noise ratio, and image artifacts as described in previous sections. Improvements in soft-tissue contrast may further reduce the use of fiducial markers or other surrogates of tumor position. Moreover,

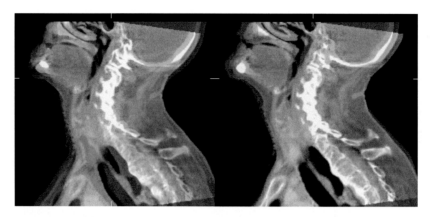

FIGURE 5.29 (See color insert)   Sagittal slices of a CBCT-to-planning CT registration using different regions of interest. In the image on the left, the top vertebrae were registered. In the image on the right, the lower vertebrae were registered. Because of posture changes occurring over the course of radiation therapy, it is important to choose the appropriate region for registration.

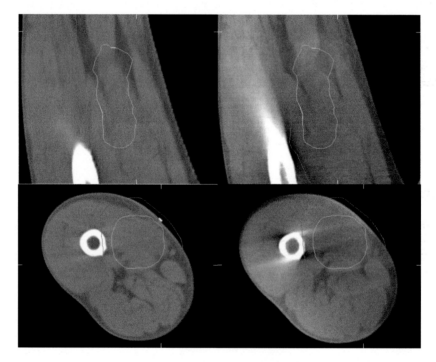

FIGURE 5.30   Coronal and axial slices of a sarcoma patient illustrating soft-tissue visibility in (left) CT and (right) CBCT.

improvements in CT number accuracy will facilitate clinical implementations of offline and online adaptive plan modifications.

5.7 Summary and Future Directions

The development and broad application of kV CBCT represents one of the most exciting developments in radiation therapy over the last decade. The scope of research associated with such activity spans a broad spectrum of expertise including 3D reconstruction, image quality assessment, radiation dosimetry,

new hardware development, system integration, image registration, quality assurance, and a tremendous spectrum of clinical application that has affected virtually every anatomical site in which radiotherapy is applied. This broad, interdisciplinary effort has involved physicists, computer scientists, engineers, and radiation oncologists in a common goal: more precise and effective delivery of radiation dose to disease while sparing normal tissue. Equal in the breadth of activities evident in the first decade of CBCT-guided radiotherapy is that the horizon for the next decade includes the development of new source-detector configurations, improved image quality, more effective integration of CBCT in online and/or adaptive guidance strategies, and the application to advanced therapeutic regimens.

Acknowledgments

The authors extend their thanks to family, friends, and colleagues for their support not only in the drafting of this chapter but over years of research and application of the techniques summarized herein. Special gratitude is owed to several individuals who contributed by way of advice, collaboration, and camaraderie: Dr. David A. Jaffray (Princess Margaret Hospital, Toronto, ON), Dr. Douglas J. Moseley (Princess Margaret Hospital, Toronto, ON), Dr. Kristy K. Brock (Princess Margaret Hospital, Toronto, ON), Dr. Michael B. Sharpe (Princess Margaret Hospital, Toronto, ON), Dr. John Wong (Johns Hopkins University, Baltimore, MD), Dr. Simon Rit (Netherlands Cancer Institute, Amsterdam, NL), Dr. Peter Remeijer (Netherlands Cancer Institute, Amsterdam, NL), Dr. Lennert Ploeger (Netherlands Cancer Institute, Amsterdam, NL), and Dr. Marcel van Herk (Netherlands Cancer Institute, Amsterdam, NL). Some of the content presented in this chapter was supported in part by research grants from the National Institutes of Health (R01-CA-89081, R21-CA-88322, R33-AG-19381, and R01-CA-112163) and research collaborations with Elekta Oncology Systems (Crawley, UK) and Varian Medical Systems (Palo Alto, CA).

Bibliography

Ali I and Ahmad S. 2009. Evaluation of the effects of sagging shifts on isocenter accuracy and image quality of cone-beam CT from kV on-board imagers. *J Appl Clin Med Phys.* 10(3):2930.

Bani-Hashemi A, Blanz E, Maltz J, Hristov D, and Svatos M. 2005. Cone beam x-ray scatter removal via image frequency modulation and filtering. *Med Phys.* 32(6):2093.

Barrett HH, Gordon SK, and Hershel RS. 1976. Statistical limitations in transaxial tomography. *Comput Biol Med.* 6(4):307–323.

Bartolac S, Clackdoyle R, Noo F, Siewerdsen JH, Moseley D, and Jaffray DA. 2009. A local shift-variant Fourier model and experimental validation of circular cone-beam computed tomography artifacts. *Med Phys.* 36(2):500–512.

Bergner F, Berkus T, Oelhafen M, Kunz P, Pan T, and Kachelriess M, 2009. Autoadaptive phase-correlated (AAPC) reconstruction for 4D CBCT. *Med Phys.* 36(12):5695–5706.

Bertram M, Wiegert J, and Rose G. 2005. Potential of software-based scatter corrections in cone-beam volume CT. *Proc SPIE Phys Med Imaging.* 5745:259–270.

Bissonnette JP, Moseley D, White E, Sharpe M, Purdie T, and Jaffray DA. 2008a. Quality assurance for the geometric accuracy of cone-beam CT guidance in radiation therapy. *Int J Radiat Oncol Biol Phys.* 71(1):S57–S61.

Bissonnette JP, Moseley DJ, and Jaffray DA. 2008b. A quality assurance program for image quality of cone-beam CT guidance in radiation therapy. *Med Phys.* 35(5):1807–1815.

Boda-Heggemann J, Walter C, Rahn A, et al. 2006. Repositioning accuracy of two different mask systems-3D revisited: comparison using true 3D/3D matching with cone-beam CT. *Int J Radiat Oncol Biol Phys.* 66(5):1568–1575.

Boellaard R, van Herk M, Uiterwaal H, and Mijnheer B. 1997. Two-dimensional exit dosimetry using a liquid-filled electronic portal imaging device and a convolution model. *Radiother Oncol.* 44:149–157.

Boggula R, Lorenz F, Abo-Madyan Y, et al. 2009. A new strategy for online adaptive prostate radiotherapy based on cone-beam CT. *Med Phys.* 19(4):264–276.

Boone JM and Lindfors KK. 2006. Breast CT: potential for breast cancer screening and diagnosis. *Future Oncol.* 2(3):351–356.

Boone JM. 2001. Determination of the presampled MTF in computed tomography. *Med Phys.* 28(3):356–360.

Borst GR, Sonke JJ, Betgen A, Remeijer P, van Herk M, and Lebesque JV. 2007. Kilo-voltage cone-beam computed tomography setup measurements for lung cancer patients; first clinical results and comparison with electronic portal-imaging device. *Int J Radiat Oncol Biol Phys.* 68(2):555–561.

Brooks RA and DiChiro G. 1976. Beam hardening in reconstructive tomography. *Phys Med Biol.* 21:390–398.

Bushberg JT, Seibert JA, Leidholdt EM and Boone JM. 2002. *The essential physics of medical imaging, 2* (Lippincott Williams & Wilkins, Hagerstown, MD).

Case RB, Sonke JJ, Moseley DJ, Kim J, Brock KK, and Dawson LA. 2009. Inter- and intrafraction variability in liver position in non-breath-hold stereotactic body radiotherapy. *Int J Radiat Oncol Biol Phys.* 75(1):302–308.

Chen B and Ning R. 2002. Cone-beam volume CT breast imaging: Feasibility study. *Med Phys.* 29(5):755–770.

Chen G-H, Tang J, and Leng S. 2008. Prior image constrained compressed sensing (PICCS): a method to accurately reconstruct dynamic CT images from highly undersampled projection data sets. *Med Phys.* 35:660–663.

Cho Y, Moseley DJ, Siewerdsen JH, and Jaffray DA, 2005. Accurate technique for complete geometric calibration of cone-beam computed tomography systems. *Med Phys.* 32:968–983.

Daly MJ, Siewerdsen JH, Cho YB, Jaffray DA, and Irish JC. 2008. Geometric calibration of a cone-beam CT-capable mobile C-arm. *Med Phys.* 35(5):2124–2136.

Daly MJ, Siewerdsen JH, Moseley DJ, Jaffray DA, and Irish JC. 2006. Cone-beam CT for image-guided head and neck surgery: assessment of dose and image quality using a C-arm prototype. *Med Phys.* 33(10):3767–3780.

De Jong R, Minkema D, Sonke J-J, van Herk M, and Remeijer R. 2004. A quality assurance protocol for cone-beam CT for the radiation therapy technologist. *Radiother Oncol.* 73 (Suppl. 1):S469 (abstract).

De Man B, Nuyts J, Dupont P, Marchal G, and Suetens P. 2001. An iterative maximum-likelihood polychromatic algorithm for CT. *IEEE Trans Med Imag.* 20:999–1008.

Desbat L, Rit S, Clackdoyle R, Mennessier C, Promayon E, and Ntalampeki S. 2007. Algebraic and analytic reconstruction methods for dynamic tomography. *Conf Proc IEEE Eng Med Biol Soc.* 2007:726–730.

Dietrich L, Jetter S, Tücking T, Nill S, and Oelfke U. 2006. Linac-integrated 4D cone beam CT: first experimental results. *Phys Med Biol.* 51(11):2939–2952.

Dixon RL, Anderson JA, Bakalyar DM, et al. 2010. *AAPM Report No. 111: Comprehensive methodology for the evaluation of radiation dose in x-ray computed tomography* (American Association of Physicists in Medicine, College Park, MD).

Dixon RL. 2003. A new look at CT dose measurement: beyond CTDI. *Med Phys.* 30:1272–1280.

Edwards M, Keller J, Larsen G, Rowberg A, Sandler B, and Whitaker R. 1981. A computed tomography radiation therapy treatment planning system utilizing a whole body CT scanner. *Med Phys.* 8:242–248.

Elbakri IA and Fessler JA. 2002. Statistical image reconstruction for polyenergetic x-ray computed tomography. *IEEE Trans Med Imaging.* 21:89–99.

Erdogan H and Fessler JA. 1999. Ordered subsets algorithms for transmission tomography. *Phys Med Biol.* 44:2835.

Fahrig R and Holdsworth DW. 2000. Three-dimensional computed tomographic reconstruction using a C-arm mounted XRII: image-based correction of gantry motion nonidealities. *Med Phys.* 27:30–38.

Fahrig R, Dixon R, Payne T, Morin RL, Ganguly A, and Strobel N. 2006. Dose and image quality for a cone-beam C-arm CT system. *Med Phys.* 33:541–550.

Fatunase T, Wang Z, Yoo S, et al. 2008. Assessment of the residual error in soft tissue setup in patients undergoing partial breast irradiation: results of a prospective study using cone-beam computed tomography. *Int J Radiat Oncol Biol Phys.* 70(4):1025–1034.

Feldkamp LA, Davis LC, and Kress JW. 1984. Practical cone-beam algorithm. *J Opt Soc Am A.* 1: 612–619.

Fessler JA and Hero AO. 1995. Penalized maximum-likelihood imagereconstruction using space-alternating generalized EM algorithms. *IEEE Trans Image Process.* 4:1417–1429.

Foroudi F, Wong J, Haworth A, et al. 2009. Offline adaptive radiotherapy for bladder cancer using cone beam computed tomography. *J Med Imaging Radiat Oncol.* 53(2):226–233.

Fujita H, Tsai DY, Itoh T, et al. 1992. A simple method for determining the modulation transfer function in digital radiography, *IEEE Trans Med Imaging.* 11(1):34–39.

Glover GH. 1982. Compton scatter effects in CT reconstructions. *Med Phys.* 9:860–867.

Grills IS, Hugo G, Kestin LL, et al. 2008. Image-guided radiotherapy via daily online cone-beam CT substantially reduces margin requirements for stereotactic lung radiotherapy. *Int J Radiat Oncol Biol Phys.* 70(4):1045–1056.

Guan H and Gordon R. 1996. Computed tomography using algebraic reconstruction techniques (ARTs) with different projection access schemes: a comparison study under practical situations. *Phys Med Biol.* 41:1727.

Guckenberger M, Baier K, Guenther I, et al. 2007. Reliability of the bony anatomy in image-guided stereotactic radiotherapy of brain metastases. *Int J Radiat Oncol Biol Phys.* 69(1):294–301.

Guckenberger M, Meyer J, Vordermark D, Baier K, Wilbert J, and Flentje M. 2006. Magnitude and clinical relevance of translational and rotational patient setup errors: a cone-beam CT study. *Int J Radiat Oncol Biol Phys.* 65(3):934–942.

Hanson KM. 1979. Detectability in computed tomographic images. *Med Phys.* 6:441–451.

Harsolia A, Hugo GD, Kestin LL, Grills IS, and Yan D. 2008. Dosimetric advantages of four-dimensional adaptive image-guided radiotherapy for lung tumors using online cone-beam computed tomography. *Int J Radiat Oncol Biol Phys.* 70(2):582–589.

Hatton J, McCurdy B, and Greer PB. 2009. Cone beam computerized tomography: the effect of calibration of the Hounsfield unit number to electron density on dose calculation accuracy for adaptive radiation therapy. *Phys Med Biol.* 54:329–346.

Hawkins MA, Brock KK, Eccles C, Moseley D, Jaffray D, and Dawson LA. 2006. Assessment of residual error in liver position using kV cone-beam computed tomography for liver cancer high-precision radiation therapy. *Int J Radiat Oncol Biol Phys.* 66(2):610–619.

Hawkins MA, Brooks C, Hansen VN, Aitken A, and Tait DM. 2010. Cone beam computed tomography-derived adaptive radiotherapy for radical treatment of esophageal cancer. *Int J Radiat Oncol Biol Phys.* 77(2): 378–383.

Hendee WR and Ritenour ER. 2002. *Medical imaging physics,* 4th Edition (Wiley, Hoboken, NJ).

Hoppe S, Dennerlein F, and Noo F. 2010. Accurate image reconstruction using real C-arm data from a circle-plus-arc trajectory. *Int J Comput Assist Radiol Surg.* (submitted).

Hoppe S, Noo F, Dennerlein F, Lauritsch G, and Hornegger J. 2007. Geometric calibration of the circle-plus-arc trajectory. *Phys Med Biol.* 52(23):6943–6960.

Hsieh J, Molthen RC, Dawson CA, and Johnson RH. 2000. An iterative approach to the beam hardening correction in cone beam CT. *Med Phys.* 27(1):23–29.

Hu H. 1999. Multi-slice helical CT: scan and reconstruction. *Med Phys.* 26:5–18.

IEC. 1998. *European standard EN 60601-2-1 medical electrical equipment Part 2-1: particular requirements for the safety of electron accelerators in the range of 1MeV to 50 MeV.* IEC 60601-2-1:1998.

Islam MK, Purdie TG, Norrlinger BD, et al. 2006. Patient dose from kilovoltage cone beam computed tomography imaging in radiation therapy. *Med Phys.* 33(6):1573–1582.

Jaffray DA and Siewerdsen JH. 2000. Cone-beam computed tomography with a flat-panel imager: initial performance characterization. *Med Phys.* 27:1311–1323.

Jaffray DA, Drake DG, Moreau M, Martinez AA, and Wong JW. 1999. A radiographic and tomographic imaging system integrated into a medical linear accelerator for localization of bone and soft-tissue targets. *Int J Radiat Oncol Biol Phys.* 45(3):773–789.

Jaffray DA, Siewerdsen JH, Wong JW, and Martinez AA. 2002. Flat-panel cone-beam computed tomography for image-guided radiation therapy, *Int J Radiat Oncol Biol Phys.* 53(5):1337–1349.

Jarry G, Graham SA, Moseley DJ, Jaffray DA, Siewerdsen JH, and Verhaegen F. 2006. Characterization of scattered radiation in kV CBCT images using Monte Carlo simulations. *Med Phys.* 33(11):4320–4329.

Jia X, Lou Y, Li R, Song WY, and Jiang SB. 2010. GPU-based fast cone beam CT reconstruction from undersampled and noisy projection data via total variation. *Med Phys.* 37(4):1757–1760.

Johns PC and Yaffe M. 1982. Scattered radiation in fan beam imaging system. *Med Phys.* 9:231–239.

Joseph PM, Spital RD. 1978. A method for correcting bone induced artifacts in computed tomography scanners. *J Comput Assist Tomogr.* 2(1):100–108.

Judy PF, Balter S, Bassano D, McCullough EC, Payne JT, and Rothenberg L. 1977. *AAPM Report No. 1: Phantoms for performance evaluation and quality assurance of CT scanners* (American Association of Physicists in Medicine, Chicago, IL).

Kak AC and Slaney M. 1988. *Principles of computerized tomographic imaging* (IEEE Press, New York, NY).

Kalender WA. 1995. Principles and performance of spiral CT. *In: Medical CT and ultrasound: current technology and applications.* LW Goldman and JB Fowlkes, Editors (Advanced Medical Publishing: Madison, WI).

Kamino Y, Takayama K, Kokubo M, et al. 2006. Development of a four-dimensional image-guided radiotherapy system with a gimbaled x-ray head. *Int J Radiat Oncol Biol Phys.* 66(1):271–278.

Katsevich A. 2002. Analysis of an exact inversion algorithm for spiral cone-beam CT. *Phys Med Biol.* 47(15):2583–2597.

Kwan AL, Boone JM, Yang K, and Huang SY. 2007. Evaluation of the spatial resolution characteristics of a cone-beam breast CT scanner. *Med Phys.* 34(1):275–281.

Lange K and Carson R. 1984. EM reconstruction algorithms for emission and transmission tomography. *J Comput Assist Tomogr.* 8(2):306–316.

Lehmann J, Perks J, Semon S, Harse R, and Purdy JA. 2007. Commissioning experience with cone-beam computed tomography for image-guided radiation therapy. *J Appl Clin Med Phys.* 8(3):2354.

Leng S, Tang J, Zambelli J, Nett B, Tolakanahalli R, and Chen GH. 2008a. High temporal resolution and streak-free four-dimensional cone-beam computed tomography. *Phys Med Biol.* 53(20):5653–5673.

Leng S, Zambelli J, Tolakanahalli R, et al. 2008b. Streaking artifacts reduction in four-dimensional cone-beam computed tomography. *Med Phys.* 35(10):4649–4659.

Létourneau D, Martinez AA, Lockman D, et al. 2005. Assessment of residual error for online cone-beam CT-guided treatment of prostate cancer patients. *Int J Radiat Oncol Biol Phys.* 62(4):1239–1246.

Létourneau D, Wong R, Moseley D, et al. 2007. Online planning and delivery technique for radiotherapy of spinal metastases using cone-beam CT: image quality and system performance. *Int J Radiat Oncol Biol Phys.* 67(4):1229–1237.

Li T, Koong A, and Xing L. 2007. Enhanced 4D cone-beam CT with inter-phase motion model. *Med Phys.* 34(9):3688–3695.

Li T, Schreibmann E, Yang Y, and Xing L. 2006a. Motion correction for improved target localization with on-board cone-beam computed tomography. *Phys Med Biol.* 51(2):253–267.

Li T, Xing L, Munro P, et al. 2006b. Four-dimensional cone-beam computed tomography using an on-board imager. *Med Phys.* 33(10):3825–3833.

Li W, Moseley DJ, Manfredi T, and Jaffray DA. 2009. Accuracy of automatic couch corrections with on-line volumetric imaging. *J Appl Clin Med Phys.* 10(4):3056.

Liu V, Lariviere NR, and Wang G. 2003. X-ray micro-CT with a displaced detector array: application to helical cone-beam reconstruction. *Med Phys.* 30(10):2758–2761.

Liu X, Shaw C, Altunbas M, and Wang T. 2005. A scanning sample measurement (SSM) technique for scatter measurement and correction in cone beam breast CT. *Med Phys.* 32(6): 2093.

Mail N, Moseley DJ, Siewerdsen JH, and Jaffray DA. 2008. An empirical method for lag correction in cone-beam CT. *Med Phys.* 35(11):5187–5196.

Manglos SH, Gagne GM, Krol A et al. 1995. Transmission maximum-likelihood reconstruction with ordered subsets for cone beam CT. *Phys. Med. Biol.* 40:1225.

Marchant TE, Moore CJ, Rowbottom CG, MacKay RI, and Williams PC. 2008. Shading correction algorithm for improvement of cone-beam CT images in radiotherapy. *Phys Med Biol.* 53(20):5719–5733.

Masi L, Casamassima F, Polli C, Menichelli C, Bonucci I, and Cavedon C. 2008. Cone beam CT image guidance for intracranial stereotactic treatments: comparison with a frame guided set-up. *Int J Radiat Oncol Biol Phys.* 71(3):926–933.

McBain CA, Henry AM, Sykes J, et al. 2006. X-ray volumetric imaging in image-guided radiotherapy: the new standard in on-treatment imaging. *Int J Radiat Oncol Biol Phys.* 64(2):625–634.

Moseley DJ, White EA, Wiltshire KL, et al. 2007. Comparison of localization performance with implanted fiducial markers and cone-beam computed tomography for on-line image-guided radiotherapy of the prostate. *Int J Radiat Oncol Biol Phys.* 67(3):942–953.

Mosleh-Shirazi MA, Swindell W, and Evans PM. 1998. Optimization of the scintillation detector in a combined 3D megavoltage CT scanner and portal imager. *Med Phys.* 25:1880–1890.

Navab N, Bani-Hashemi A, and Mitschke M. 1996. Dynamic geometric calibration for 3-D cerebral angiography. *Proc SPIE*. 3708:361–370.

Navab N, Bani-Hashemi A, and Nadar M. 1998. 3D reconstruction from projection matrices in a C-arm based 3D-angiography system. *MICCAI* 1496:119–129.

Neitzel U. 1992. Grids or air gaps for scatter reduction in digital radiography: a model calculation. *Med Phys*. 19:475–481.

Nguyen TN, Moseley JL, Dawson LA, Jaffray DA, and Brock KK. 2009. Adapting liver motion models using a navigator channel technique. *Med Phys*. 36(4):1061–1073.

Nielsen T, Manzke R, Proksa R, and Grass M. 2005. Cardiac cone-beam CT volume reconstruction using ART. *Med Phys*. 32:851.

Nijkamp J, de Jong R, Sonke JJ, Remeijer P, van Vliet C, and Marijnen C. 2009. Target volume shape variation during hypo-fractionated preoperative irradiation of rectal cancer patients. *Radiother Oncol*. 92(2):202–209.

Nijkamp J, Pos FJ, Nuver TT, de Jong R, Remeijer P, Sonke JJ, and Lebesque JV. 2008. Adaptive radiotherapy for prostate cancer using kilovoltage cone-beam computed tomography: first clinical results. *Int J Radiat Oncol Biol Phys*. 70(1):75–82.

Ning R, Tang X, and Conover D. 2004. X-ray scatter correction algorithm for cone beam CT imaging. *Med Phys*. 31(5):1195–1202.

Ning R, Tang X, Yu R, Zhang D, and Conover D. 1999. Flat panel detector-based cone beam volume CT imaging: detector evaluation. *Proc. SPIE*. 3659:192–203.

Noo F, Clackdoyle R, Mennessier C, White TA, and Roney TJ. 2000. Analytic method based on identification of ellipse parameters for scanner calibration in cone-beam tomography. *Phys Med Biol*. 45(11):3489–3508.

Noo F, Pack J, and Heuscher D. 2003. Exact helical reconstruction using native cone-beam geometries. *Phys Med Biol*. 48:3787–3818.

Pack J and Noo F. 2005. Cone-beam reconstruction using 1D filtering along the projection of M-lines. *Inverse Prob*. 21:1105–1120.

Payne WH, Waggener RG, McDavid WD, and Dennis MJ. 1978. Treatment planning in cobalt-60 radiotherapy using computerized tomography techniques. *Med Phys*. 5:48–51.

Pos F, Bex A, Dees-Ribbers HM, Betgen A, van Herk M, and Remeijer P. 2009. Lipiodol injection for target volume delineation and image guidance during radiotherapy for bladder cancer. *Radiother Oncol*. 93(2):364–367.

Purdie TG, Moseley DJ, Bissonnette JP, et al. 2006. Respiration correlated cone-beam computed tomography and 4DCT for evaluating target motion in stereotactic lung radiation therapy. *Acta Oncol*. 45(7):915–922.

Remeijer P, Minkema D, Betgen A, and Dewit L. 2007. Frameless radiosurgery on a conventional linac utilizing cone-beam CT image guidance. *Radiother Oncol*. 84:S13 (abstract).

Rit S, Wolthaus JW, van Herk M, and Sonke JJ. 2009. On-the-fly motion-compensated cone-beam CT using an a priori model of the respiratory motion. *Med Phys*. 36(6):2283–2296.

Rougee, C. Picard, C. Ponchut, and Y. Trousset. 1993. Geometrical calibration of x-ray imaging chains for three-dimensional reconstruction. *Comput Med Imaging Graph*. 17(4–5):295–300.

Saw CB, Yang Y, Li F, et al. 2007. Performance characteristics and quality assurance aspects of kilovoltage cone-beam CT on medical linear accelerator. *Med Dosim*. 32(2):80–85.

Schreibmann E, Elder E, and Fox T. 2009. Automated quality assurance for image-guided radiation therapy. *J Appl Clin Med Phys*. 10(1):2919.

Sharpe MB, Moseley DJ, Purdie TG, Islam M, Siewerdsen JH, and Jaffray DA. 2006. The stability of mechanical calibration for a kV cone beam computed tomography system integrated with linear accelerator. *Med Phys*. 33(1):136–144.

Shepard SJ, Lin P-JP, Boone JM, et al. 2002. *AAPM Report No. 74: Quality control in diagnostic radiology*, 1st Edition (Medical Physics Publishing. Madison, WI).

Sidky EY and Pan XC. 2008a. Image reconstruction in circular cone-beam computed tomography by constrained, total-variation minimization. *Phys Med Biol*. 53(17):4777–4780.

Sidky EY and Pan XC. 2008b. Image reconstruction in circular cone-beam computed tomography by constrained, total-variation minimization. *Phys. Med. Biol*. 53:4777–4807.

Siewerdsen JH and Jaffray DA. 1999. Cone-beam computed tomography with a flat-panel imager: effects of image lag. *Med Phys*. 26(12):2635–2647.

Siewerdsen JH and Jaffray DA. 2000a. Cone-beam CT with a flat-panel imager: Noise considerations for fully 3D computed tomography. *Proc SPIE* 3977:408–416.

Siewerdsen JH and Jaffray DA. 2000b. Optimization of x-ray imaging geometry (with specific application to flat-panel cone-beam computed tomography. *Med Phys*. 27(8):1903–1914.

Siewerdsen JH and Jaffray DA. 2001. Cone-beam computed tomography with a flat-panel imager: magnitude and effects of x-ray scatter. *Med Phys*. 28(2):220–231.

Siewerdsen JH and Jaffray DA. 2003. Three-dimensional NEQ transfer characteristics of volume CT using direct and indirect-detection flat-panel imagers. *Proc SPIE*. 29(11):2655–2671.

Siewerdsen JH, Bakhtiar B, Moseley DJ, Richard S, and Jaffray DA. 2004. The influence of anti-scatter grids on soft-tissue detectability in cone-beam CT. *Med Phys*. 31(12):3506–3520.

Siewerdsen JH, Cunningham IA, and Jaffray DA. 2002. A framework for noise-power spectrum analysis of multidimensional images. *Med Phys*. 29(11):2655–2671.

Siewerdsen JH, Daly MJ, Bakhtiar B, et al. 2006. A simple, direct method for x-ray scatter estimation and correction in digital radiography and cone-beam CT. *Med Phys*. 33(1):187–197.

Siewerdsen JH, Moseley DJ, Burch S, et al. 2005. Volume CT with a flat-panel detector on a mobile, isocentric C-arm: Pre-clinical investigation in guidance of minimally invasive surgery. *Med Phys*. 32:241–254.

Silverman J, Paul NS, and Siewerdsen JH. 2009. Low-dose limits of lung nodule detection in 320-slice volume CT. *Med Phys.* 36(5):1700–1710.

Smitsmans MH, de Bois J, Sonke JJ, et al. 2005. Automatic prostate localization on cone-beam CT scans for high precision image-guided radiotherapy. *Int J Radiat Oncol Biol Phys.* 63(4):975–984.

Smitsmans MH, Pos FJ, de Bois J, et al. 2008. The influence of a dietary protocol on cone beam CT-guided radiotherapy for prostate cancer patients. *Int J Radiat Oncol Biol Phys.* 71(4):1279–1286.

Sonke JJ, Lebesque J, and van Herk M. 2008. Variability of four-dimensional computed tomography patient models. *Int J Radiat Oncol Biol Phys.* 70(2):590–598.

Sonke JJ, Rossi M, Wolthaus J, van Herk M, Damen E, and Belderbos J. 2009. Frameless stereotactic body radiotherapy for lung cancer using four-dimensional cone beam CT guidance. *Int J Radiat Oncol Biol Phys.* 74(2):567–574.

Sonke JJ, Zijp L, Remeijer P, and van Herk M. 2005. Respiratory correlated cone beam CT. *Med Phys.* 32(4):1176–1186.

Spies L, Ebert M, Groh BA, Hesse BM, and Bortfeld T. 2001. Correction of scatter in megavoltage cone-beam CT. *Phys Med Biol.* 46(3):821–833.

Stock M, Pasler M, Birkfellner W, Homolka P, Poetter R, and Georg D. 2009. Image quality and stability of image-guided radiotherapy (IGRT) devices: A comparative study. *Radiother Oncol.* 93(1):1–7.

Taguchi K. and Aradate H. 1998. Algorithm for image reconstruction in multislice helical CT. *Med Phys.* 25:550–561.

Tward DJ and Siewerdsen JH. 2008. Cascaded systems analysis of the 3D noise-power spectrum of flat-panel cone-beam CT. *Med Phys.* 35(12):5510–5529.

Tward DJ and Siewerdsen JH. 2009. Noise aliasing and the 3D NEQ of flat-panel cone-beam CT: effect of 2D/3D apertures and sampling. *Med Phys.* 36(8):3830–3843.

van Herk M, Betgen A, Remeijer P, et al. 2004. Comparison of setup error determined with EPID and with cone beam CT for lung cancer patients—how accurate is EPID image analysis in clinical practice for a difficult site? International Workshop Electronic Portal Imaging, Brighton, UK (abstract).

Von Smekal L, Kachelrieß M, Stepina E, and Kalender WA. 2004. Geometric misalignment and calibration in cone-beam tomography. *Med Phys.* 31:3242–3266.

Voogt J, de Bois J, van Herk M and Sonke J-J. 2007. Cone beam CT motion artifact reduction by projection image selection. *International conference on the use of computers in radiation therapy (ICCR)* (Novel Digital Publishing, Toronto, ON, Canada).

Wagner RF, Brown DG, and Pastel MS. 1979. Application of information theory to the assessment of computed tomography. *Med Phys.* 6:83–94.

Wang J, Li T, and Xing L. 2009. Iterative image reconstruction for CBCT using edge-preserving prior. *Med Phys.* 36:252.

Wang Z, Nelson JW, Yoo S, et al. 2009. Refinement of treatment setup and target localization accuracy using three-dimensional cone-beam computed tomography for stereotactic body radiotherapy. *Int J Radiat Oncol Biol Phys.* 73(2):571–577.

White EA, Cho J, Vallis KA, et al. 2007. Cone beam computed tomography guidance for setup of patients receiving accelerated partial breast irradiation. *Int J Radiat Oncol Biol Phys.* 68(2):547–554.

Wong J, Armour E, Kazanzides P, et al. 2008. High-resolution, small animal radiation research platform with x-ray tomographic guidance capabilities. *Int J Radiat Oncol Biol Phys.* 71(5):1591–1599.

Wu Q, Chi Y, Chen PY, Krauss DJ, Yan D, and Martinez A. 2009. Adaptive replanning strategies accounting for shrinkage in head and neck IMRT. *Int J Radiat Oncol Biol Phys.* 75(3):924–932.

Yan D, Vicini F, Wong J, and Martinez A. 1997. Adaptive radiation therapy. *Phys Med Biol.* 42(1):123–132.

Yang TI, Minkema D, Elkhuizen PH, Heemsbergen W, van Mourik AM, and van Vliet-Vroegindeweij C. 2010. Clinical applicability of cone-beam computed tomography in monitoring seroma volume change during breast irradiation. *Int J Radiat Oncol Biol Phys.* (in press).

Ye YB, et al. 2005. A general exact reconstruction for cone-beam ct via backprojection-filtration. *IEEE Trans Med Imaging.* 24:1190–1198.

Yee D, Parliament M, Rathee S, Ghosh S, Ko L, and Murray B. 2010. Cone beam CT imaging analysis of interfractional variations in bladder volume and position during radiotherapy for bladder cancer. *Int J Radiat Oncol Biol Phys.* 76(4):1045–1053.

Yoo S, Kim GY, Hammoud R, et al. 2006. A quality assurance program for the on-board imagers. *Med Phys.* 33(11):4431–4447.

Yu HY and Wang G. 2004. Studies on implementation of the Katsevich algorithm for spiral cone-beam CT. *J X-Ray Sci Technol.* 12:96–117.

Yu H, Zhao S, Ye Y, et al. 2005. Exact BPF and FBP algorithms for nonstandard saddle curves. *Med Phys.* 32:3305–3312.

Zeng R, Fessler JA, and Balter JM. 2007. Estimating 3-D respiratory motion from orbiting views by tomographic image registration, *IEEE Trans Med Imaging.* 26(2):153–163.

Zhu L, Strobel N, and Fahrig R. 2005. X-ray scatter correction for conebeam CT using moving blocker array. *Proc. SPIE Phys. Med. Imaging* 5745:251–258.

Zijp L, Sonke J.-J, and van Herk M. 2004. Extraction of the respiratory signal from sequential thorax cone-beam x-ray images. Proceedings of the 14th ICCR, Seoul, Korea, pp. 507–509.

Zou Y and Pan XC. 2004. An extended data function and its generalized backprojection for image reconstruction in helical cone-beam CT. *Phys Med Biol.* 49:N383–N387.

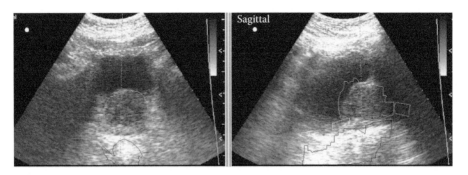

FIGURE 2.9 The user interface displays quasiorthogonal US images with the isocenter indicators (blue lines) and CT-derived contours of the prostate (orange), urethra (green), rectum (red), and seminal vesicles (yellow). (J. A. Molloy, S. Srivastava, and B. F. Schneider, *Med Phys.* 31, 433–442, 2004. With permission.)

(a)   (b)

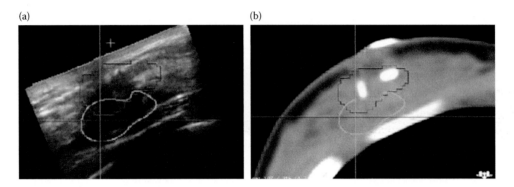

FIGURE 2.10 The potential difference in target definition for a breast seroma as indicated by US imaging (a) (green contour) versus CT imaging and surgical clips (b) (red contour) is illustrated. Soft tissue differentiation on the CT image is not feasible and reliance on surgical clips can produce a systematic positioning error. The seroma cavity is readily identifiable on the US image. (Illustration courtesy of Elekta Medical Systems [formally Resonant].)

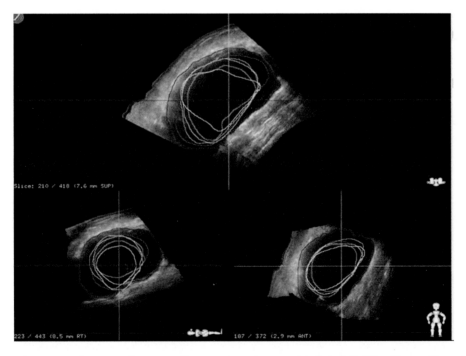

FIGURE 2.11 Changes in seroma volume over the course of treatment may be appreciated via daily US guidance. The various colored contours represent the seroma volume as determined via daily US. (Illustration courtesy of Resonant Medical.)

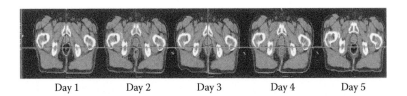

Day 1   Day 2   Day 3   Day 4   Day 5

FIGURE 3.8 Prostate and rectum position for five consecutive treatment days. Prostate outlined in red; rectum in green. (From Wong, J. R., et al., *Phys. Med.*, (XVII) 4: 272–276, 2001. With permission.)

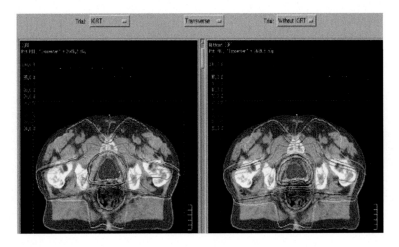

FIGURE 3.9 Dose comparison for treatment with and without image-guided intensity-modulated radiotherapy (IGRT). (From Wong, J. R., et al., *Int. J. Radiat. Oncol. Biol. Phys.*, (75) 1: 49–55, 2009. With permission.)

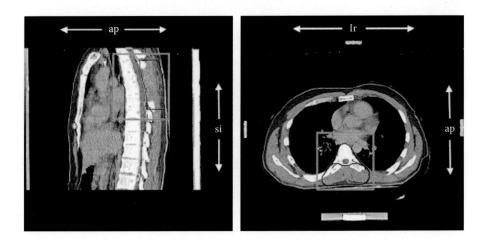

FIGURE 3.11 Example case with a thoracic paraspinal tumor. Outlined are the target and boost volume (magenta), the spinal cord (yellow), and the registration box (green) in sagittal view (left) and axial view (right). lr = left–right axis; ap = anterior–posterior axis; si = superior–inferior axis. (From Stoiber, E. M., et al., *Int. J. Radiat. Oncol. Biol. Phys.*, (75) 3: 933–940, 2009. With permission.)

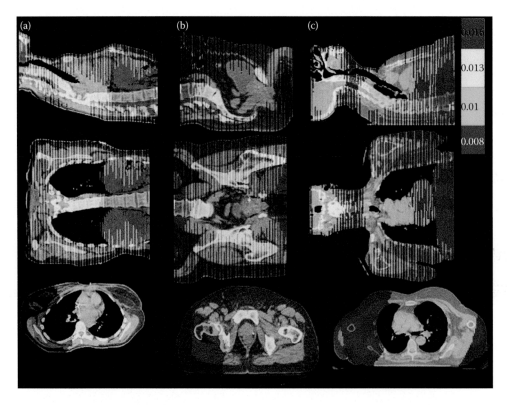

FIGURE 4.8 MV CT Dose for normal setting in Gy for different anatomical sites: A Breast, B Prostate, C lung (courtesy of Sanford Meeks, M.D. Anderson Hospital Orlando FL)

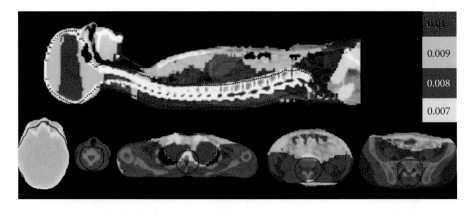

FIGURE 4.9 MV CT Dose for coarse setting in Gy for a craniospinal case (courtesy of Sanford Meeks, M.D. Anderson Hospital Orlando FL).

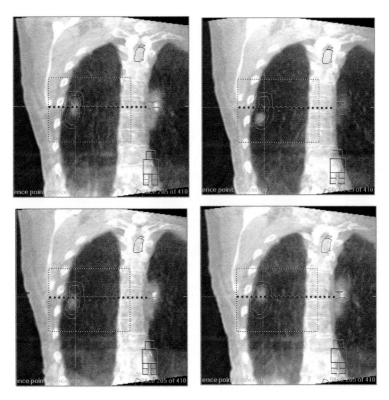

FIGURE 9.10 IGRT of a lung lesion. Coronal views of reconstructed CBCT data acquired on four different fractions. Baseline shift of the target relative to the bony anatomy.

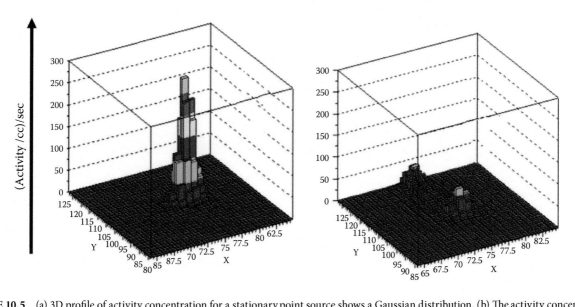

FIGURE 10.5 (a) 3D profile of activity concentration for a stationary point source shows a Gaussian distribution. (b) The activity concentration of the same point source is stretched due to the motion. The two peaks correspond to the end points of the oscillating motion.

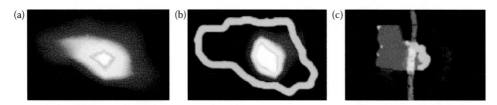

FIGURE 10.12 Transaxial ^{18}F-FDG PET image through a patient's lesion in nongated mode (a) and the corresponding image in gated mode acquired in the first bin (b). (c) Planning target volume in nongated (light blue) and gated (pink) modes. Note that light blue extends under whole pink area. Gating, in this particular case, has mainly spared left lung tissues from high dose regions.

40 degree DTS

40 degree RDTS

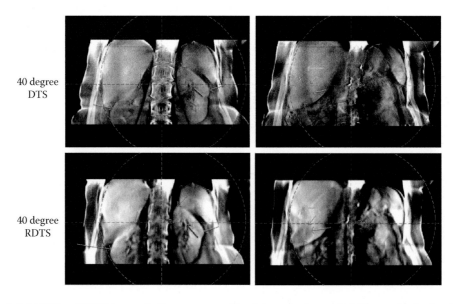

FIGURE 11.10 Breath-hold DTS and RDTS images for liver treatment. The pink arrows denote the kidney and lesion borders, and the red arrows point to the more detailed soft-tissue markings.

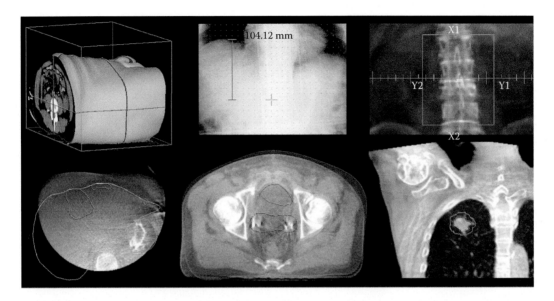

FIGURE 12.3 Examples of surrogates in radiotherapy include: the external body and alignment of skin marks with room lasers (top-left); registration based on neighboring organs may include the diaphragm (top-center) or bony-anatomy (top-right); tumor bearing organ alignment such as the liver (bottom-left); registration based on implanted markers in or near the tumor (bottom-center); direct alignment of the tumor itself (bottom-right).

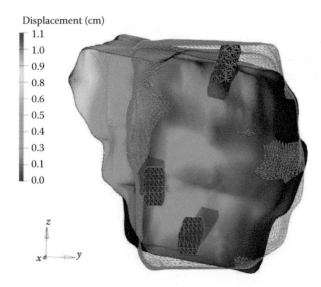

FIGURE 12.4 Sagittal slice showing the interior surface of a repeated MR (displacement colorwash) and initial MR mesh (pink). Residual error due prostate deformation over 1 cm was observed even after rigid registration based on translations and rotations of the implanted seeds.

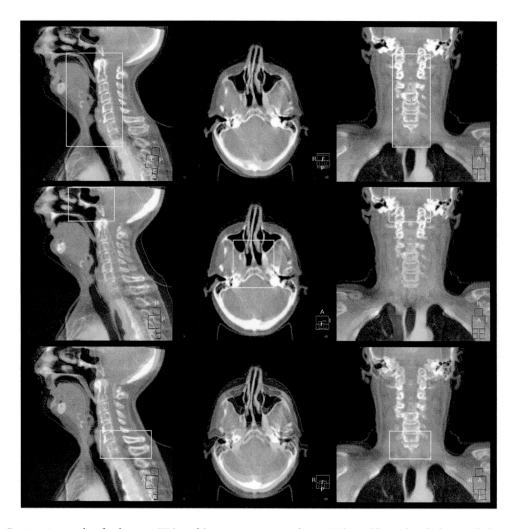

FIGURE 12.5 Registration results of a planning CT (purple) to a treatment cone-beam CT (green) limited to clipboxes. Clipbox around the entire cervical neck (top) resulted in translations (mm) of 0.2 left–right (LR), 4.5 superior–inferior (SI) 3.4 anterior posterior (AP), and rotations (°) of 6.0 pitch, −0.4 roll, and −0.3 yaw. Clipbox centered over the sphenoid bone (middle) resulted in −0.6 LR, 2.7 SI, −7.3 AP, and −0.9 pitch, −0.8 roll, and 0.4 yaw. Clipbox around the C6-C7 vertebrae (bottom) resulted in 1.4 LR, 3.3 SI, 5.8 AP, and 1.3 pitch, 0.9 roll, and −0.7 yaw.

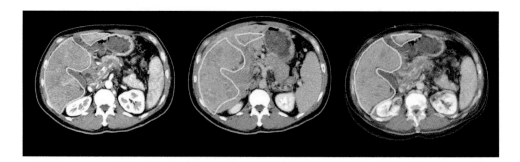

FIGURE 12.6 Exhale breath-hold CT (left) and inhale breath-hold CT (middle) is acquired in the same position with the exhale liver contour overlaid. Results (right) of mutual information-based registration limited to the liver, between exhale CT (gray scale) and inhale CT (thermal scale).

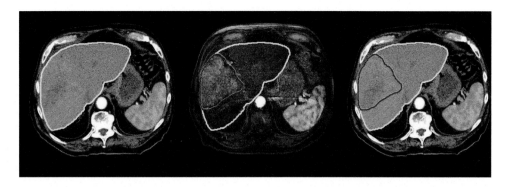

FIGURE 12.8 Registration of the liver (yellow) between noncontrast CT (left) and MR (middle) allows the segmented MR tumor (red) to be mapped onto the planning CT (right).

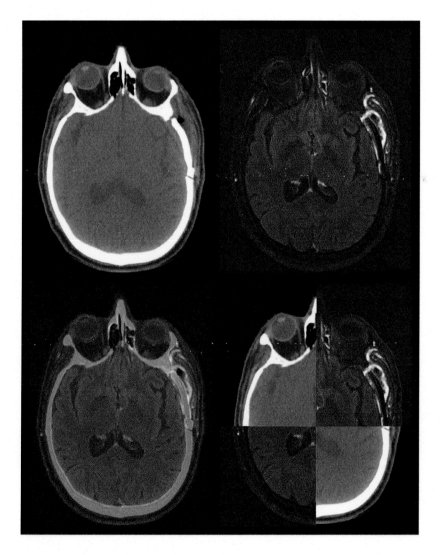

FIGURE 12.10 CT shown in gray-scale (top-left) and MR in thermal-scale (top-right). The registered images can be displayed in color overlay, (bottom-left), or checkerboard (bottom-right).

6

Megavoltage Cone-Beam IGRT

Olivier Morin
University of California

Jean Pouliot
University of California

6.1 Introduction

Less than 15 years ago, a linear accelerator equipped with multileaf collimators and portal imaging capability was considered state-of-the-art technology for external beam radiation treatment. Today, imaging plays a much bigger role in managing the patient position and anatomy over the entire course of treatment. With three-dimensional (3D) imaging increasingly becoming available in the treatment room, new image-guided radiation treatment (IGRT) techniques are being developed. This chapter focuses on megavoltage cone-beam CT (MVCBCT), the most recent addition to the in-room 3DCT imaging systems. The main objectives of this chapter are to review MVCBCT technological features and to provide guidelines on the effective implementation of IGRT procedures based on the MVCBCT system.

Primary motivations for developing the MVCBCT system were those common to all IGRT technologies: to achieve better positioning accuracy with volumetric information and the possibility to observe not only bony anatomy but also soft-tissue structures to assess patient setup and anatomical changes occurring over the course of therapy (Barker et al., 2004). An advantage to the MVCBCT technique compared with kV IGRT techniques is the use of the megavoltage x-ray beam produced by the linear accelerator for treatment. Thus, a second x-ray source (the kV x-ray source) is not required. Although MVCBCT does not require major hardware modification to conventional linear accelerator designs, it makes available a wealth of information about an individual patient in the radiation treatment position, thus paving the way for more personalized treatment. Specialized staff training with detailed procedures is the key in taking full advantage of this new information.

One could argue that IGRT is not such a new concept. After all, megavoltage two-dimensional (2D) projection images produced by a linear accelerator on film or electronic portal imaging device (EPID) have been used to guide radiation treatment for decades (Balter et al., 1995). However, the term IGRT only started being used with the recent development of 3D imaging capabilities integrated with the radiation treatment machine. It was, as if, the capability of 3D imaging in the treatment room was bringing major changes to the practice of radiation oncology. This book is a testament that 3D in-room imaging has already fundamentally changed how radiotherapy is administered. Perhaps the term IGRT now represents the in-room imaging technologies (2D or 3D) along with the new procedural requests, software tools, and quality assurance (QA) checks to improve the efficiency of radiation treatment. In today's IGRT, patient images are used to a broader extent, which may have global effects on a department's workflow. Several IGRT technologies have been developed in recent years and each has its own physical performance and software tools, which affect the possible clinical applications and the new skills that must be learned by radiation oncology workers. This book clarifies what is possible with each of these technologies.

MVCBCT refers to the imaging modality that uses the linear accelerator to produce a cone of megavoltage x-rays and an opposed planar detector to capture 2D projection images of the patient anatomy from different gantry angles. These low-dose portal images (< 0.05 monitor units) are then used for 3D reconstruction of the patient anatomy on the treatment table immediately before dose delivery. The image on the left of Figure 6.1 shows the major hardware components of an MVCBCT system. In addition, an MVCBCT system consists of software applications for 3D image reconstruction, display and analysis, and specialized phantoms for calibration and quality assurance. The term MVCBCT is used throughout the text to represent both the imaging modality and the actual reconstructed 3D image of the patient on the treatment couch. Similar to CT, MVCBCT reconstructions consist of a volumetric set of voxels representing attenuation properties of the patient anatomy for the x-ray source used for imaging. When using a grayscale intensity map to visualize CT and MVCBCT, bony structures and air cavities appear white and black, respectively. The images obtained from each modality can be visualized in the axial, sagittal, and coronal views. For clarity, it may be more appropriate to use the term kilovoltage fan-beam CT (kVFBCT) to describe conventional CT. Indeed, early generation CT scanners used a single row of detectors and a fan beam of kV x-rays to image a cross-section of the anatomy. The patient couch had therefore to be translated in the scanner in order to reconstruct a volumetric dataset (i.e., consecutive 2D slices). Modern CT scanners now have several rows of detectors for higher scanning efficiency and could therefore be described as a form of kVCBCT in which the cone-beam dimensions are smaller in the z direction compared with the radial direction. For MVCBCT, an approximately 27×27 cm^2 megavoltage cone beam and appropriately matched large 2D planar detector are used to capture the raw data required for 3D image reconstruction, and there is no need for couch movement. Although CT and MVCBCT share the mathematical concepts required for image reconstruction, the x-ray sources (energy, scatter, and source size), detector geometries (ring vs. flat panel), and acquisition modes differ greatly. The two imaging modalities therefore exhibit different physical performance and clinical utility. Using MV photons for imaging is a departure from conventional preferences of using kilovoltage (kV) photons, which have resulted in superior image quality for diagnostic purposes. Advantages and disadvantages of using MV systems over kV systems for the specific tasks of image guidance will be discussed.

The objective of this chapter is to introduce the MVCBCT system along with details on how to implement successful IGRT procedures. First, the literature on MVCBCT is reviewed to gain historical perspective on the first clinical MVCBCT systems in radiation oncology, and technical challenges associated with the

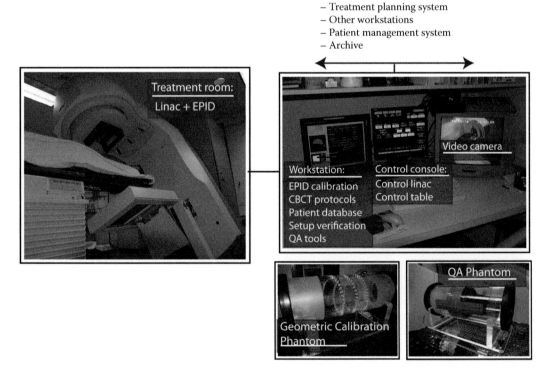

FIGURE 6.1 Major system components for MVCBCT imaging. Inside the treatment room, the system consists of a modern linear accelerator with an electronic portal imaging device (EPID) adapted for megavoltage imaging. Nearly all the imaging calibrations and online clinical tasks are performed with the computer workstation. The linear accelerator and patient table positions are modified at the control console, which is connected to the workstation. The system is connected to the department network giving automatic access to other workstations, the treatment planning system and the archiving system. A geometric calibration phantom and a quality assurance phantom are included with the system.

development of MVCBCT are discussed. Second, the major hardware and software components and functions of MVCBCT are described. In addition, the commissioning and calibration of the first commercial MVCBCT system is briefly presented. An overview of the steps involved in creating, delivering, and optimally registering MVCBCT with CT is described. The physical performance of the first-generation MVCBCT system is summarized in order to set realistic expectations in the clinic. Next, a sample QA program is proposed. The rest of this chapter then focuses on IGRT clinical applications using MVCBCT, presented through selected examples of prostate, spine, lung, esophagus, and head and neck (H&N) patients. Finally, recent advances for the next-generation MVCBCT system are discussed.

6.2 Historical perspective

Almost 30 years ago, shortly after the invention of CT, a group (Swindell et al., 1983) used for the first time an MV x-ray beam from a linear accelerator for 3D imaging. Eight years later, Nakagawa et al. (1991) investigated using a similar MV imaging system for routine patient setup verification. Both of these early systems used MV fan-beam radiation geometries, produced using slit collimators and linear accelerator gantry rotation, to collect intensity projection profiles for the reconstruction of anatomical information. As the detector technology of EPIDs advanced (Mosleh-Shirazi et al., 1998), cone-beam reconstruction systems became increasingly feasible. Subsequently, researchers acquired MVCBCT images using standard linear accelerators and liquid-filled ionization chamber detectors (Midgley et al., 1998), video-based EPIDs (Midgley et al., 1998; Spies et al., 2001), and amorphous silicon (a-Si) flat panel

detectors (Ford et al., 2002; Groh et al., 2002). In much of the early work, high doses (50–200 cGy per MVCBCT) were utilized to maximize detector signal. Strategies such as the development of more sensitive detectors (Ghelmansarai et al., 2005; Seppi et al., 2003) and the restriction of the imaging volume to the treatment volume (Anastasio et al., 2003; Sidhu et al., 2003) have reduced these imaging doses to clinically acceptable values, which are generally higher in radiotherapy than for diagnostic applications given the potential benefits of avoiding geometrical miss with large amount of radiation received by the patients for treatment. Other developments included the adaptation of MVCBCT for lung tumor visualization by synchronizing image acquisition with respiration (Sillanpaa et al., 2005), which also resulted in improved image quality while reducing radiation dose to the patient.

The development of the first clinical MVCBCT system and its applications has been quite rapid following these early investigations. Starting in 2001, the University of California, San Francisco, worked in collaboration with Siemens (Siemens Medical Systems, Concord, CA) on the first clinical implementation of an MVCBCT system using a 6-MV x-ray beam. Figure 6.2 presents a timeline showing key technical and clinical milestones since 2001. The very first (H&N) patient was imaged in 2003. Visualization of soft-tissue structures was obtained soon after in the same year. In less than 10 years, the improvements in image quality have been remarkable. New clinical applications such as dose calculations are starting to emerge.

Several publications covered the development of MVCBCT imaging for the clinic. A first proof of feasibility was demonstrated with a low-dose 6-MV x-ray MVCBCT acquisition and sufficient image quality for 3D registration with the CT reference

Evolution of MVCBCT image quality

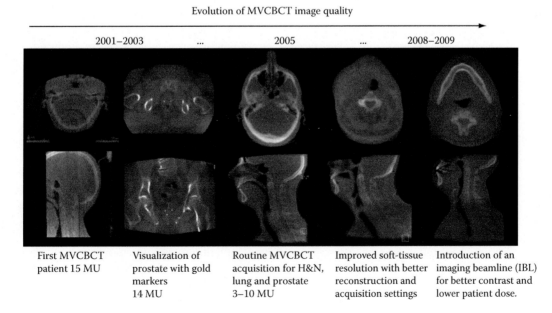

| 2001–2003 | ... | 2005 | ... | 2008–2009 |

First MVCBCT patient 15 MU

Visualization of prostate with gold markers 14 MU

Routine MVCBCT acquisition for H&N, lung and prostate 3–10 MU

Improved soft-tissue resolution with better reconstruction and acquisition settings

Introduction of an imaging beamline (IBL) for better contrast and lower patient dose.

FIGURE 6.2 Evolution of the MVCBCT system and image quality. The system improvements have been remarkable since the acquisition of the first clinical images in 2003. Recently, the development of a new imaging beam line for MVCBCT has reduced the patient dose and improved the soft-tissue resolution.

planning image (Pouliot et al., 2002). The first MVCBCT system approved by the US Food and Drug Administration for market was described in 2005 (Pouliot et al., 2005). An overview of the initial IGRT clinical applications with the first-generation MVCBCT system was presented (Morin et al., 2006). The unique performance of MVCBCT in the presence of metallic structures, because of use of megavoltage photons for imaging, and the resulting application for complementing the planning CT has been proposed (Aubin et al., 2005). The dose delivered to patients from MVCBCT imaging was thoroughly reviewed and discussed by two independent groups (Gayou et al., 2007; Miften et al., 2007; Morin et al., 2007a, 2007b, 2007c). Two methods to incorporate the patient dose in the treatment plan were also described for cases where routine high-quality images are needed. The feasibility of performing dose calculation using MVCBCT was demonstrated in 2007 (Morin et al., 2007a, 2007b, 2007c). The image quality obtained from a limited set of image acquisition protocols available in the first generation of MVCBCT system has also been evaluated (Gayou et al., 2007). Commissioning of the first commercial product based on MVCBCT was described (Gayou et al., 2007). A set of recommendations on how to optimize image quality with the first generation of MVCBCT system for given clinical applications and body sites was recently published (Morin et al., 2009a, 2009b). Finally, two groups have discussed implementations of QA programs for their MVCBCT systems (Gayou et al., 2007; Morin et al., 2007a, 2007b, 2007c).

Recently, the development of MVCBCT and its applications has been primarily on two fronts. Considerable work has been done to correct and calibrate MVCBCT images for dose calculation (Aubry et al., 2008a, 2008b, 2008c; Morin et al., 2007a, 2007b, 2007c). Large amount of data has been collected to investigate the dosimetric impact of observed anatomical and position changes (Cheung et al., 2009). In addition, there has been significant improvement of the MVCBCT image quality and a reduction of the patient dose with the introduction of a new MV imaging beam line (Faddegon et al., 2008). These recent developments are discussed in this chapter, as they will likely become part of the next generation of MVCBCT system.

6.3 System Development, Technical Description, and Clinical Workflow

6.3.1 Overview of Components and Acquisition

A conventional linear accelerator equipped with an EPID optimized for MV imaging and a computer workstation are all that is needed for MVCBCT imaging. The megavoltage x-ray source used for imaging is produced by the linear accelerator, and the transmitted beam intercepts the EPID with inline geometry. Figure 6.1 presents the MVCBCT main components as well as important computer connections for transfer of information, for the first generation, first commercially available MVCBCT system, called MVision™, which was integrated with the Primus™ (or ONCOR™) linear accelerator (both from

Siemens Medical Systems). The computer workstation (with Coherence™ RTT or Syngo® RTT software) is responsible for nearly all tasks related to 2D and 3D imaging. The workstation is directly connected to the linear accelerator control console to transfer the acquisition parameters needed to setup the machine for imaging. The workstation is also directly connected to the EPID and controls the acquisition of 2D projection images required for reconstruction. In addition, the workstation is used for detector calibration and image registration and serves as the local patient database for MVCBCT image review. Two phantoms are provided with the system for geometric calibration and QA.

6.3.2 System Development and Technical Challenges

There were key technological challenges to make the clinical acquisition of MVCBCT images possible. The initial objective was to obtain a 3D image with sufficient image quality for registration with the planning CT while keeping the patient dose as low as reasonably possible. This was not a small task given that linear accelerators were not designed for stable low-dose radiation delivery (Sillanpaa et al., 2005). Initial strategies were to simultaneously work on a new x-ray beam output mode and to optimize current flat panel EPID to be more sensitive to MV photons.

First, a function controller for the linear accelerator was designed specifically for MVCBCT x-ray delivery. Although the initial MVCBCT beam line was identical to the 6-MV beam line used for treatment, the actual x-ray delivery modes were quite different. A machine x-ray output of 300 MU per minute is generally utilized for a 6-MV treatment beam. Such a high beam current and dose rate beam cannot be easily and rapidly switched on and off for imaging and would deliver too much patient dose per electron pulse reaching the target. To produce an instantaneous beam and reduce the patient dose, the dose rate needed to be reduced for the MVCBCT mode. A lower dose rate of 50 MU per minute for MVCBCT was initially utilized by reducing the injector current at the electron gun and by increasing the pulse repetition frequency. Therefore, the MVCBCT x-ray delivery mode presently consists of a large number of small dose pulses that can be rapidly switched on and off. Output calibration factors were introduced to allow the user to specify the total exposure desired for an arc acquisition in MVCBCT mode. Ultimately, these output factors define the beam-on time needed per projection for a total MVCBCT exposure. Therefore, given a fixed dose-rate of 50 MU per minute, the gantry speed in MVCBCT mode slows down with higher exposure.

Following this early work on defining the linear accelerator x-ray delivery mode for MVCBCT imaging, a number of flat panel EPIDs were tested with the hope of improving the detector sensitivity to MV photons. The evaluated detectors had different buildup and scintillator material designs (Ghelmansarai et al., 2003, 2005). As a result of this early work, current EPID models used for MVCBCT imaging are approximately 10 times more sensitive than other MV EPID conventionally used in the radiation oncology community (Ghelmansarai et al., 2005). The EPID used for MVCBCT has also been designed such that key electronic components are not irradiated during imaging. With these developments, it became possible to acquire MVCBCT images with an average dose about 2 cGy, which is less than that delivered for single beam, double exposure portal imaging in most radiation oncology clinics.

Another considerable technical challenge for MVCBCT imaging was that linear accelerators were not designed for perfect isocentric geometry, which is a necessary requirement for CT reconstruction using analytical equations. Linear accelerators are heavy apparatus with intricate weight balance for rotation, with a typical rotational accuracy of approximately 1 mm diameter at the isocenter. Additionally, the rotation of the EPID, which is located opposite to the x-ray source, is not perfectly symmetric as the accelerator gantry rotates. An approximately sinusoidal deviation from agreement with the x-ray beam central axis is observed during gantry rotation. Previous work on geometric calibration for CBCT imaging on a C-arm scanner has demonstrated that any system geometrical behavior in rotation, such as sagging or twisting of mechanical supports, can be calibrated with projection matrices (Wiesent et al., 2000). The theoretical description of projection matrices is introduced in the next section. For this geometric calibration (i.e., projection matrices) to remain valid, the source-detector relationship in rotation only needs to be reproducible over time. A geometric calibration phantom consisting of a helical pattern of tungsten balls (Figure 6.1) was designed to calibrate the linear accelerator geometry for MVCBCT imaging. Using this phantom, it became possible to define where a point in space (as defined by the phantom ball pattern) is projected on the detector (as measured by each ball projected on the detector). With this calibration, it became possible to correctly reconstruct quality MVCBCT images on the first investigational MVCBCT system, despite a measured flat panel positioning sag of up to several centimeters. Although the current MVCBCT system is much more rigid, geometrical variations under gantry rotation are still captured and compensated for by following the same geometric calibration method.

6.3.3 Image Reconstruction

The reconstruction of MVCBCT is briefly presented here to introduce parameters that are mentioned in the chapter. Not all the steps in the MVCBCT reconstruction are presented. The theory of CT reconstruction of 3D functions from their 2D projections is well-documented (Kak and Slaney, 1988; Turbell, 2001). As illustrated in Figure 6.3, the 3D coordinate system (volumetric object to be reconstructed) represented by (x, y, z) is fixed in space. The detector coordinate system rotates with the gantry at a projection angle θ around the y-axis and is represented by the coordinate system (u, v). The acquisition consists of collecting projection images I(u, v, θ) around the patient. Next, projection filtering using either pixel averaging or diffusion

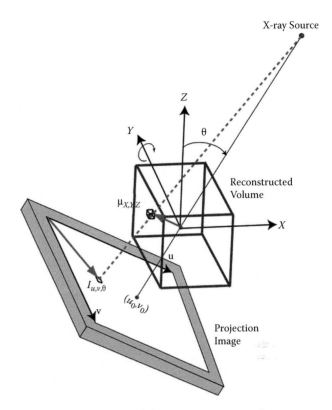

FIGURE 6.3 Geometry of the MVCBCT system. The reconstruction volume (X, Y, Z) is fixed in space. Projection images are acquired at a gantry angle θ around the Y axis. A reconstructed voxel (X, Y, Z) is obtained by backprojecting and adding filtered, weighted, and processed intensity values (u, v) on the detector. Smaller voxels for a given reconstruction volume results therefore in a larger sampling of processed projection data on the detector and better image quality.

(Perona and Malik, 1990) filtering is applied on I to reduce noise. This MV-specific step of noise reduction is followed by a logarithmic conversion and intensity normalization described in

$$p(u,v,\theta) = \ln\left(\frac{I_0(\theta)}{I(u,v,\theta)}\right). \quad (6.1)$$

The detector intensity for the nonattenuated x-ray beam at an angle is represented by $I_0(\theta)$. This factor is obtained in Equation 6.2 by multiplying a system calibration factor $I_{0\,\text{per MU}}$ (the detector sensitivity to 1 MU exposure of the nonattenuated x-ray beam) by $MU(\theta)$, the fractional x-ray exposure per projection

$$I_0(\theta) = I_{0\,\text{per MU}} \cdot MU(\theta). \quad (6.2)$$

Pixels on p are then combined in a step called binning to reduce image noise. Backprojection filtering is performed on rows u separately using different filters (Ram-lak, Shepp-Logan, or Gaussian) that have been developed for CT reconstruction. These filters were designed to produce edge enhancing, edge preserving, and smoothing, respectively. Finally, for each volume element (voxel) of the reconstruction volume, the voxel is projected on the detector plane, and the processed projection data are added to the voxel. This voxel driven step of backprojection is repeated for each projection angle θ of the acquisition. Backprojection of projection data in the reconstruction volume is accomplished using projection matrices $P_{mat}(\theta)$ in Equation 6.3, which determine the relationship between a point in the reconstruction volume $\vec{S}_{3d}$ and a point on the detector $\vec{s}_{2d}$ for a projection angle θ.

$$\vec{s}_{2d}(u,v) = P_{mat}(\theta) \cdot \vec{S}_{3d}(x,y,z). \quad (6.3)$$

The set of projection matrices $P_{mat}(\theta)_{3 \times 4}$ is obtained from geometric calibration of the imaging system. More details about the calibration procedure can be found in the literature (Wiesent et al., 2000).

The MVCBCT algorithm produces a reconstruction volume containing a large number of small voxels representing the attenuation coefficient $\mu(x, y, z)$ at position (x, y, z). The float values (32 bits) obtained for μ are converted to unsigned integer 16 bits to represent the CT numbers of the MVCBCT image. CT numbers can then be converted to Hounsfield unit by simply normalizing them to the CT number of water. Finally, other postprocessing filtering such as uniformity correction or thick multiplanar reconstruction may be applied to the MVCBCT reconstruction.

6.3.4 Commissioning and Calibration

Following the hardware and software installation of MVCBCT, there are a number of steps that must be taken prior to using the system clinically. First, control console "soft-pots" of the MVCBCT x-ray beam delivery mode are adjusted to deliver the desired dose rate. The total MVCBCT imaging exposure is adjusted using output calibration factors that are obtained by running a number of MVCBCT arcs with different exposures (2-5-15-30-60 MU). Interpolation of output calibration factors is then utilized to allow MVCBCT acquisition of any exposure between 2 and 60 MU. These initial adjustments are followed by calibrations of the x-ray detector. EPID images need to be corrected for dark current, gain and dead pixels. Calibration of these panel defects is performed semiautomatically with the computer workstation. In addition, MVCBCT requires a gain calibration that is computed through a complete MVCBCT arc. A detector sensitivity factor ($I_{0\,per}$ MU introduced in Equation 6.2) required for CT number normalization of the MVCBCT is calculated during this gain calibration. Finally, a geometric calibration acquisition is delivered with a geometric phantom centered at isocenter. The projection matrices required for reconstruction are automatically calculated and saved in the workstation. The manufacturer's installer generally completes all of these steps over the weekend of MVCBCT installation.

Following the initial calibrations, the user can evaluate the image quality and the overall system workflow for specific IGRT needs. An image quality phantom (see Figure 6.1) is provided with the system to obtain quantitative metrics of image quality. The phantom contains sections to evaluate the positioning accuracy, uniformity, spatial resolution and contrast-to-noise performances. This initial evaluation and familiarization with the system is critical in developing a successful IGRT program. One important commissioning task is to simulate the complete treatment workflow (CT scanning, treatment planning, data export, MVCBCT imaging, etc.) using the image quality phantom. This global end-to-end clinical test with the system is crucial to find possible sources of data corruption that may render the complete system unusable. For instance, potential problems due to incorrect data may occur each time patient specific information is entered manually. It is important for staff to follow their normal clinical procedure at all stages of a patient treatment to identify sources of problems, and ultimately adjust the internal procedures. MVCBCT images of the QA phantom at different exposures may also be useful as a baseline for future imaging performance comparisons. At our institution, MVCBCT image quality is evaluated on a monthly basis using an in-house graphical user interface that was developed with MATLAB® (Morin et al., 2007a,b,c) to rapidly quantify and monitor the image quality metrics.

6.3.5 MVCBCT Acquisition and Clinical Workflow for Patient Setup

An MVCBCT acquisition is similar to an arc treatment in which x-ray exposure is delivered as the treatment unit continuously rotates around the patient. An image acquisition field is created in the computer workstation using one of the predefined MVCBCT protocols, which contain the information needed by the system to perform the acquisition (field size, start and end angles, total exposure, flat panel distance, reconstruction filters, etc.). There have been so far two major commercial implementations of MVCBCT (MVision™ Siemens Oncology Care Systems, Concord, CA) system by the manufacturer. The first-generation MVision system can be installed on Primus™ and Oncor™ linear accelerators. The new-generation MVision system can only be installed on the Artiste™ linear accelerator, which has greater flexibility and capabilities. Figure 6.4 summarizes the key differences between the implementations of MVCBCT system. On top of a higher performing EPID detector, which translates to better image quality and/or less patient dose, the second-generation MVCBCT system has an increased field of view (using half beam acquisition mode implemented for kVCBCT systems) in the transverse plane. Small modifications were also applied to the reconstruction algorithm to improve image quality and speed. The start and end angles as well as the detector position for MVCBCT imaging can be easily modified. The maximum field size allowed was chosen to protect sensitive components of the detector. The primary collimators (Y jaws) in the head of the linac can be moved independently to reduce the amount of tissue being irradiated in the longitudinal direction. The craniocaudal imaging length can be specified to have a value between 5 and 27 cm located anywhere within a 27-cm window centered at the isocenter. Next, the MVCBCT field parameters are directly transferred to the control console

	ARTISTE	ONCOR/PRIMUS

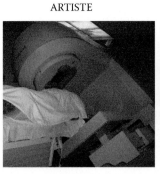 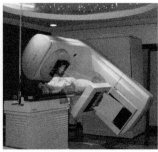

Detector Model	Perkin Elmer AG9, adjustable gain	Perkin Elmer AG9
Scintillator/thickness	Lanex Fast	Lanex Fast
Build-up plate/thickness	Yes	Yes
Beamline	6 MV TBL, 4 MV IBL	6 MV TBL
Possible Arc	Full rotation	270 to 110
Maximum transverse FOV	40 cm	27 cm
Flat panel lateral offset	9.1 cm	no
Cranio-caudal imaging length	27 cm	27 cm
Typical patient dose @ iso	0.7 X	X
Head and neck	~3.4 cGy	~4.5 cGy
Thorax	~5 cGy	~7 cGy
Pelvis	~5 cGy	~7 cGy
CNR on Emma Phantom	1.3 Y	Y
Uniformity	>98%	>95%
Time to reconstruct 512^3	60 s	105 s
Software	Syngo RTT	Coherence RTT

FIGURE 6.4 Side-by-side comparison of the two generations of MVCBCT system. The first generation introduced in 2005 was designed for Primus and Oncor linear accelerators. It utilized the 6 MV treatment beam line (TBL) for imaging. The newer generation installed on Artiste includes several improvements including; a more flexible acquisition, a faster and better reconstruction, a larger transverse field-of-view, less patient dose and better image quality. The new imaging beam line (IBL), which has a dedicated target and no flattening filter for improved soft-tissue contrast resolution can be installed on Artiste (see Figure 6.9).

of the linac (see Figure 6.1) to place the system in position for imaging. The linac gantry then rotates while acquiring low-exposure EPID images. For each projection image, the exposure is measured by the dosimetry system and recorded in the header of the DICOM file containing the raw projections. Section 2.1 describes the role of the exposure per projection of the 3D reconstruction. The duration of the acquisition procedure increases with the total exposure specified. For a typical 5 MU, the acquisition lasts approximately 45 s. The image reconstruction starts immediately after the acquisition of the first portal image, with a typical 512 × 512 × 274 voxels completed

in 55 s. The reconstructed MVCBCT and the raw projection images are saved in the patient database of the computer workstation as DICOM images.

Next, the MVCBCT image is automatically loaded in a 3D alignment application along with its reference planning CT data. A software application called adaptive targeting (AT) showed in Figure 6.5 is used to perform the registration of two 3D images (reference CT and MVCBCT in this case). An automatic alignment based on an algorithm of maximization of mutual information is performed immediately after the two 3D dataset are loaded in the software. Manual registration is generally required

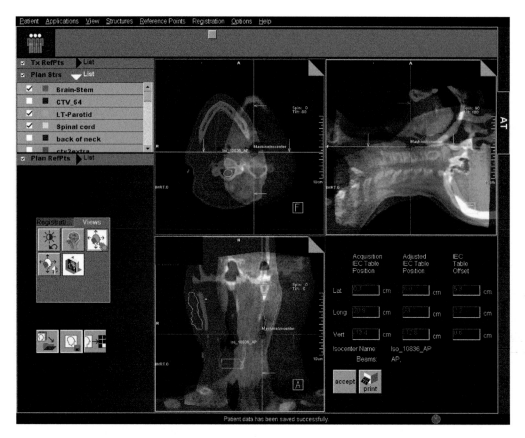

FIGURE 6.5 Software used in the computer workstation for alignment of 3D images. The CT and MVCBCT are displayed using hot (heated object spectrum) and grayscale colormaps, respectively. The images are displayed at 50% transparency each. Points of interest and contours are displayed on the reference CT. The transparency of CT can be set to 0%, with the CT contours still visible on the MVCBCT for easier manual alignment. After alignment, the adjusted IEC table position is accepted and transferred to the control console for couch position correction.

since the automatic algorithm uses the complete image information for alignment. Therefore, the automatic alignment is generally based on predominant features such as water–air, water–lung, and water–bone interfaces. It is strongly advised to verify and adjust the alignment manually as it is expected that the algorithm will perform alignment on air cavities and bones predominantly.

To facilitate simultaneous visualization of CT and MVCBCT, a blending tool is used to display 70% of the MVCBCT image and 30% of the planning CT. Figure 6.6 shows how AT is utilized to perform image-guided alignment for a lung patient. Anatomical contours may be a useful means for physicians to communicate to the therapist their choice of predominant anatomical feature for setup. For example, the carina is often drawn by physicians for alignment of lung tumors located close to the midline. The window and level of the dataset are adjusted such that anatomical features (mostly bones or soft tissue) have the same overall appearance. The MVCBCT is displayed with 3 mm thick multislice projection reconstruction (MPR). Finally, the reference CT and MVCBCT are displayed using an inverse grayscale and grayscale colormap, respectively. The blending tool is then used to confirm the manual registration. The couch position is modified remotely and the treatment begins.

6.4 Physical Performance

The clinical applications of an IGRT system are defined based on the physical characteristics and performance of that system. As a general definition, the physical characteristics of an imaging system include measures of performance and stability with respect to spatial positioning accuracy, reconstruction time, field of view, dose delivered to patients, and image quality. Two groups have evaluated the initial physical characteristics of MVCBCT (Gayou et al., 2007; Morin et al., 2009a, 2009b). The main results and the clinical implications are discussed here.

6.4.1 Positioning Accuracy

The absolute positioning accuracy and stability of MVCBCT evaluated with gold markers and a Rando anthropomorphic head phantom was showed to be better than 1 mm over a period of 12 months (Morin et al., 2007a, 2007b, 2007c, 2009a, 2009b). Such accuracy and stability is largely sufficient for patient setup. However, the overall accuracy of patient positioning using MVCBCT may be reduced (less accurate than 1 mm) because of other sources of positioning error such as laser alignment, isocenter placement, and couch motor precision. For this reason,

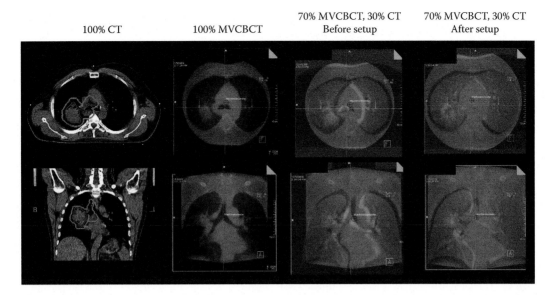

FIGURE 6.6 (See color insert)   Example of lung patient setup using CT and MVCBCT. MVCBCT images clearly show the tumor mass in the lung, the vertebral column and the carina. Contours on the CT were obtained from 4DCT imaging. These contours can be displayed on MVCBCT to facilitate the alignment. Inverse grayscale and grayscale color maps are used for CT and MVCBCT, respectively. The images are registered by using a level of transparency. The MVCBCT is displayed at 70% and the CT at 30%. The window and levels are set to similar values. Discontinuous levels of gray (light or dark) show areas that are not aligned. The last images on the right show a good alignment of the carina although some regions on the lung-tissue interface are not perfectly aligned.

our institution uses a threshold of 2 mm (in any direction) for couch adjustment based on MVCBCT images. A physician should therefore expect to achieve an alignment accuracy of at least 2 mm when guiding the registration on high-contrast structures such as bony anatomy or fiducial markers. To date, there has not been any study showing the MVCBCT setup accuracy using soft-tissue anatomical structures.

6.4.2 Patient Alignment Time, Operator Training, and Decision Thresholds

Elapsed treatment time is an important consideration in determining the implementation of new IGRT procedures. It is our clinical experience that a complete positioning procedure with MVCBCT can be done in less than 5 min. Initially, an extra 15 min was added to the regular treatment schedule of all patients undergoing online setup with MVCBCT but over time, staff became more comfortable with the system and new processes. At first, only chief therapists responsible for the clinical transfer of new technologies were trained with the system. Over time, the training was rapidly transferred from the chief therapists to all therapists in the department. The time required for physician review of daily MVCBCT images is also an important aspect to consider for IGRT. Some centers have introduced the physician-of-the-day ("POD") concept for IGRT coverage, such that on a given day, one doctor, the POD, is in charge of reviewing all patient setup images acquired that day. Threshold values for setup errors may be specified to clarify when treatment can proceed ($\Delta < 3$ mm), physics assistance should be requested (3 mm $< \Delta < 6$ mm), or the patient's doctor should be

notified ($\Delta > 6$ mm). Although this approach seam ideal, its feasibility may be limited for most clinics. Not long ago most clinics had similar discussions on the evaluation of EPID images. Over time, clear protocol and training will help improve the IGRT workflow with increased participation of the therapists.

6.4.3 Reconstructed Field of View

The maximum volume of tissue that can be fully included in the MVCBCT image, also called the field of view (FOV) is limited by detector size and source-detector-distance. To have maximum clearance of the EPID and gantry during MVCBCT acquisition, the source-detector-distance is often set to 145 cm. Given the current detector size of 41 × 41 cm², the MVCBCT reconstruction volume forms a right cylinder of about 27 cm in length (craniocaudal) and diameter, centered at isocenter. For most setup cases, this FOV performance is not a limitation. The clearance may however become a problem for patients that have a treatment isocenter placed several centimeters away from the midline. The most recent generation of MVCBCT system offers an additional acquisition mode, similar to the half-beam scan for kVCBCT (Smitsmans et al., 2005), which uses an off-set position for the EPID image receptor and should achieve a reconstruction diameter of roughly 40 cm. In addition, the detector distance as well as the gantry start and end positions of the acquisition will be adjustable such that clearance is never an issue. Finally, one practical feature with MVCBCT is the capability to change the craniocaudal imaging length by independently moving the upper jaws. One can therefore exclude the patient eyes from the radiation field during an H&N MVCBCT acquisition while still capturing the anatomy needed to evaluate patient positioning. As far as image quality is concerned, it was demonstrated that reducing the craniocaudal imaging length only slightly improves the image uniformity and contrast-to-noise ratio (Morin et al., 2009a, 2009b). Therefore, the decision of closing the imaging length in the craniocaudal direction should be motivated by a reduction of patient dose and not an improvement in image quality.

6.4.4 Dose Delivered to Patients

The dose delivered to patients during MVCBCT acquisition was measured on phantom and simulated on patient images using the treatment planning system (Morin et al., 2007a, 2007b, 2007c). The MVCBCT acquisition is simulated using an arc treatment with a 6-MV x-ray treatment beam of proper field size. Most treatment planning systems can compute a full MVCBCT imaging dose distribution in a few minutes. For typical MVCBCT settings (arc: 270°–110°), the dose delivered to patients forms a small anterior–posterior gradient ranging from 1.2 to 0.6 cGy per MVCBCT unit of exposure (per MU). In addition, the stability of patient dose, using ionization chamber measurements, was found to be on the order of 3% over a period of 12 months. Overall, studies on the dose delivered by IGRT techniques showed that imaging dose for routine IGRT is small compared to the treatment dose (<4% of the prescription). However, patient dose should always be minimized because higher dose to normal tissue may increase the risk of side effects and radiation induced cancers (Amemiya et al., 2005), thus potentially hindering the benefits of using IGRT techniques in the first place. For this reason, research groups of all IGRT technologies are studying ways to further reduce the imaging dose delivered by their system. Taking into account the variation in radiobiological efficiency (RBE) of the x-ray energy, one of the kVCBCT systems commercially available and MVCBCT deliver the most dose equivalent for imaging (Ding et al., 2008; Gayou et al., 2007; Islam et al., 2006; Meeks et al., 2005; Morin et al., 2007a, 2007b, 2007c). Both systems routinely deliver maximum point doses that are higher than 5 cGy. Fortunately, there are easy ways to reduce the MVCBCT dose. First, a user can reduce the number of MU for MVCBCT acquisition down to a value that provides sufficient image quality for the particular clinical situation. This option is of great use to visualize lung tumors where contrast is high or for easy setup based on bony anatomy and fiducial markers. In addition, the MVCBCT dose can be incorporated explicitly in the patient treatment plan (Miften et al., 2007; Morin et al. 2007a, 2007b, 2007c), thus insuring the dose is accounted for and nearly eliminating the concern for "extra dose" caused by IGRT procedures.

6.4.5 Image Quality

Image quality is a generic concept that helps quantify what can be expected from a clinical imaging system. The principal components are uniformity, contrast, spatial resolution, and noise. Studies of MVCBCT image quality demonstrate that soft-tissue visualization can be substantially improved with proper system settings (Morin et al., 2009a, 2009b). The main factors affecting the image quality of MVCBCT are the radiation exposure (dose, or number of photons), the voxel size, the reconstruction filters, the displayed slice thickness, and the body site imaged. Using an optimal MVCBCT reconstruction protocol, large adipose and muscular structures (e.g., with dimensions of greater than 2–3 cm) are differentiated at an exposure of 9 MU (~9 cGy). For the same protocol, the spatial resolution was approximately 2 mm. This latter result indicates that high-contrast objects (fiducials) smaller than 2 mm would be difficult to identify on MVCBCT. The study also demonstrated that large adipose and muscular structures could be differentiated with reasonable accuracy at an exposure of 9 MU. The uniformity of MVCBCT images using built-in correction filters was better than 90% in all directions. The clinical applications of MVCBCT presented in the next sections have different requirements for imaging quality. Table 6.1 specifies parameters of the MVCBCT acquisition and reconstruction used at our institution for specific clinical applications and body sites. For example, the proposed exposure varies based on the anatomical structure (bone or soft tissue) used for setup. These parameters were selected from the work done to optimize image quality and our clinical experience of the last 5 years. The table should help guide users to obtain the

TABLE 6.1   Example of MVCBCT Imaging Protocols Used for Patient Alignment of Different Body Sites. The Required Exposure Varies Based on the Type of Anatomical Feature Used for Alignment

	Head and Neck	Pelvis	Breast or Thorax	Extremities
Exposure (MU)	5–10 (bone)	3–5 (seeds), 5–10 (bone), 10–15 (soft tissue)	3–5 (carina), 5–10 (bone or soft tissue)	5–10 (bone)
Reconstruction size	512 × 512	512 × 512	512 × 512	512 × 512
Reconstruction slice thickness	1 mm	1 mm	1 mm	1 mm
Craniocaudal imaging length	Exclude eyes if possible	Exclude bowel if possible	Full field	Full field
Kernel	Smoothing	Smoothing	Smoothing	Smoothing
Uniformity correction model	Head and neck	Pelvis	Pelvis	Head and neck
Displayed slice thickness	3–5 mm MPR	3–5 mm MPR	3–5 mm MPR	3–5 mm MPR

best image quality from the MVCBCT system while minimizing patient dose for a given situation. Some users may find the need to increase the imaging exposure based on their need. Because the reconstruction algorithm is voxel driven, image quality is further improved by using a large number of voxels (512 versus 256) for reconstruction, followed by a resample or filter to a larger slice thickness. Finally, it is critical to set proper window and level values for display when comparing MVCBCT and CT images. Figure 6.7 shows the importance of selecting optimal acquisition, reconstruction, and display settings. The user should select the same window levels for both images such that the "visual texture" of anatomical features is similar. This is an important step to limit possible errors generated by how a user visualizes gray levels on computer monitors.

6.4.6 Megavolatge Versus Kilovoltage X-ray for Soft-Tissue CBCT Imaging

The shared use of the linac beam for treatment and imaging is inexpensive and convenient. However, the use of MeV photons for imaging is a departure from the general preference for keV beams in diagnostic imaging. The basic physics of x-ray interactions with matter can be used to explain the tradeoffs between using keV or MeV beams for imaging in radiotherapy. The visibility of large low-contrast objects in tomographic images, for example, the prostate, depends on the contrast-to-noise ratio (CNR). Contrast is determined by the differential attenuation of the beam through different bodily tissues. In the MeV range, Compton scattering provides the majority of the beam attenuation. Because of the small energy dependence of Compton interaction, the contrast in MeV imaging is thus relatively constant over a large energy range. However, the greater dose per photon deposited by MeV photons reduces the imaging beam intensity that may be applied given patient dose constraints, thus reducing the signal. Moreover, the attenuation coefficient differences between various body tissues are smaller for MeV energies and vary approximately linearly with tissue physical density, diminishing image contrast compared to that obtained with keV photons, where image contrast strongly depends on number of photoelectric interactions. The other important parameter, noise, includes the statistical fluctuation of photon detection as well as any source of unwanted radiation (i.e., radiation containing no imaging information). In transmission imaging, the x-rays reaching the detector consist of unscattered (primary) and scattered (secondary) components. The primary fluence produces the signal in the resulting image, while the secondary fluence introduces noise and image artifacts and produces quantitative inaccuracies in the reconstructed CT numbers. The magnitude of scatter reaching the detector depends on the photon energy, the field size, the object (size and composition), and the object-to-detector distance. The fan beam geometry rejects a considerable amount of scattered radiation, while the cone-beam geometry exposes the detector to a much larger fraction of scattered radiation. For a typical kVCBCT pelvic image (cone angle ~10°) acquired with the optimal air gap, the scatter-to-primary ratio (SPR) is greater than 170%, leading to CT number inaccuracies on the order of 40% (Siewerdsen and Jaffray, 2001). Methods of reducing the effects of scatter include changing the acquisition parameters (dose, field-of-view, voxel size, etc.), using an antiscatter grid, performing preprocessing of the 2D projection raw images, and applying postprocessing scatter correction algorithms on the 3D reconstruction. Antiscatter grids have been studied for kV images but, so far, have not greatly improved the CNR for high scatter acquisitions (Siewerdsen et al., 2004). For an MV projection image of a pelvis (cone angle ~14°), the SPR is much smaller, on the order of 20–40% (Jaffray et al., 1994). The small energy dependence of MeV photon interaction also makes the scatter fluence less dependent on the patient internal anatomy. The reduced effect of scatter for MeV images narrows the difference in kV and MV

(a) Varying reconstruction filters

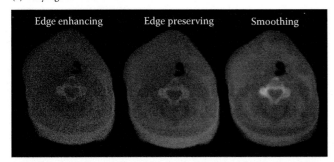

(b) Varying window and levels and slice thickness

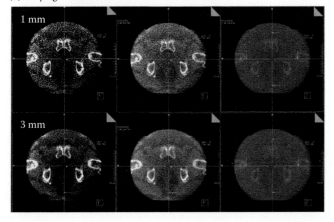

FIGURE 6.7 MVCBCT images of a head and neck patient and prostate showing the importance of selecting optimal reconstruction and display settings for a given clinical application. (a) MVCBCT images of the same acquisition obtained with different reconstruction kernels (edge enhancing, edge preserving, and smoothing) show substantial differences in image quality. Smoothing generally provides the best soft-tissue contrast-to-noise ratio. (b) MVCBCT images of the same reconstruction showing the importance of selecting proper display settings. A compromise between bony and soft-tissue window and levels is generally easier to use for alignment with CT. The MVCBCT images should also be displayed using a 3-mm thick multiplanar reconstruction or averaging filter.

cone-beam imaging quality. The lower dependence of the scatter on the exact patient anatomy may also make it easier to correct MVCBCT for scatter and allows for the accurate calibration of the voxel intensities into electron or physical densities.

6.5 Quality Assurance

MVCBCT is now widely used in the radiation oncology community and optimal quality of the system must be insured. The challenge is to define a QA program that produces useful assessments while keeping the amount of work to a reasonable level for the staff. At our institution, a QA program was defined following a complete evaluation of the MVCBCT system stability. Two MVCBCT systems were followed for a period of 12 months. The MVCBCT systems were fully calibrated (geometry, CT number normalization factor, and flat panel corrections) and analyzed daily on the first week, weekly for a month and monthly thereafter. The study specifically investigated the MVCBCT system stability with respect to the beam output, the absolute positioning and the image quality. To investigate how frequently calibration of the MVCBCT system is needed, phantom images were reconstructed on each day of QA using the original calibration obtained at installation and freshly acquired calibrations of the complete system.

6.5.1 Beam Output

The x-ray beam intensity output in MVCBCT mode needs to be characterized and confirmed for stability for patient safety and to conserve CT number calibration. A Farmer chamber (Model BC 2581 A 0.6 cc, CNMC Company Inc., TN) was utilized to verify that the exposure in MVCBCT mode is equivalent to the exposure in standard treatment mode, where 1 MU MVCBCT = 1 MU 6 MV photon treatment, under normal treatment conditions (1 MU = 1 cGy at d_{max} = 1.5 cm for a 10 × 10 cm^2 field size and 6 MV). The results showed that the treatment and MVCBCT exposures remained within 3% of each other for a period of 12 months. The maximum variation in exposure for 10 consecutive MVCBCT acquisitions was 2%. Therefore, excellent stability was confirmed for the linac output in MVCBCT mode.

6.5.2 Absolute Positioning

To investigate absolute positioning accuracy, system stability and a simple method for positioning QA, MVCBCT projection images of a gold seed placed at isocenter with the room lasers were routinely acquired. An exposure of 20 MU was selected for MVCBCT acquisition to minimize the image reconstruction noise near the gold seed. For each day of QA, the reconstructed position of the seed using the initial geometric calibration was compared to the reconstruction position using newly acquired geometric calibration. The position of the gold seed relative to the central voxel of the reconstruction was obtained using the tools available in the software application AT (Figure 6.5) of the computer workstation. The results showed great accuracy and

stability of the system absolute positioning. The reconstructed seed position remained within 1 mm of the laser point (treatment isocenter) over the 12 month duration. Using only the initial geometric calibration of the system did not cause noticeable reduction in absolute positioning accuracy or image quality.

6.5.3 Image Quality

Assuming that a specific, automated image quality application will be provided in the near future, it may be useful to acquire and analyze monthly images of the QA phantom to establish a baseline of performance for the main components of image quality (CT#, CNR, spatial resolution, uniformity, and noise). More than one image of the phantom should be acquired every month to assure a proper analysis of the system imaging performance that day. At our institution, we currently acquire two images (using the most popular MVCBCT protocol and exposure) of the QA phantom per MVCBCT system each month. These two images can then be analyzed and compared to the performance baseline of a typical imaging protocol used in the clinic. Measurements so far have demonstrated that image quality measures do not vary greatly over a period of 1 year. Therefore, monthly recalibration of the MVCBCT system may not be necessary.

6.5.4 Example of QA Program

The following QA program has been successfully implemented in our clinic and has showed to produce quantifiable results that can be documented and followed over time. Here is a list of tasks with frequency of the QA program: *Daily*—Every morning of the week, the therapists perform a verification of the flat panel position by taking a portal image with the physical graticule accessory. The projection of the graticule is compared to the calibrated software reticule. The hardware graticule and the reticule should agree within 2 mm. This agreement is needed to prevent flat panel positioner failure that could cause error in the deployment of the detector. *Monthly*—The monthly checks include the MVCBCT absolute positioning, image quality and dose output. The MVCBCT absolute positioning is verified by imaging a gold marker or small fiducial (~2 mm) centered at isocenter with the room lasers. As previously stated, position of the seed is compared with the calibrated machine isocenter for MVCBCT. The MVCBCT image quality is monitored by acquiring two MVCBCT images (5 MU) of the QA phantom. Portal images of the PIPSpro QC3 phantom are also acquired. Images are analyzed using in-house software capable of analyzing the CT#, CNR, and uniformity. Finally, the dose is evaluated with a calibrated ionization chamber at standard monthly dose verification settings (100 SSD, 10 × 10 cm^2, 5 cm depth). *Annual*—Flat panel calibrations (gain, dead pixel map, and geometric calibration) should be acquired once a year unless noticeable image quality degradation is observed in data acquired with the QA phantom. Safety interlocks such as collision sensors on the detector's cover are also tested on a yearly basis.

6.6 Clinical Applications

With recent literature on in-room imaging systems and their IGRT applications, including those systems reviewed in this book, it is somewhat difficult to define the gold standard for the management of cancer patients treated with external radiation treatment. IGRT has fundamentally changed how radiation treatment is delivered for some cases, while for other cases, new techniques are still not offering great improvements over previous methods. This section focuses on the implementation and development of IGRT techniques using MVCBCT. The simple imaging system presented in this chapter opens the possibility for several new mechanisms of verification and feedback into the clinical processes of radiation oncology. The opportunities with MVCBCT are numerous because the management of cancer patients with eternal beam still "relies" on a perfect scenario (ideal patient setup day-to-day with no anatomical changes) that is rarely observed. The clinical applications of MVCBCT can be divided in four main categories: patient setup, monitoring of anatomical changes, delineation of anatomical structures for planning, and dose calculation. Each application brings its own requirements on the imaging technology and level of complexity for the adjustment of treatment parameters.

The development of clear internal procedures are the key for the successful implementation of new IGRT techniques. The list of important questions in the implementation of new IGRT procedures includes

- What is the clinical objective?
- Anatomical structures of most importance.
- Margin of error in setup and/or anatomical changes?
- What planning data (points, contours, etc.) is required at the treatment machine?
- What are the roles of therapists, doctors, dosimetrists and physicists?
- What are the technical requirements for MVCBCT?
  - Frequency of imaging
  - Imaging exposure
  - Include patient dose in the treatment plan
- Who needs to be present and approve the images?
- What is the mechanism by which the treatment will be modified?

Our experience with the implementation of new IGRT procedures is that the logistic aspect of new clinical processes is just as important as the technology. For this reason, new IGRT protocols are introduced carefully and deliberately in the clinic by following clear procedures for the staff involved. Every clinic should define and answer their own list of questions as the level of staff and technical support very greatly between institutions.

As presented before, the image quality of MVCBCT depends on a number of acquisition and reconstruction parameters that can be selected by the user. The selection of suboptimal parameters may render the application of new IGRT techniques difficult. Table 6.1 summarizes the MVCBCT parameter

selections at our institution for patient alignment. The selected MVCBCT exposure varies based on the anatomical site and the anatomical structure used for alignment. For example, the alignment based on the visualized prostate volume requires more radiation exposure that an alignment based on gold markers. The MVCBCT image quality is further improved by increasing the total x-ray exposure thus giving more patient radiation for imaging. The values listed in the table represent our attempt at providing a good compromise of image quality and patient dose. Exposures as high as 18 MU have been used for applications such as soft tissue contouring in the presence of metallic hardware. Each clinic should define their level of satisfaction for the exposure and image quality, with Table 6.1 providing a good starting point.

6.6.1 Patient Setup

Patient setup verification was the primary reason for developing volumetric imaging capability on the linear accelerator. There is no doubt that 3D imaging provides more information about the patient than conventional 2D projection imaging techniques used for setup (film or portal imaging), but it is not always clear that this additional information directly translates into clinical benefits for the patients. To clarify this question, the first generation MVCBCT system and portal imaging were used on different cases treated with external beam including patients with cancers in the H&N, prostate, lung, spine, breast, and extremities. More than 400 patients have been imaged to date with MVCBCT at our institution. In the majority of cases, MVCBCT provided valuable information which was not visible with conventional 2D methods. However, at first this additional information came with an additional workload that impacted clinic logistics and efficiency. Clear procedures have helped reduce the workload for optimal use of the new information provided by MVCBCT.

In the next sections, MVCBCT IGRT techniques are presented for four anatomic sites, with each technique designed to correct any significant systematic errors in the patient setup while keeping the workload as small as possible. For example, MVCBCT may be the only possible option if the setup requires an assessment of soft-tissue structures. In the case where bony alignment is sufficient, portal imaging may be a simpler option than MVCBCT. Through our experience, it has become clear that portal imaging, though useful for confirming patient position, is somewhat disruptive given the fact that nearly every piece of patient information for planning is 3D in nature. Having 3D images for setup naturally exposes patient errors that were not visible before.

6.6.1.1 Head and Neck

Tumors in the H&N area are some of the most difficult to treat because of the close proximity of several important anatomical structures. For this reason, highly conformal IMRT plans have been the gold standard to provide high dose to the tumor while keeping the dose of critical structures as far as possible from their tolerance values. Small systematic errors (a few millimeters) in the daily setup could result in significant increase of patient complications. Therefore, patients are usually immobilized with thermoplastic mask covering the head, neck, and shoulders. For years, portal images (film or EPID) acquired on a weekly basis have been the standard. Recent studies have showed that although the mean setup errors of H&N are small (<2 mm, <1°), there are a small number of patients that simply do not setup well on a day-to-day basis (up to 5 mm random errors). In addition, there are patients that continue treatment with systematic errors in the order of 3 mm in their setup (Lawson et al., 2007). Finally, a large percentage of H&N patients will suffer from significant weight loss that may cause severe dosimetric errors (Barker et al., 2004). Such soft-tissue changes are difficult or nearly impossible to see on portal images. These results suggest that (1) weekly imaging is not adequate to assure an accurate setup for all patients, and (2) portal imaging is not adequate to observe anatomical changes that occur over time. For these reasons, there has been a trend to increasingly verify the position and anatomy of H&N patients using MVCBCT. Studies on the imaging frequency for H&N IGRT (Zeidan et al., 2007) suggest to image everyday for the first week of treatment to quantify systematic (mean of errors in each direction) and random (standard deviation in each direction) errors. Systematic errors are then corrected by changing the table position or the reference marks on the patient's skin or mask. The magnitude of random errors may be used to determine the type of imaging schedule for the remaining treatment fractions or if change of treatment plan is required. Large random errors may indeed necessitate replanning with larger CTV to PTV margins. The frequency of MVCBCT imaging is finally reduced only when the correction of a positioning problem is confirmed.

6.6.1.2 Prostate

It is well documented that the prostate gland position varies day to day due to bladder and rectum filling (Langen and Jones, 2001). For this reason, it has been the gold standard to image and adjust the position of prostate patients on a daily basis. Gold markers implanted in the prostate have been showed to be an accurate surrogate for the prostate. They were initially proposed because the prostate itself could not be seen on portal images. Adjusting the daily position of prostate patient with portal imaging has been used at our institution with great results since 2000. However, a recent study demonstrated that distended rectum at the time of planning is likely to be less distended at the time of treatment (de Crevoisier et al., 2005). For this reason, local control and side effects to the rectum are often compromised. With MVCBCT, these changes are now clearly visible and can at least be quantified and documented. One strategy could be to image with MVCBCT daily for the first week of treatment and then with portal imaging if no major day-to-day nonrigid anatomical changes are observed. MVCBCT could also be used for soft-tissue alignment without the need of gold markers. There are some patients that simply are not good candidates for either gold marker implantation and/or portal imaging. The presence of hip prostheses, for example, hinders the alignment with portal images since

the gold seeds are often not visible on the lateral film or portal image. It may also be difficult to identify gold markers from surgical clips for patients who underwent prostatectomy. Finally, alignment on soft tissue with MVCBCT could be attractive for clinics that did not implement the use of gold markers. Recent MVCBCT images acquired on prostate patients with the new imaging beam line for MVCBCT suggest that daily alignment with the prostate is possible.

6.6.1.3 Lung

There are several factors that make the treatment of lung tumors challenging. First, retrospective analysis of 4DCT acquisitions has demonstrated that tumor motion may vary significantly between patients (Keall et al., 2006). Also, the tumor location and size may not be good predictors of tumor motion. Therefore, the general approach has been to use fairly generous margins, which inevitably increase the dose to the normal lung tissue. Second, the common methods used for immobilization (vacuum bag or wing board) are either not sufficiently reproducible or too uncomfortable for the patient. Finally, portal images are of limited utility to accurately visualize structures of interest other than bony anatomy. The carina has been proposed as a good guide for tumors located close to the midline. However, the carina is difficult to align using a lateral portal image. A new research protocol at our institution is comparing the alignment of lung patients using portal imaging and MVCBCT. Daily images are acquired for the first five days of treatment to identify potential systematic errors. Then, images are acquired on a weekly basis. Although images have been acquired only on a limited number of patients, it is already clear that alignment of the carina is much easier to achieve with MVCBCT. Figure 6.6 shows a nongated treatment technique with MVCBCT that can help assure patient setup and tumor coverage. The tumor intrafractional mobility affected by both respiration and heart activity was evaluated using 4DCT for contouring. A maximum intensity projection (MIP) is generated from the 4DCT phases and represents the internal target volume. A MIP image is optimal for generating contours since it represents where the tumor volume was at one point in time in the breathing cycle. Additional margin (5–10 mm) is usually added from ITV to PTV to account for positioning error. Both the ITV (red) and PTV (green) are displayed on the planning CT of Figure 6.6. At the time of treatment, an MVCBCT is then acquired for setup. Generally, MVCBCT represents a timed-average version of the ITV because the image acquisition takes roughly 45 s. It is arguably a better representation of the tumor position during treatment than a free-breathing CT. The image registration is performed using the CT data set used for planning along with the ITV and PTV target volumes displayed on MVCBCT. First, on each day of treatment, the carina (or bony anatomy depending on the case) reconstructed on MVCBCT is aligned with CT. Then, the blurred tumor lesion position visible on MVCBCT is inspected such that it is centered in the ITV. Larger scale studies are needed to determine the clinical values of MVCBCT compared to other conventional techniques.

6.6.1.4 Spine

The treatment of paraspinous tumors is challenging due to several factors. First, surgery plays the primary management role of the disease and implanted orthopedic hardware is often in proximity to the target volume. This metallic hardware hinders the quality of CT images used for treatment planning. In addition, the dose prescribed to the target volume is limited by the maximum dose tolerance of the spinal cord. Without special techniques that allow highly accurate contouring, setup, and treatment, some patients who might benefit from radiotherapy may remain untreated or may be treated with a dose unlikely to provide long-term local control. Thus, the use of MVCBCT, with its positioning accuracy and imaging performance in the presence of metallic structures, may allow the administration of more aggressive treatment for the treatment of paraspinous tumors. For example, the case of a woman with a tumor wrapped around the spinal cord was reported by our group (Hansen et al., 2006). The treatment objective was changed from palliative to curative because of the suitable image quality of MVCBCT in the presence of metallic hardware. First, a high-quality MVCBCT was obtained to delineate the target volume, orthopedic hardware, and spinal cord. The reconstructed hardware displayed via MVCBCT was used on a daily basis to assure patient alignment. Dosimetric simulations indicated that without the imaging, the spinal cord maximum dose would have increased beyond spinal cord tolerance. In this case, MVCBCT has proven to be an invaluable tool for the treatment of a difficult case.

6.6.2 Monitoring the Anatomical Changes

Patients experience different types of anatomical changes occur over the course of therapy. It is well documented that a fair percentage (~33%) of H&N patients will suffer weight loss due to radiation side effects that compromise nutrition (Barker et al., 2004). The overall position and size of organs such as the bladder and rectum of patients treated in the pelvic area will certainly change slightly day to day. Another important change is direct tumor shrinkage in response to radiation, which often occurs with certain types of cancers such as lymphomas (Hindorf et al., 2003). Because these changes could not be observed before, it is not clear which are clinically significant. Certainly, changes such as weight loss and tumor shrinkage, which translates into systematic dosimetric errors, should be taken into account especially if they occur early in the treatment course (Aubry et al., 2008a, 2008b, 2008c). The general approach in the past has been to reimage and replan based on physical examination or at halfway through the treatment fractions. With the availability of 3D imaging in the treatment room, all those possible changes can now be quantified and documented. Following patient positioning with MVCBCT, the overall anatomy can be inspected for anatomical changes. Figure 6.8 shows two patients that suffered severe weight loss and/or tumor shrinkage only two weeks into treatment. In Figure 6.8a, an H&N patient treated with IMRT lost up to 4 cm of soft tissue around the neck. In Figure 6.8b, a patient treated for a lymphoma showed great tumor response

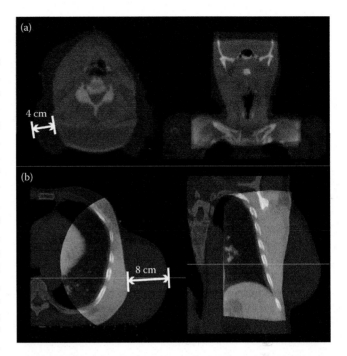

FIGURE 6.8 Images of two patients showing substantial weight loss and/or tumor shrinkage. The patients' planning CT (grayscale) was registered with an MVCBCT image (color) acquired two weeks after the start of treatment. In (a), a head and neck patient treated with IMRT for a base of tongue carcinoma lost up to 4 cm of soft tissue on both sides of the neck. Lymph nodes in the target volume also reduced in size. In (b), a chest patient treated for a large lymphoma showed great tumor response after only few days of treatment. Nearly all the tumor volume disappeared after only 10 days of radiation. The anatomical changes can easily be quantified at the treatment workstation.

resulting in a clinically significant reduction in tumor volume. In these two examples, MVCBCT was critical in quantifying the anatomical changes and the patients were replanned halfway through the treatment course.

6.6.3 Organ Delineation in Presence of Metallic Structures

The presence of high atomic number (Z) materials such as metallic implants complicate the use of conventional kV CT images for treatment planning due to severe imaging artifact that may affect both contouring and dose calculation. Several postprocessing algorithms have been developed to reduce the image degradation (Mahnken et al., 2003). However, the level of artifact reduction is still only adequate on images affected by small metal objects, such as gold seeds, and cannot resolve artifacts that accompany the use of larger metallic structures such as femoral and spinal implants, dental fillings, and arterial stents. In comparison, the image quality of MVCBCT is nearly unaffected by high-Z materials due to the predominance of Compton interactions in the MV x-ray energy range. In fact, MVCBCT CT numbers scale linearly with electron density, a unique physical characteristic to predict dose deposition. For these reasons, MVCBCT images have been used for prostate delineation in presence of bilateral hip prostheses (Aubin et al., 2006). Megavoltage imaging has also been used in brachytherapy to facilitate the digitization of catheters in the presence of metallic implants (Descovich et al., 2006). Finally, the presence of metal artifact in kV CT makes it difficult to use the image quantitatively for dose calculation. Not only do the image artifacts produce errors in the measured tissue electron density, but the superposition convolution algorithm use for dose calculation does not perform well in such circumstances (Huang et al., 2002). For these cases, the treated volume is usually assumed to be water-equivalent in the treatment plan calculations. Treating the volume as water and ignoring the presence of metal may cause severe deviations between the planned dose distribution and the real dose delivered. Increasingly, MVCBCT is being proposed as an alternative for measuring the true tissue electron density. Optimal dose simulation could be obtained using a Monte Carlo calculation engine that better reproduces the physical interactions of high-energy x-ray in metal. MVCBCT and Monte Carlo are being used to evaluate the dosimetric implications for x-ray beams entering through metallic structures before reaching the target volumes of different treatment plans (Morin et al., 2009a, 2009b).

6.6.4 Dose Recalculation with MVCBCT

Variations in target volume and anatomy presented in Figure 6.8 may have dosimetric consequences that require replanning. At what point during treatment a patient needs to be replanned is currently difficult to determine. Commonly, treatment plans are revised only when the set up is no longer reproducible, the mask used to positioning the patient no longer fits, or significant weight loss is noted. Weekly physical examination and total body weight measurements are performed but are unable to quantify changes that occur locally at the target or along the treatment beams. Most importantly, these methods do not quantify the dosimetric impact of the changing anatomy or patient positioning inaccuracies. While MVCBCT was primarily developed for setup, the images obtained could also be used to perform dose calculations. This would open the possibility to monitor the dosimetric impact of changes in anatomy or position as compared to the reference CT by applying the initial treatment plan on the MVCBCT images. A 3D image data set has to fulfill two requirements before being used for dose calculation. First, the image volume has to include all the patient tissue along the treatment beams. Second, the treatment planning system requires the image to be calibrated for electron density, the relevant radiological parameter related to dose deposition in radiotherapy. Prior to image calibration, any artifact inherent to the imaging modality must be minimized. The feasibility of performing dose calculations on H&N MVCBCT images has been demonstrated (Cheung et al., 2009; Morin et al., 2007a, 2007b, 2007c). Dose calculation on weekly H&N MVCBCT images is now routinely done in our clinic to evaluate the dosimetric impact of observed

changes. Patients that suffer large anatomical changes are now given the best chance of cure with a plan that is routinely adapted based on personal biophysical response to treatment.

6.7 Summary and Future Development

New IGRT treatment techniques have been one of the main driving forces of change in the administration of radiation treatment in recent years. This book is one of the first attempts

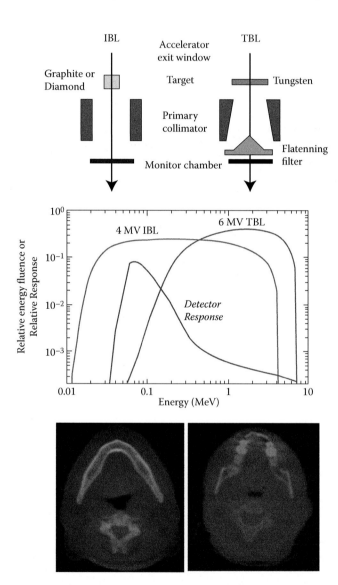

FIGURE 6.9 Comparison of the treatment and imaging beam line for MVCBCT. The treatment beam line (TBL) on the right is identical to the beam used for 6 MV treatment with photons. In the case of the imaging beam line (IBL) on the left, the tungsten target is replaced by carbon or diamond to produce a larger number of low-energy photons. In addition, the flattening filter is removed to avoid beam hardening and conserve the low-energy photon spectrum. These changes in the beam line result in a beam with relative energy fluence that is closer to the detector response. MVCBCT images with the IBL show substantially improved contrast-to-noise ratio and a reduction in patient dose.

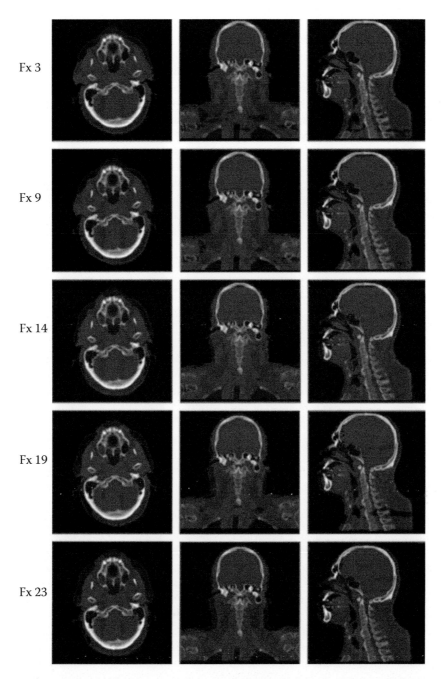

FIGURE 6.10 (See color insert) Weekly MVCBCT images showing the dosimetric impact of anatomical changes. Green corresponds to areas where the calculated dose is within 3% of the initial plan. The blue and red areas show dosimetric differences greater than −3% and +3%, respectively. These maps of dosimetric differences are being used to assess if and when modification of the original plan should be ordered. The maps could also be used at the treatment machine to reoptimize the treatment plan and therefore remove the potential treatment quality reduction caused by anatomical changes.

at summarizing the technicalities in implementing successful IGRT procedures. This chapter has focused on MVCBCT, an imaging technology that uses the megavoltage treatment x-ray beam combined with an EPID flat panel detector to acquire a 3D image of the patient anatomy prior to treatment. The system implementation, its initial physical performance, and some clinical examples have been presented. With the introduction of an MVCBCT acquisition mode, it is now possible to perform 3D setup based on bony anatomy and soft tissues to determine patient-specific anatomical variations. The MVCBCT system has been used mostly for setup of H&N, prostate, spine and lung patients. So far, the most common imaging frequency has been both patient and anatomical site dependent. While daily imaging is preferable for prostate patients, weekly imaging may be sufficient for most H&N patients positioned with thermoplastic masks. Another strategy has been to image everyday with MVCBCT for the first week of treatment to assess systematic setup error, and then continue with weekly imaging once an observed setup problem is resolved. This last strategy could be of great use for the setup of complex H&N cases. In addition, the wealth of information in 3D imaging can now expose slow temporal changes in the anatomy. Two cases were presented where both tumor responses to radiation and weight loss resulted in clinically significant reduction in the amount of soft tissue along the treatment beams. MVCBCT images have also enabled unique applications in complementing the conventional kV CT for contouring in the presence of metallic structures. The capability of MVCBCT to render better estimates of the tissue electron density may provide for more accurate dose calculations in the presence of high atomic number materials.

MVCBCT has improved tremendously in a short time and the system advantages for patient setup accuracy now largely outweigh initially perceived weaknesses in image quality and patient dose. New developments using an MV beam line optimized for imaging and more sensitive flat-panel detector have demonstrated that significant improvements can be made in image quality for the next-generation MVCBCT system (Faddegon et al., 2008). Figure 6.9 shows the details of this new imaging beam line. The tungsten x-ray target is replaced by carbon or diamond, which produces more low energy photons. In addition, the flattening filter is removed to prevent beam hardening and therefore conserve the low energy photons produced in the new target. The resulting beam has an energy fluence distribution that matches more with the detector response. Figure 6.9 shows the improvement in both soft tissue and bone contrast compared to the conventional treatment beam line used for MVCBCT. Using this new MVCBCT imaging beam line, soft-tissue structures in the H&N were resolved with a dose of only 1 cGy. This relatively low imaging dose has opened the possibility for imaging pediatric cases (Kun and Beltran, 2009). The new 3D anatomical information for patients over their course of treatment can be used to tailor the treatment plan for future fractions to account for individual variations. In addition, software tools and image corrections are being developed to apply the original plan to MVCBCT images (Cheung et al., 2009). The deposited dose on treatment day, obtained within minutes and compared with the planned dose distributions either within specific volumes or as an overall distribution, will provide an accurate estimate of the dosimetric impact of observed anatomical changes. Figure 6.10 shows typical dosimetric maps generated for H&N patients treated at UCSF. Over time, weight loss and/or tumor response result in large dosimetric differences compared to the original plan. These dosimetric considerations could be used to determine the most effective time for patient replanning. Additionally, tumor response and radiation side effects can be understood based on actual absorbed dose during treatment. With these new developments, MVCBCT could become a crucial component in personalized treatment strategies and adaptations.

References

Amemiya, K., Shibuya, H., Yoshimura, R., and Okada, N. 2005. The risk of radiation-induced cancer in patients with squamous cell carcinoma of the head and neck and its results of treatment. *British Journal of Radiology* 78: 1028–33.

Anastasio, M. A., Daxin, S., Xiaochuan, P., Pelizzari, C., and Munro, P. 2003. A preliminary investigation of local tomography for megavoltage CT imaging. *Medical Physics* 30: 2969–80.

Aubin, M., Morin, O., Bucci, K., et al. 2005. Megavoltage cone beam CT to complement planning CT in the presence of "non-compatible CT" objects. *International Journal of Radiation Oncology, Biology, Physics* 63, p. S561.

Aubin, M., Morin, O., Chen, J., et al. 2006. The use of megavoltage cone-beam CT to complement CT for target definition in pelvic radiotherapy in presence of hip replacement. *British Journal of Radiology* 79: 918–21.

Aubry, J.-F., and Pouliot, J. 2008a. Imaging changes in radiation therapy: does it matter? *Imaging Decision MRI* 12: 3–13.

Aubry, J.-F., Cheung, J., Gottschalk, A. R., Morin, O., Beaulieu, L., and Pouliot, J. 2008b. Correction of megavoltage cone-beam CT images of the pelvic region based on phantom measurements for dose calculation purposes. *Journal of Applied Clinical Medical Physics* 10: 2852.

Aubry, J.-F., Pouliot, J., and Beaulieu, L. 2008c. Correction of megavoltage cone-beam CT images for dose calculation in the head and neck region. *Medical Physics* 35: 900–7.

Balter, J. M., Lam, K. L., Sandler, H. M., Littles, J. F., Bree, R. L., and Ten Haken, R. K. 1995. Automated localization of the prostate at the time of treatment using implanted radiopaque markers: technical feasibility. *International Journal of Radiation Oncology, Biology, Physics* 33: 1281–6.

Barker, J. L. J., Garden, A. S., Ang, K. K., et al. 2004. Quantification of volumetric and geometric changes occurring during fractionated radiotherapy for head-and-neck cancer using an integrated CT/linear accelerator system. *International Journal of Radiation Oncology, Biology, Physics* 59: 960–70.

Cheung, J., Aubry, J.-F., Yom, S. S., Gottschalk, A. R., Celi, J. C., and Pouliot, J. 2009. Dose recalculation and the dose-guided radiation therapy (DGRT) process using megavoltage cone-beam CT. *International Journal of Radiation Oncology, Biology, Physics* 74: 583–92.

de Crevoisier, R., Tucker, S. L., Dong, L., et al. 2005. Increased risk of biochemical and local failure in patients with distended rectum on the planning CT for prostate cancer radiotherapy. *International Journal of Radiation Oncology, Biology, Physics* 62: 965–73.

Descovich, M., Morin, O., Aubry, J.-F., et al. 2006. Megavoltage cone-beam CT to complement CT-based treatment planning for HDR brachytherapy. *Brachytherapy* 5: 85–6.

Ding, G. X., Duggan, D. M., and Coffey, C. W. 2008. Accurate patient dosimetry of kilovoltage cone-beam CT in radiation therapy. *Medical Physics* 35: 1135–44.

Faddegon, B. A., Wu, V., Pouliot, J., Gangadharan, B., and Bani-Hashemi, A. 2008. Low dose megavoltage cone beam computed tomography with an unflattened 4 MV beam from a carbon target. *Medical Physics* 35: 5777–86.

Ford, E. C., Chang, J., Mueller, K., et al. 2002. Cone-beam CT with megavoltage beams and an amorphous silicon electronic portal imaging device: potential for verification of radiotherapy of lung cancer. *Medical Physics* 29: 2913–24.

Gayou, O., and Miften, M. 2007. Commissioning and clinical implementation of a mega-voltage cone beam CT system for treatment localization. *Medical Physics* 34: 3183–92.

Gayou, O., Parda, D. S., Johnson, M., and Miften, M. 2007. Patient dose and image quality from mega-voltage cone beam computed tomography imaging. *Medical Physics* 34: 499–506.

Ghelmansarai, F. A., Misra, S., and Pouliot, J. 2003. Electronic readout of a-Si EPIDs for optimum signal-to-noise ratio. *SPIE-Int. Soc. Opt. Eng. Proceedings of Spie – The International Society for Optical Engineering. Medical Imaging* 5030: 788–98.

Ghelmansarai, F., Bani-Hashemi, A., Pouliot, J., et al. 2005. Soft tissue visualization using a highly efficient megavoltage cone beam CT imaging system. *SPIE-Int. Soc. Opt. Eng. Proceedings of Spie – The International Society for Optical Engineering. Medical Imaging* 5745: 159–70.

Groh, B. A., Siewerdsen, J. H., Drake, D. G., Wong, J. W., and Jaffray, D. A. 2002. A performance comparison of flat-panel imager-based MV and kV cone-beam CT. *Medical Physics* 29: 967–75.

Hansen, E. K., Larson, D. A., Aubin, M., et al. 2006. Image-guided radiotherapy using megavoltage cone-beam computed tomography for treatment of paraspinous tumors in the presence of orthopedic hardware. *International Journal of Radiation Oncology, Biology, Physics* 66, p. 323.

Hindorf, C., Linden, O., Stenberg, L., Tennvall, J., and Strand, S.-E. 2003. Change in tumor-absorbed dose due to decrease in mass during fractionated radioimmunotherapy in lymphoma patients. *Clinical Cancer Research* 9: 4003S–4006S.

Huang, C.-Y., Chu, T.-C., Lin, S.-Y., Lin, J.-P., and Hsieh, C.-Y. 2002. Accuracy of the convolution/superposition dose calculation algorithm at the condition of electron disequilibrium. *Applied Radiation and Isotopes* 57: 825–30.

Islam, M. K., Purdie, T. G., Norrlinger, B. D., et al. 2006. Patient dose from kilovoltage cone beam computed tomography imaging in radiation therapy. *Medical Physics* 33, p. 1573.

Jaffray, D. A., Battista, J. J., Fenster, A., and Munro, P. 1994. X-ray scatter in megavoltage transmission radiography: physical characteristics and influence on image quality. *Medical Physics* 21: 45–60.

Kak, A.C. & Slaney, M., 1988, *Principles of computerized tomographic imaging*, Society of Industrial and Applied Mathematics, 2001.

Keall, P. J., Mageras, G. S., Balter, J. M., et al. 2006. The management of respiratory motion in radiation oncology report of AAPM Task Group 76. *Medical Physics* 33: 3874–900.

Kun, L., and Beltran, C. 2009. Radiation therapy for children: evolving technologies in the era of ALARA. *Pediatric Radiology* 39: 65–70.

Langen, K. M., and Jones, D. T. L. 2001. Organ motion and its management. *International Journal of Radiation Oncology, Biology, Physics* 50: 265–78.

Lawson, J. D., Elder, E., Fox, T., Davis, L., and Crocker, I. 2007. Quantification of dosimetric impact of implementation of on-board imaging (OBI) for IMRT treatment of head-and-neck malignancies. *Medical Dosimetry* 32: 287–94.

Mahnken, A. H., Raupach, R., Wildberger, J. E., et al. 2003. A new algorithm for metal artifact reduction in computed tomography: In vitro and in vivo evaluation after total hip replacement. *Investigative Radiology* 38: 769–75.

Meeks, S. L., Harmon, J. F. J., Langen, K. M., Willoughby, T. R., Wagner, T. H., and Kupelian, P. A. 2005. Performance characterization of megavoltage computed tomography imaging on a helical tomotherapy unit. *Medical Physics* 32: 2673–81.

Midgley, S., Millar, R. M., and Dudson, J. 1998. A feasibility study for megavoltage cone beam CT using a commercial EPID. *Physics in Medicine & Biology* 43: 155–69.

Miften, M., Gayou, O., Reitz, B., Fuhrer, R., Leicher, B., and Parda, D. S. 2007. IMRT planning and delivery incorporating daily dose from mega-voltage cone-beam computed tomography imaging. *Medical Physics* 34: 3760–7.

Morin, O., Aubin, M., Aubry, J. F., Chen, J., Descovich, M., and Pouliot, J. 2007a. TH-D-L100J-5: Quality assurance of megavoltage cone-beam CT. *Medical Physics* 34: 51-61.

Morin, O., Aubry, J.-F., Aubin, M., et al. 2009a. Physical performance and image optimization of megavoltage cone-beam CT. *Medical Physics* 36: 1421–32.

Morin, O., Chen, J., Aubin, M., et al. 2007b. Dose calculation using megavoltage cone-beam CT. *International Journal of Radiation Oncology, Biology, Physics* 67: 1201–10.

Morin, O., Gillis, A., Chen, J., Aubin, M., Bucci, K., and Pouliot, J. 2006. Megavoltage cone-beam CT: system description and clinical applications. *Medical Dosimetry* 31: 51–61.

Morin, O., Gillis, A., Descovich, M., et al. 2007c. Patient dose considerations for routine megavoltage cone-beam CT imaging. *Medical Physics* 35: 1819–27.

Morin, O., Sawkey, D., Cheung, J., Yom, S., Faddegon, B., and Pouliot, J. 2009b. TU-E-BRC-02: Combined Use of CT and MVCBCT for Optimal Dose Calculation in Presence of High-Z Material. *Medical Physics* 36: 2744.

Mosleh-Shirazi, M. A., Evans, P. M., Swindell, W., Webb, S., and Partridge, M. 1998. A cone-beam megavoltage CT scanner for treatment verification in conformal radiotherapy. *Radiotherapy & Oncology* 48: 319–28.

Nakagawa, K., Akanuma, A., Aoki, Y., et al. 1991. A quantitative patient set-up and verification system using megavoltage CT scanning. *International Journal of Radiation Oncology, Biology, Physics* 21, p. 228.

Perona, P., and Malik, J. 1990. Scale-space and edge detection using anisotropic diffusion. *IEEE Transactions on Pattern Analysis and Machine Intelligence* 12: 629–39.

Pouliot, J., Aubin, M., Verhey, L., et al. 2002. Low dose megavoltage cone Beam CT reconstruction for patient alignment. *7th International Workshop on Electronic Portal Imaging.*

Pouliot, J., Bani-Hashemi, A., Chen, J., et al. 2005. Low-dose megavoltage cone-beam CT for radiation therapy. *International Journal of Radiation Oncology, Biology, Physics* 61: 552–60.

Seppi, E. J., Munro, P., Johnsen, S. W., et al. 2003. Megavoltage cone-beam computed tomography using a high-efficiency image receptor. *International Journal of Radiation Oncology, Biology, Physics* 55: 793–803.

Sidhu, K., Ford, E. C., Spirou, S., et al. 2003. Optimization of conformal thoracic radiotherapy using cone-beam CT imaging for treatment verification. *International Journal of Radiation Oncology, Biology, Physics* 55: 757–67.

Siewerdsen, J. H., and Jaffray, D. A. 2001. Cone-beam computed tomography with a flat-panel imager: Magnitude and effects of X-ray scatter. *Medical Physics* 28: 220–31.

Siewerdsen, J. H., Moseley, D. J., Bakhtiar, B., Richard, S., and Jaffray, D. A. 2004. The influence of antiscatter grids on soft-tissue detectability in cone-beam computed tomography with flat-panel detectors. *Medical Physics* 31: 3506–20.

Sillanpaa, J., Chang, J., Mageras, G., et al. 2005. Developments in megavoltage cone beam CT with an amorphous silicon EPID: reduction of exposure and synchronization with respiratory gating. *Medical Physics* 32: 819–29.

Smitsmans, M. H. P., De Bois, J., Sonke, J.-J., et al. 2005. Automatic prostate localization on cone-beam CT scans for high precision image-guided radiotherapy. *International Journal of Radiation Oncology, Biology, Physics* 63: 975–84.

Spies, L., Ebert, M., Groh, B. A., Hesse, B. M., and Bortfeld, T. 2001. Correction of scatter in megavoltage cone-beam CT. *Physics in Medicine & Biology* 46: 821–33.

Swindell, W., Simpson, R. G., Oleson, J. R., Chen, C. T., and Grubbs, E. A. 1983. Computed tomography with a linear accelerator with radio therapy applications. *Medical Physics* 10: 416–20.

Turbell H. *Thesis: Cone-Beam Reconstruction using Filtered Backprojection.* Linkoping Studies in Science and Technology. (2001).

Wiesent, K., Barth, K., Navab, N., et al. 2000. Enhanced 3-D-reconstruction algorithm for C-arm systems suitable for interventional procedures. *IEEE Transactions on Medical Imaging* 19: 391–403.

Zeidan, O. A., Langen, K. M., Meeks, S. L., et al. 2007. Evaluation of image-guidance protocols in the treatment of head and neck cancers. *International Journal of Radiation Oncology, Biology, Physics* 67: 670–7.

7

Kilovoltage X-Ray IMRT and IGRT

Hiroki Shirato
Hokkaido University

Masayori Ishikawa
Hokkaido University

Shinichi Shimizu
Hokkaido University

Gerard Bengua
Hokkaido University

Ken Sutherland
Hokkaido University

Rikiya Onimaru
Hokkaido University

Hidefumi Aoyama
Hokkaido University

7.1 Introduction

In radiotherapy, it is essential to give sufficient dose to cancer without harming the normal tissue. Computed tomography (CT) has made it possible to see the position of the tumor deep in the body and has addressed the image-based radiotherapy in the 1980s. Three-dimensional (3D) radiotherapy planning (RTP) systems were first quickly developed and then greatly expanded to use CT anatomical information to concentrate radiation dose to the tumor, using approaches such as 3D conformal radiotherapy (3D CRT), stereotactic body radiotherapy (SBRT), and intensity-modulated radiotherapy (IMRT). In the early 1990s, image guidance in the setup of patients on the treatment couch was realized to be an important step to register the virtual world in the treatment planning computer to the real world. However, tumors move in the body with physiological functions such as respiration, cardiac beat, digestion, and urination. The reliability of the tumor position as observed on static CT images and magnetic resonance imaging (MRI) has been questioned in the light of tumor motion studies performed in the late 1990s. For instance, in two studies, lung cancers and liver cancers near the diaphragm were shown to move not only in the craniocaudal direction but also in the anterodorsal and right–left lateral directions with amplitudes of 10–30 mm (Shimizu et al. 1999; 2000a, 2000b). Precise investigations in the early 2000s showed that the magnitude and trajectory of the motion differs among

patients, changes day by day in the same patient, and shifts its baseline position even in a relatively short time such as one minute (Seppenwoolde et al. 2002; Shirato et al. 2004a, 2004b, 2006). These results apparently imply that sharp dose gradients designed during the RTP phase for 3D CRT, SBRT, and IMRT approaches may be different from the real situation for tumors in moving organs.

7.2 Background and Rationale

To achieve precise conformal radiotherapy for mobile tumors, in the early 1990s, we started investigating four-dimensional (4D) radiotherapy. After verifying that precise prediction of tumor motion is impractical in nature, we concluded that real-time estimation of the tumor position during radiotherapy is required. To this end, we proposed a gating system to shoot the therapeutic beam to the planned position only when the tumor or its fiducial marker is located within the gating window. We called this as the real-time tumor-tracking radiotherapy (RTRT) system (Shirato et al. 1999) (Figure 7.1).

In the RTRT approach, a linear accelerator is synchronized with a multisource x-ray fluoroscopic real-time tumor-tracking system by which 3D coordinates of a 2.0-mm gold marker in or near the tumor can be determined automatically (Figure 7.1b). Before RTRT, the 3D relationships between the marker and the tumor at different respiratory phases are evaluated using CT imaging at

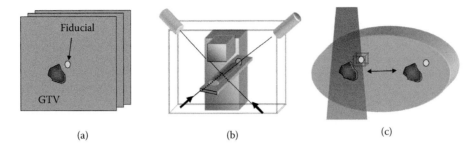

(a)   (b)   (c)

FIGURE 7.1   Concept of real-time tumor-tracking radiotherapy (RTRT). (a) Four-dimensional treatment planning registering fiducial marker position relative to the center of GTV at the end of expiration respiratory phase. (b) Fluoroscopic real-time tracking of the fiducial marker at set-up and during irradiation. (c) Schematic of gated radiotherapy: irradiation only occurs when the gold marker is within the gating window.

each respiratory phase, whereby the optimum phase to synchronize with irradiation can be selected, a process of 4D treatment planning (Shirato et al. 2000a). The linac is triggered to irradiate the tumor only when the marker is located within the region of the planned coordinates relative to the isocenter (Figure 7.1c). A phantom experiment showed the coordinates of the marker could be detected with an accuracy of ± 1 mm during radiotherapy. The time delay between recognition of the marker position and the start or stop of megavoltage x-ray irradiation was 0.033 s.

7.3 Geometry of Imaging and Treatment System

The prototype fluoroscopic real-time tumor-tracking system consists of four sets of diagnostic x-ray television systems, a

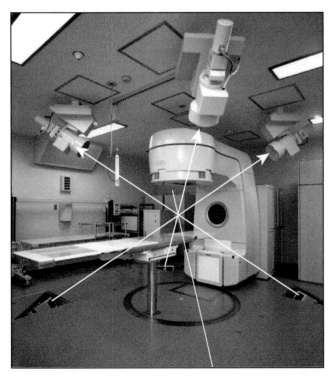

FIGURE 7.2   Prototype real-time tumor-tracking radiotherapy (RTRT) system.

moving object recognition system, and a carbon fiber patient couch placed in the linear accelerator room (Figure 7.2) (Shirato et al. 2000b). Each of the diagnostic x-ray television systems is composed of a 1.5 MHU x-ray tube embedded under the floor, a 9-inch image intensifier mounted on the ceiling, and a high-voltage x-ray generator. All four system geometries were adjusted such that the central axis of the diagnostic x-rays would cross at the isocenter of the linear accelerator. Equipment for calibration was used to maintain the geometric accuracy of the multisource system. Two of the four x-ray television systems are selected to display the gold marker in the patient's body during radiotherapy for each treatment of beam geometry. When the appropriate two sets are used, the gantry of the linear accelerator does not interfere with the fluoroscopic fields. Two fluoroscopic images are displayed on a liquid crystal display (LCD) monitor adjacent to the treatment console of the linear accelerator.

The second-generation RTRT system has two sets of diagnostic x-ray television systems rather than four sets (Figure 7.3). The position of two x-ray sources and two image intensifiers can be changed by mechanical remote control by a rotation along a ceiling mounted track to cover the same four positions as the prototype system (Figure 7.3b). This new system has 5-mm-wide multileaf collimators (leaf width projected at the isocenter) to make it possible to perform step-and-shoot IMRT with RTRT. At this moment, there are only these two types of RTRT systems in the world by which the real-time tracking of fiducial marker during the delivery of radiotherapy can be performed (Jiang 2006).

Coordinates of the tumor center and the gold marker are electronically transferred from the 3DRTP system to the fluoroscopic real-time tumor-tracking system through a network. The information is transformed using projection geometry and overlapped with the two x-ray television images displayed on the LCD monitor to enable analysis and interpretation.

7.4 Imaging Principles and Algorithms

The imaging principles of the RTRT system and its algorithms are as follows. First, in the treatment room, the patient is positioned on the treatment couch using laser beam localizers and skin markings were grossly determined by the CT simulation. The operator confirms that the gold marker can be visualized on the two x-ray

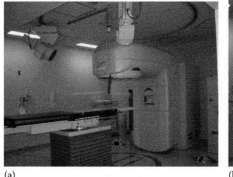
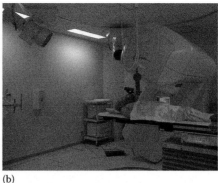

(a)   (b)

FIGURE 7.3 Second-generation RTRT system. (a) Basic position of the image intensifiers. (b) Position of the image intensifiers and treatment coach for a treatment field directed from the oblique inferior direction.

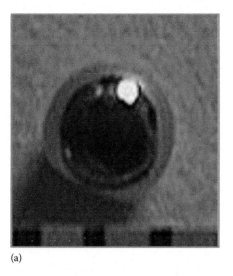
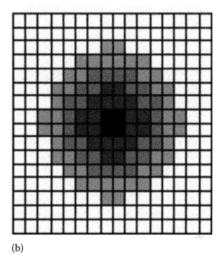

(a)   (b)

FIGURE 7.4 (a) A fiducial gold marker and (b) its image template for pattern matching.

TV images using the LCD monitor, and that the marker is crossing over the planned coordinates. If necessary, the location of the patient couch is adjusted such that the marker will cross over the planned target coordinates. When the moving gold marker is satisfactorily visible on the two x-ray images on the LCD monitor, the operator clicks the mouse to start an automatic search for it. The pattern of the gold marker in the x-ray image is already registered as a template in the computer of the fluoroscopic real-time tumor-tracking system (Figure 7.4). Once the computer recognizes the pattern of marker as matching the template, the marker is surrounded by a white square and the square moves in accordance with the movement of the marker every 0.033 s; that is, approximately 30 times a second. Recognition score, derived from the regression coefficient between the searched area and the template, is shown on the LCD every 0.033 s.

If the recognition score is less than the predetermined level, or if recognition is less than satisfactory, the fluoroscopic real-time tumor tracking system prevents the linear accelerator from irradiating the patient. If the recognition score is satisfactory and the coordinates of the marker are within the limits of predetermined "accepted" dislocation, the system allows the linear accelerator

to irradiate the patient. The time delay from the matching of the coordinates to the start of irradiation is 0.05 s (Figure 7.5).

The markers are first found in the digital images by means of a template matching algorithm, which is performed using special hardware. The correlation function, Q, is given by

$$Q_{xy} = \frac{\sum_{i,j}^{n} F_{x+i\,y+j} G_{i,j} - n\overline{F}\,\overline{G}}{\sqrt{\sum_{i,j}^{n} F_{x+i,\,y-j}{}^2 - n\overline{F}^2}\,\sqrt{\sum_{i,j}^{n} G_{i,j}{}^2 - n\overline{G}^2}} \quad (7.1)$$

and this function is evaluated for all $1{,}024 \times 1{,}024$ possible pixel positions x,y. In Equation 7.1, $G_{i,j}$ is a predefined template image, $F_{i,j}$ is a digitized fluoroscopic image, and n is the total number of pixels. A bar over the symbols F and G denotes an average over all pixels. For reasons of speed, the cost function is only evaluated for those pixels in $G_{i,j}$, which are nonzero. The template image has 24×24 pixels with a pixel size of 0.09×0.09 mm². A fixed template image is used because the marker is always approximately in the same position and therefore has an identical shape and size. The location x, y, which gives the highest

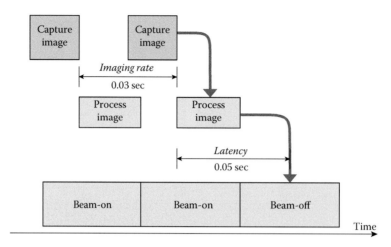

FIGURE 7.5   Imaging rate and latency in RTRT system.

correlation, is considered to be the marker position in the image. Because the marker is spherical, no matching for rotation has to be performed. If the correlation function Q is below a certain value, a machine interlock is issued. The threshold of Q is determined in the commissioning of the RTRT system to minimize the risk of tracking errors (Sharp et al. 2004b).

The same procedure is applied to both x-ray system images, rendering tumor marker coordinates A (X_A, Y_A) and B (X_B, Y_B). In the central processing unit, the tumor marker coordinates are converted to two straight lines, A and B, using fluoroscopic transformation matrices M_A and M_B, which were obtained during the calibration procedure and stored in advance.

The fluoroscopic transformation matrix M is calculated as follows. A spatial coordinate calibrator is used which consists of acrylic cube with sides of 58 mm in which eight markers with a diameter of 2 mm which are precisely centered on the vertexes of the cube. The isocenter is indicated with precise markers in the center of the faces of the cube. After aligning the calibrator with the room lasers, fluoroscopic images are taken and the operator gives commands to the system such that six out of eight markers are detected. The fluoroscopic transformation matrix M gives the equation of a straight line passing through the marker and the isocenter, that is, [aM] 5 [b], where [b] is the 2D marker position expressed in homogeneous coordinates (i.e., the third coordinate is set to one), [a] is any position on the line (in homogeneous coordinates), and M is a [4 3 3] matrix M of rank 3. By measuring the image marker locations [a] with two x-ray systems for six known marker positions [b], one obtains 12 equations with 12 unknowns and the matrix M can be solved.

The 3D coordinates of the tumor marker are calculated by intersecting these two lines, M_A and M_B. However, in most cases, the two lines will not intersect exactly due to small geometric inaccuracies. In that case, the center of the shortest connection between both lines is used as the marker position. A machine interlock is issued when the distance between both lines exceeds a certain distance, such 1.0 mm, which can be determined beforehand.

The x-ray images are normally digitized at a video rate of 30 frames/s, although lower frame rates can be used to reduce the

x-ray dose. The process of image acquisition and processing causes a small delay between the actual marker position and the gating of the treatment machine. A correction algorithm has been implemented, which is based on the speed of the tumor marker motion. The speed is calculated from the difference in 3D coordinates between two image frames. With an assumption of constant linear marker speed, the position correction is the speed of the tumor multiplied by the delay time (which is about 0.05 s). The predicted marker position, y, is thus given by

$$y = y_2 + (y_1 - y_2) . (t - t_1)/(t_2 - t_1),   (7.2)$$

where t_1 is time of previous image frame, t_2 is the time of the present image frame, t, is the anticipated time of gating (t_2 plus the measured delay), y_1 is the recognized marker coordinate in the previous frame (pair), and y_2 is the recognized marker coordinate in the present frame (pair).

The gating of the accelerator can be based on the predicted position. However, reduction of frame rates with this straightforward prediction model can deteriorate the accuracy of the irradiation for moving tumors. Thus, the prediction model of target motion must be evaluated in clinical trials where more complex motions may occur besides the simple assumption of cyclical respiration only. More complex prediction models have been investigated to improve the prediction (Ren et al. 2007; Sharp et al. 2004a).

7.5 Treatment Principles

At the time of May, 2010, the following treatment principles are used at Hokkaido University Hospital.

(1) Three or four 1.5-mm gold markers (99.9% Au) are inserted into the tumor or placed near the tumor to be detected by CT scanning for treatment planning and also by fluoroscopy during radiotherapy for lung cancers.

(2) The treatment planning CT scan is obtained with a 1.0-mm slice thickness and a 1.0-mm interval. Since it is so apparent that tumor position is stable at the end of exhale phase but

not at the end of inspiration, we have adapted the former as the optimal respiration phase for intercepting (gated) radiotherapy. CT scanning of the exhalation phase at a normal depth of breath is performed simply by asking patients to hold their breath at the exhalation phase.

(3) CT data are all transferred to the 3DRTP system. The coordinates of the gold marker at the inhalation phase are registered also and are used during fluoroscopic RTRT.

(4) A margin of 5 mm is added for suspected microscopic tumor extensions to obtain the clinical target volume (CTV). The planning target volume (PTV) margin for movement and setup error ranges from 1.0 to 9.0 mm, depends on the distance between the CTV and critical organs, and may be different in the lateral, craniocaudal, and anterior–dorsal directions, respectively. If there are no critical organs around the target volume, slight dislocation may be permitted without apparent injury to the patient. If a critical structure, such as the spinal cord, is situated closely to the tumor, perhaps several millimeters away, maximum accuracy is required for use of high-dose irradiation. Radiation oncologists can specify the "allowed" dislocation of the treatment isocenter from ±1.0 mm to ±9.0 mm but usually they use ±2.0 mm. The "allowed" dislocation is determined during treatment planning, depending on the distance to the critical organ and the volume of the irradiated portion of the organ. If the PTV margin of 1.0 mm was used, "allowed displacements" are set at 1.0 mm in the tumor-tracking system.

(5) The treatment planning process is finished using conventional methods, that is, the beams are setup in the beam's eye view, and dose calculation is performed. If one uses IMRT, inverse planning for static multiple leaf collimators is used. The planned position of the markers will be displayed as an overlay on the fluoroscopic images from the RTRT system.

(6) The patient is positioned on the treatment couch using the conventional method based on tattoos and localizing lasers. The coach top is made of carbon fiber reinforced plastic which is transparent for diagnostic x-ray imaging.

(7) With the patient positioned, by briefly switching on the x-ray sources, the operator confirms that the gold markers are visible on the selected two x-ray images, that the reference markers coincide with their planned coordinates, and that the moving tumor marker passes through its planned position in the gating window. By calculating the set-up discrepancy, the patient couch is adjusted from outside the treatment room by remote control of the patient couch (4D set-up) (Shirato et al. 2006).

(8) The tumor tracking system is switched on and starts to search automatically for the markers in the x-ray images.

(9) Once the computer recognizes a tumor marker, a white square is centered on the marker on the x-ray images. This square follows the movement of the marker in real time. The 3D coordinates of the tumor marker are calculated from the pair of images. The image recognition system will interlock the linac when the quality of the match is poor.

(10) The linac is enabled during the period when the detected location of the tumor marker is within the gating window, the accepted volume. In fluoroscopic RTRT, the accuracy of irradiation can be controlled by the selection of the accepted volume, which is a cube-shaped volume of "allowed dislocation." These procedures to determine the optimum timing of irradiation and the "permitted" dislocation in 3D coordinates is called *4D treatment planning.*

Fluoroscopic x-ray imaging has the additional merit compared to CT in terms of real-time visualization of the internal fiducial markers. However, fluoroscopic imaging, which uses 2D projection images that integrate information along ray trajectories, has the limitation in the evaluation of the relationship between tumor mass and the fiducial markers—the target volume is likely not visible. CT before each RT set-up is a logical procedure but requires considerable time in routine practice. Alternatively, if three or four markers were inserted around the tumor and used for the daily set-up, the possibility of misalignment due to marker migration can be minimized without obtaining daily CT images (Imura et al. 2005). In clinical practice, if the distance between three markers differs from the original planned position by more than 2.0 mm, marker and/or target position changes are assumed and replanning with a new CT scanning is required. Therefore, for prostate and lung cancer, three to four markers are to be inserted around the tumor as a minimal requirement in practice. For IMRT of the lung with a treatment period of more than 2 weeks, weekly CT examination is mandatory for adaptive radiotherapy (Imura et al. 2005).

7.6 Additional Dose from the Fluoroscopic Imaging during Radiotherapy

Unlike the general situation with diagnostic imaging and image-guided surgery, IGRT adds imaging dose to an already high level of therapeutic radiation. Therefore, if the use of image guidance can reduce potential high doses to organs at risk, the small dose from the image guidance, in this case fluoroscopic imaging for RTRT, is meaningful and of benefit to be added (Murphy et al. 2007). In earlier work, the dose due to the diagnostic x-ray monitoring ranged from 0.01% to 1% of the target (tumor) dose for a 2.0-Gy irradiation of a chest phantom using an RTRT system, which utilizes pulsed generation of the imaging x-rays (Shirato et al. 2000b). The ~100 kilovoltage (kV) diagnostic x-ray beams used in fluoroscopy in IGRT have lower energy than the megavoltage (MV) x-ray beams used for therapy (6 MV or higher) and can deliver high entrance skin (surface) doses. Synchronization of the kV and MV techniques in RTRT and IMRT is expected to be useful for the treatment of tumors in motion (Shirato et al. 2004a, 2004b), such that imaging and treatment irradiations are alternated during a treatment fraction to optimize the dose delivery. A goal for one study was to estimate the feasibility of the synchronization of RTRT and IMRT from the viewpoint of possible excessive dose resulting from the use of fluoroscopy. Using an ionization chamber for diagnostic x-rays, measurements were made of the air kerma rate, surface dose with backscatter, and dose distribution in depth in a solid phantom from a fluoroscopic RTRT system (Shirato 2004a, 2004b). Nominal 50–120 kV x-ray energies and nominal 1–4 ms of pulse width were used in the measurements. The mean ± SD in-air kerma rate from one fluoroscope was 238.8 ± 0.54 mGy/h at 100 kV and 2.0 ms pulse width at the isocenter of the linear accelerator. The air kerma rate increased steeply with increase in x-ray beam energy. The surface dose rate was 28–980 mGy/h. The absorbed dose at a 5.0-cm depth in the phantom was 37–58% of the maximum dose, depending on x-ray energy. The estimated patient skin surface dose from one x-ray system in RTRT was 29–1,182 mGy/h and was strongly dependent on the x-ray energy (kV) and pulse width of the fluoroscope, and slightly dependent on the distance between the skin and isocenter. In short, the skin surface dose and absorbed dose at depth resulting from fluoroscopic imaging during RTRT is not high when used for conventional 3D CRT and SBRT but can be significant when RTRT is synchronized with IMRT using a multileaf collimator. Additionally, skin dose can be strikingly changed by the manner of x-ray generation, for example, pulsed or not pulsed. More thorough analyses are required to determine whether fluoroscopic imaging dose in RTRT is useful for improving (optimizing) the delivered dose distribution of IMRT for moving tumors. Investigation to reduce fluoroscopic dose is an important matter in IGRT (Wang et al. 2009).

7.7 Insertion of Fiducial Markers

The feasibility and reliability of insertion of internal fiducial markers into various organs is essential for precise setup and real-time tumor-tracking using fluoroscopy. Equipment and techniques for the insertion of 1.5- or 2.0-mm-diameter gold markers into or near the tumor were developed for spinal/paraspinal lesions, prostate tumors, and liver and lung tumors and have been evaluated for accuracy (Shirato et al. 2003). Insertion of gold markers for RTRT of the lung is carried out using a bronchial endoscope (Olympus Co Ltd., Japan) (Figure 7.6). Three 2.0-mm gold markers are implanted near the prostate gland using a similar device made by Medikit Co. Ltd., Japan.

Three markers are used to guide the center of the mass of the target volume to the planned position in spinal/paraspinal lesions and prostate tumors (the three-marker method). The feasibility of the marker insertion and the stability of the position of markers were tested using stopping rules in the clinical protocol (i.e., the procedure was abandoned if 2 of 3 or 3 of 6 patients experienced marker dropping or migration). After the feasibility evaluation, the stability of the marker positions was monitored in those patients who entered a dose-escalation study (Shirato et al. 2003). Each of the following placement sites was shown to be feasible: bronchoscopic insertion for the peripheral lung; image-guided transcutaneous insertion for the liver; cystoscopic and image-guided percutaneous insertion for the prostate; and surgical implantation for spinal/paraspinal lesions. Transcutaneous insertion of markers for spinal/paraspinal lesions and bronchoscopic insertion for central lung lesions were abandoned. Overall, marker implantation was successful and was used for RTRT in 90 (90%) of 100 lesions, with no serious complications related to the marker insertion noted for any of the 100 lesions. Using three markers surgically implanted into the vertebral bone, the mean ± standard deviation in distance among the three markers was within 0.2 ± 0.6 mm (range –1.4 to 0.8) through the treatment period of 30 days. The distance between the three markers gradually decreased during RT in five of six prostate cancers, consistent with a mean rate of volume

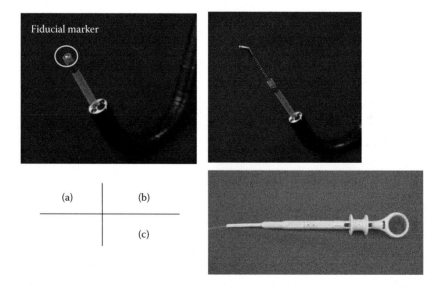

FIGURE 7.6 (a) Olympus transbronchial insertion kit for gold fiducial markers, (b) guiding wire for small bronchi, and (c) a disposable introducer.

regression of 9.3% (range 0.015–13%) in 10 days. Thus, internal 2.0-mm-diameter gold markers can be safely inserted into various organs for real-time tumor-tracking in RT using the prescribed equipment and techniques. The three-marker method has been shown to be a useful technique for precise setup for spinal/paraspinal lesions, prostate tumors, and lung tumors.

The fixation rate of the markers for lung cancer using the bronchial insertion technique, reliability of the setup using markers around the target volume, dislocation of the markers after real-time tumor-tracking RT, and long-term toxicity of marker insertion have been investigated (Imura et al. 2005). Between July 2000 and April 2004, 154 gold markers were inserted into 57 patients with peripheral lung cancer. The distances between the implanted markers in 198 measurements in 71 set-ups in 11 patients were measured using two sets of orthogonal diagnostic x-ray images of the RTRT system. The distance between the markers and the chest wall was also measured in a transaxial CT image on 186 occasions in 48 patients during treatment planning and during follow-up. The median treatment time was 6 days (range, 4–14 days). In 115 (75%) of the 154 inserted markers, the gold marker was detected throughout the treatment period. In 122 markers detected at CT planning, 115 (94%) were detected until the end of treatment. The variation in the distances between the implanted markers was within ± 2 mm in 95% and ± 1 mm in 80% during treatment. The variation in the distances between the implanted markers was > 2 mm in at least one direction in 9% of the setups for which reexamination with a CT scan was indicated. The fixation rate in the left upper lobe was lower than in the other lobes. A statistically significant relationship was found between a shorter distance between the markers and the chest wall and the fixation rate, suggesting that the markers in the smaller bronchial lumens fixed better than those in the larger lumens. A learning curve among the endoscopists was suggested in the fixation rate. The distance between the markers and the chest wall changed significantly within a median of 44 days (range, 16–181 days) after treatment. The fixation of markers into the bronchial tree was useful for the setup for peripheral lung cancer and had an accuracy of ±2 mm during the 1–2-week treatment period. The relationship between the markers and tumor can change significantly after 2 weeks, suggesting that adaptive radiotherapy with replanning is required for the IMRT using the treatment period 2 weeks or longer. Histopathologic findings at several points after the insertion of the gold markers have also been investigated (Imura et al. 2008). Sixteen gold markers were inserted for preoperative marking in seven patients who subsequently underwent partial resection of tumors by video-assisted thoracoscopic surgery within 7 days. Fibrotic changes and hyperplasia of type 2 pneumocytes around the markers were seen 5 or 7 days after insertion, and fibrin exudation without fibrosis was detected 1 or 2 days after insertion. Because fibroblastic changes start approximately 5 days after gold-marker insertion, RTRT should be started >5 days after insertion. Percutaneous insertion of the marker near the

lung cancer using CT guidance is known to be often harmful (Kothary et al. 2009; Yousefi et al. 2007). Endoscopic insertion is strongly recommended if feasible.

Hashimoto et al. (2005) have evaluated the feasibility of real-time monitoring of a fiducial marker in/near the digestive tract and analyzed the motion of organs at risk to determine a reasonable internal margin (Hashimoto et al. 2005). They developed two methods to insert a fiducial marker into/near the digestive tract adjacent to the target volume. One method involves an intraoperative insertion technique, and the other involves endoscopic insertion into the submucosal layer of the normal digestive tract. The fluoroscopic RTRT system was used to monitor the single, implanted marker. Fourteen markers (2 in the mediastinum and 12 in the abdomen) were implanted intraoperatively in 14 patients with no apparent migration. Seventeen of 20 markers (13/14 in the esophagus, 1/2 in the stomach, and 3/4 in the duodenum) in 18 patients were implanted using endoscopy without dropping. No symptomatic adverse effects related to insertion were observed. Thus, both intraoperative and endoscopic insertions of a fiducial marker into/near the digestive tract for monitoring of organs at risk is feasible. They concluded that the margin for internal motion can be individualized using this system.

7.8 Image Fidelity (Phantom Experiment)

7.8.1 Static Accuracy

The localization accuracy of the RTRT system was evaluated using a calibration and quality assurance phantom, which consists of an acrylic cube with sides of 58 mm in which 8 markers with a diameter of 2 mm are precisely centered on the cube vertices (Shirato 2000b). The isocenter is indicated with precise markers in the center of the faces of the cube. After aligning the cube with the room lasers, fluoroscopic images were taken, and the system calculated the 3D coordinates of the eight markers. Discrepancy of the calculated 3D coordinates of the eight markers from real 3D coordinates were then determined. The accuracy of the calculation for static markers in a human phantom was evaluated with known marker displacements in an Alderson RANDO Phantom (Radiology Support Devices, Inc., Long Beach, CA). A single gold marker with a diameter of 2 mm was placed in the prostate, to simulate a poor signal-to-noise ratio (the pelvis is the thickest part of the body). The marker was first positioned at the isocenter of the linac using the conventional laser-beam localizer and the diagnostic x-rays of the RTRT system. After that, the couch was moved to one of several predetermined positions from the isocenter (1, 2, 3, 10, 20, and 30 mm from the isocenter for lateral, craniocaudal, and anterodorsal directions) using a couch motion controller with an accuracy of 0.1 mm. The known displacements were compared with the marker displacements detected by the real-time tumor-tracking system. The x, y, and z coordinate deviations (room coordinates) for the eight markers at the corners of the cubic phantom were

0.24, 6.0, and 0.34 mm, respectively, with a mean 3D distance deviation of 0.5 mm.

7.8.2 Dynamic Accuracy

Next we performed a study to estimate the accuracy of the real-time tracking irradiation for a moving subject. A 2.0-mm gold marker was embedded in a 5×5 cm^2 plastic plate that was connected to the axis of a small rotating motor. The marker was placed at 5.0 mm from the axis of rotation. A 5×5 cm^2 x-ray film (X-OMAT V; Kodak Co., Ltd.) was fixed to the 5×5 cm^2 plate directly and sandwiched by 1-cm plastic plates. The motor was placed on the linac treatment couch, with the center of the plastic plate at 10 mm from the isocenter. A 4-MV x-ray beam with a small square field size of 5×5 mm^2 was centered on the isocenter axis. The linac was set to 200-monitor units per minute during irradiation. In this experimental model, the direction of the movement of the gold marker is constantly changing. Although the circular motion utilized here does not realistically reproduce the motion of an actual human organ, it is useful for testing the accuracy of the tracking for various speeds. At first, the film was irradiated without using the RTRT system giving 500 monitor units. The motor rotated with angle speeds of 68°/s or higher in the plane perpendicular to the linac beam axis. The corresponding speed of the gold marker was 6 mm/s or higher. This film was compared with the film exposed using RTRT in which the treatment beam, using gated mode, was set to irradiate the isocenter only when the marker was located at the planned position. The planned position did not correspond with the isocenter for practical reasons. The allowed displacement was set to 1 mm. After 50 monitor units of irradiation, the film was developed, and the displacement of the irradiated spot was measured. The system was tested for the following speeds of the gold marker: 6, 10, 12, 22, 32, and 40 mm/s, defined by varying the rotation speed of the motor. The discrepancy of the irradiated position from the planned position was measured with calipers on the film.

Figure 7.7a shows the developed film after the conventional irradiation of a RANDO phantom, which moves assuming respiratory cycles (12 times per minute). The irradiation beam has a round transaxial shape with a radius of 15 mm. Figure 7.7b shows the resulting irradiated volume when RTRT is used for the same phantom with a 2.0-mm gold marker embedded 3.0 cm apart from the isocenter. It is apparent that the RTRT approach can reduce the irradiated volume compared to the conventional radiotherapy that does not accommodate some form of motion tracking.

Tracking these implanted markers gives highly accurate position information, except when tracking fails due to poor or ambiguous imaging conditions. We investigated methods for automatic detection of tracking errors and assessed the frequency and impact of tracking errors on treatments using the prototype real-time tumor tracking system (Sharp et al. 2004b). We investigated four indicators for automatic detection of tracking errors and found that the distance between corresponding

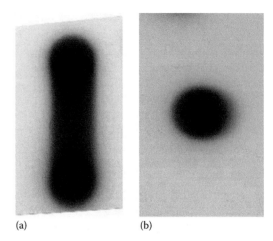

(a)   (b)

FIGURE 7.7 (a) Irradiation without RTRT and (b) with RTRT detected by x-ray film on the moving phantom. (From Shirato H, Shimizu S, Shimizu T, et al., *Lancet* 353: 1331–2, 1999. With permission.)

rays (the ray trajectories from the source through each marker) was most effective. We also found that tracking errors cause a loss of gating efficiency of between 7.6% and 10.2%. The incidence of treatment beam delivery during tracking errors was estimated at between 0.8% and 1.25%.

In general, IMRT is expected to be useful for cancers in moving organs. Effects of intrafraction motion on IMRT has been investigated, assuming regular respiratory motion (Bortfeld et al. 2002), but our precise study on respiratory motion suggests that this hypothesis is not valid for many patients. Step-and-shoot IMRT can be performed using the RTRT system when irregular respiratory motion is not a problem for deterioration of the dose distribution, although the additional fluoroscopic dose must be carefully monitored as mentioned above. We call this treatment *intensity-synchronized radiotherapy* (ISRT) (Shirato et al. 2005). Figure 7.8 shows the integrated dose distribution of lung IMRT for (a) a static phantom and then for a phantom moving with simulated respiratory motion (b) without RTRT and (c) with RTRT to enable ISRT. It is readily observed that ISRT can provide a well-delivered dose distribution under conditions of respiratory motion.

7.9 Clinical Applications

Real-time tracking radiotherapy was investigated to assess its usefulness in precise localization and verification of prostate and bladder cancers (Shimizu et al. 2000a, 2000b). The position of the patient was corrected by adjusting the actual marker position to the planned marker position, which had been transferred from the 3DRTP system and superimposed on the fluoroscopic image on the display unit of the RTRT system. Marker positions are visualized during irradiation and after treatment delivery to verify the accuracy of the localization. Ten patients with prostate cancer and five patients with bladder cancer were examined using this system for the treatment setup on 91 occasions. After manual setup using skin markers, the median of absolute value

Static phantom   Moving phantom

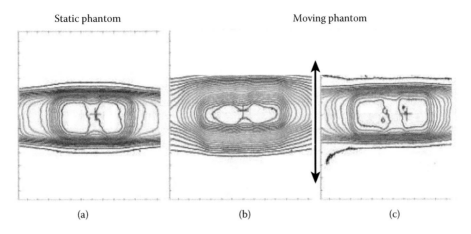

(a)   (b)   (c)

FIGURE 7.8 Dose distribution of IMRT for (a) static phantom, (b) nongated IMRT and (c) ISRT for a moving phantom.

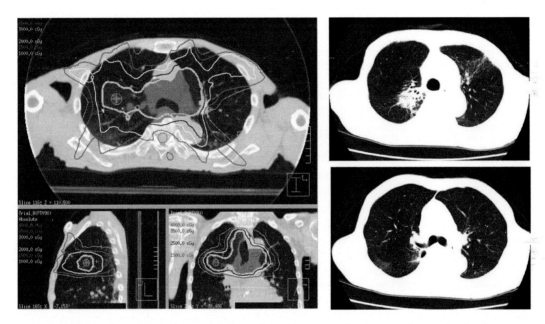

FIGURE 7.9 Dose distribution of ISRT for a patient with lung adenocarcinoma and CT images showing localized asymptomatic radiation pneumonitis detected 12 months after the radiotherapy. The pneumonitis was observed at the high dose region consistent with IMRT dose distribution for a static phantom.

of discrepancies between the actual position of the marker and the planned position of the marker for prostate cancer was 3.4 (0.1–8.9) mm, 4.1 (0.2–18.1) mm, and 2.3 (0.0–10.6) mm for the lateral, anteroposterior, and craniocaudal directions, respectively. The 3D median distance between the actual and planned positions of the marker was 6.9 (1.1–18.2) mm for prostate cancer and 6.9 (1.7–18.6) mm for bladder cancer. After relocation using RTRT, the 3D distance between the actual and planned position of the marker was 0.9 ± 0.9 mm. Median 3D distances between actual positions after treatment delivery and planned positions were 1.6 (0.0–6.3) mm and 2.0 (0.5–8.0) mm during daily radiotherapy for the markers in patients with prostate cancer and bladder cancer, respectively. Clinical outcome was excellent although the follow-up period was short and the number of patients was small at the time of analysis (Kitamura et al. 2003b).

Shimizu et al. have also investigated the 3D movement of lung tumors through an inserted internal marker using a real-time tumor-tracking system and evaluated the efficacy of this system at reducing the internal margin (Shimizu et al. 2001). The range of marker movement during the beam-off period was 5.5–10.0 mm in the lateral direction, 6.8–15.9 mm in the craniocaudal direction and 8.1–14.6 mm in the ventrodorsal direction. The range during the beam-on period was reduced to within 5.3 mm in all directions in all four patients. A significant difference was found between the mean of the range during the beam-off period and the mean of the range during the beam-on period in the x ($p = 0.007$), y ($p = 0.025$), and z ($p = 0.002$) coordinates, respectively.

After these studies, patients with various tumors were treated by conformal radiotherapy with a "tight" PTV margin. The following studies have shown that the RTRT system has significantly improved the accuracy of irradiation of targets in motion at the expense of an acceptable amount of diagnostic x-ray exposure (Ahn et al. 2004; Hashimoto et al. 2005; Katoh 2008; Kinoshita et al. 2008; Kitamura et al. 2003a, 2003b; Onimaru et al. 2002; Oita et al. 2006; Seppenwoolde et al. 2002; Taguchi et al. 2007; Yamamoto et al. 2004).

Onimaru et al. have investigated the clinical outcomes of patients with pathologically proven, peripherally located, stage I nonsmall-cell lung cancer (NSCLC) who had undergone SBRT using RTRT during the developmental period (Onimaru et al. 2008). A total of 41 patients (25 with stage T1 and 16 with stage T2) were admitted to the study between February 2000 and June 2005. A 5-mm PTV margin was added to the CTV, determined with CT acquired at the end of the expiratory phase. The gating window ranged from ± 2 to 3 mm. The dose fractionation schedule was 40 or 48 Gy in four fractions within 1 week. The dose was prescribed at the center of the PTV, giving more than an 80% dose at the PTV periphery. For 28 patients treated with 48 Gy in four fractions, the overall actuarial survival rate at 3 years was 82% for those with stage IA and 32% for those with stage IB. For patients treated with 40 Gy in four fractions within 1 week, the overall actuarial survival rate at 3 years was 50% for those with stage IA and 0% for those with stage IB. A significant difference was found in local control between those with stage IB who received 40 Gy vs. 48 Gy ($p = 0.0015$) but not in those with stage IA ($p = 0.5811$). No serious radiation morbidity was observed with either dose schedule. The results of this study show that 48 Gy in four fractions within 1 week is a safe and effective treatment for peripherally located, stage IA NSCLC. A steep dose-response curve between 40 and 48 Gy using a daily dose of 12 Gy delivered within 1 week was identified for stage IB NSCLC patients receiving SBRT using RTRT. A dose-escalation study of SBRT for stage IB NSCLC has been underway in Japan since 2007 based on the results of this study. Hashimoto et al. have evaluated the motion of esophagus to reduce adverse effects in radiotherapy for thoracic tumors (Hashimoto 2005). The mean/standard deviation of the range of motion of the esophagus was 3.5/1.8, 8.3/3.8, and 4.0/2.6 mm for the lateral, craniocaudal, and anteroposterior directions, respectively, in patients with intrafractional tumor motion less than 1.0 cm.

RTRT clinical outcomes have been studied for patients with hepatocellular carcinoma who were untreatable with other modalities because the tumors were adjacent to crucial organs or located too deep beneath the skin surface (Taguchi et al. 2007). Eighteen tumors, with a mean diameter of 36 mm, were studied in 15 patients. All tumors were treated on a hypofractionated schedule with a tight margin for setup and organ motion using a 2.0-mm fiducial marker in the liver and the RTRT system. The most commonly used radiotherapy dose was 48 Gy in eight fractions. Sixteen lesions were treated with a BED(10) of 60 Gy or more (median, 76.8 Gy). With a mean follow-up period of 20 months (range, 3–57 months), the overall survival rate was 39% at 2 years after RTRT. The 2-year local control rate was 83%

for initial RTRT but was 92% after allowance for reirradiation using RTRT, with a grade 3 transient gastric ulcer in one patient and grade 3 transient increases of aspartate amino transaminase in two patients. Intercepting radiotherapy using RTRT provided effective focal high doses to liver tumors. Because the fiducial markers for RTRT need not be implanted into the tumor itself, RTRT can be applied to hepatocellular carcinoma in patients who are not candidates for other surgical or nonsurgical treatments.

Katoh et al. have investigated the 3D movement of internal fiducial markers near adrenal tumors (metastases to the adrenal gland) using the RTRT system and examined the feasibility of high-dose hypofractionated radiotherapy for these tumors (Katoh et al. 2008). The subjects considered in this study were the 10 implanted markers in 9 patients treated with RTRT. A total of 72 days in the prone position and 61 treatment days in the supine position for nine of the 10 markers were analyzed. All but one patient were prescribed 48 Gy in eight fractions at the isocenter. The average absolute amplitude of the marker movement in the prone position was 6.1 ± 4.4 mm (range, 2.3–14.4), 11.1 ± 7.1 mm (3.5–25.2), and 7.0 ± 3.5 mm (3.9–12.5) in the left–right (LR), craniocaudal (CC), and anterior–posterior (AP) directions, respectively. The average absolute amplitude in the supine position was 3.4 ± 2.9 mm (0.6–9.1), 9.9 ± 9.8 mm (1.1–27.1), and 5.4 ± 5.2 mm (1.7–26.6) in the LR, CC, and AP directions, respectively. Of eight markers that were examined in both the prone and supine positions, there was no significant difference in the average absolute amplitude between the two positions. No symptomatic adverse effects were observed within the median follow-up period of 16 months (range, 5–21 months). The actuarial freedom-from-local-progression rate was 100% at 12 months. Thus, hypofractionated RTRT for adrenal tumors was feasible.

7.10 Intensity-Synchronized Radiotherapy (ISRT): An Example

A lung cancer patient case serves as an example to demonstrate the application of ISRT in the delivery of step-and-shoot IMRT using the RTRT image-guided system. The patient was a 72-year-old male with good performance status with a T3N2M0 squamous cell carcinoma of the right lung, referred for radiotherapy because of partial response (PR) after chemotherapy. Dose volume statistics showed that the V20 (volume of lung which would receive 20Gy) was too large with conventional 3D CRT radiotherapy, and that use of the ISRT approach would be of benefit for a satisfactory V20. Informed consent was obtained and ISRT (30Gy in 15 fractions at D95 of PTV) was given after conventional 3D CRT (30 Gy in 15 fractions) to keep the V20 less than 30% in total. The ISRT dose distribution for this case, 30 Gy in 15 fractions, is shown in Figure 7.9.

Because of possible changes in the target volume or patient and fiducial marker geometry, we had planned to do revise the IMRT plan at the midpoint of the 15 fractions. The three fiducial

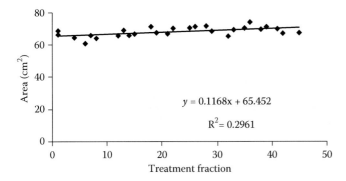

FIGURE 7.10 Area (cm²) of a triangle formed by three fiducial markers near the tumor in the patient during 48 days of treatment. The area was measured at the start of each treatment.

TABLE 7.1 Elapsed time required to deliver the same number of monitor units for each beam*

Beam No.	Units	Day 1	Day 2
Beam 1	Seconds	188	210
Beam 2	Seconds	177	374
Beam 3	Seconds	201	213
Beam 4	Seconds	89	146
Total	Minutes	13.9	18.3

* The elapsed time changes every day due to the irregularities in daily respiratory motion and the required amount of intensity synchronization needed. A total of 13.9 min was required to deliver 2 Gy on the initial day and 18.3 min on the second day.

markers distances near the tumor were measured every day to detect the deformation of lung structures due to tumor shrinkage. However, as shown in Figure 7.10, there was no systematic change during the treatment in the intermarker distances or the total area of the triangle defined by the three markers. Therefore, IMRT replanning was not performed.

Table 7.1 shows the elapsed time required to deliver the same monitor units for each beam. The elapsed time changes every day due to irregularities in daily respiratory motions and the required amount of intensity synchronization needed. These irregular motions can be substantial, as seen in Figure 7.11. A total of 13.9 min was required to irradiate 2 Gy on the initial day and 18.3 min on the second day.

7.11 Future Perspective

7.11.1 Real-Time Tracking Technology as a Tool for Tumor Motion Analysis

Precise knowledge about internal organ motion is an important issue both in scientific meaning and translational research and remains an area for further investigation. In previous work, we have precisely analyzed the trajectory of internal fiducial markers for various organs (Seppenwoolde et al. 2002; Shirato et al. 2004a, 2004b, 2006, 2007). The recorded lung tumor motions of 20 patients with 21 lung tumors were analyzed in terms of the amplitude and curvature of the tumor motion in three directions, the differences in breathing level during treatment, hysteresis (the difference between the inhalation and exhalation trajectories of the tumor), and the amplitude of tumor motion induced by cardiac motion. The average amplitude of the tumor motion was greatest (12 ± 2 mm [SD]) in the cranial–caudal direction for tumors situated in the lower lobes and not attached to rigid structures such as the chest wall or vertebrae. For the lateral and anterior-posterior directions, tumor motion was small both for upper- and lower-lobe tumors (2 ± 1 mm). The time-averaged tumor position was closer to the exhale position, because tumors spent more time in the exhalation phase than in the inhalation phase. The tumor motion was modeled as a sinusoidal movement with varying asymmetry. The tumor position in the exhale phase was more stable than the tumor position in the inhale phase during individual treatment fields. However, in many patients, shifts in the exhale tumor position were observed intra- and interfractionally. These shifts are the result of patient relaxation, gravity (posterior direction), setup errors, and/or patient movement. The 3D trajectory of the tumor showed hysteresis ranging from 1 to 5 mm for 10 of the 21 tumors. The extent of hysteresis and the amplitude of the tumor motion remained fairly constant during the entire treatment. Changes in shape of the trajectory of the tumor were observed between subsequent treatment days for only one patient. Fourier analysis revealed that for 7 of the 21 tumors, a measurable motion in the range 1–4 mm was caused by the cardiac beat. These tumors were located near the heart or attached to the aortic arch. The motion due to the heartbeat was greatest in the lateral direction. Tumor motion due to hysteresis and heartbeat can lower treatment efficiency in real-time tumor tracking-gated treatments or lead to a geographic miss in conventional or active breathing controlled treatments.

Prediction of the tumor position is an important issue to find the optimal frame rate and consider new radiotherapy machines. Many studies have been undertaken following to the study by Seppenwoolde et al. (2007). Sharp et al. evaluated various predictive models for reducing tumor localization errors for the RTRT approach with moving tumors under the conditions of a slow imaging rate and with large system latencies (Sharp 2004a). They considered 14 lung tumor cases where the peak-to-peak motion was greater than 8 mm and compared the localization error using linear prediction, neural network prediction, and Kalman filtering, against a system which uses no prediction. The beam tracking prediction accuracy was evaluated using the root mean squared error between the predicted and actual 3D motion. This work found that the prediction algorithms improved the root mean squared error for all latencies and all imaging rates evaluated. To evaluate prediction accuracy for use in gated treatment, they presented a new metric that compares a gating control signal based on predicted motion against the best possible gating control signal. They found that using prediction improves gated treatment accuracy for systems that have latencies of 200 ms or greater, and for systems that have imaging rates of 10 Hz or slower (Sharp 2004a).

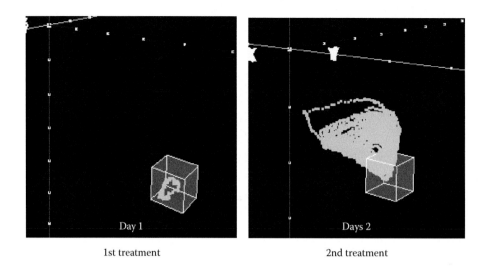

FIGURE 7.11 Interfractional change of trajectory of the same gold marker near a lung tumor: (a) first day of treatment and (b) second day of treatment.

Ren et al. evaluated the performance of an autoregressive-moving average (ARMA) model-based prediction algorithm for reducing tumor localization error due to system latency and slow imaging rate (Ren et al. 2007). This algorithm has components to accommodate the likelihood of irregular respiratory motions. For this study, they used 3D motion data from ten lung tumor cases where the peak-to-peak motion is greater than 8 mm. Some strongly irregular traces with variation in amplitude and phase were included. To evaluate the prediction accuracy, the standard deviations between predicted and actual motion position were computed for three system latencies (0.1, 0.2, and 0.4 s) at several imaging rates (1.25–10 Hz) and compared against the situation of no prediction. The simulation results indicated that the implementation of the prediction algorithm in real-time target tracking can improve the localization precision for all latencies and imaging rates evaluated. From a common initial setting of model parameters, the predictor can quickly provide an accurate prediction of the position after collecting 20 initial data points. In this retrospective analysis, they calculated the standard deviation of the predicted position from the twentieth position data point to the end of the session at 0.1 s intervals. For both regular and irregular lung tumor motions, with prediction the range of average errors was 0.4–2.5 mm in the SI direction from shorter to longer latency periods, corresponding to a range of 0.8–4.3 mm without prediction. For the AP direction a range of 0.3–1.6 mm was obtained with prediction, corresponding to a range of 0.6–3.0 mm without prediction. For 0.2 s and 0.4 s system latencies, with prediction the localization based on a relatively slow imaging rate (2.5 Hz) achieves a better or similar precision compared with no prediction on a fast imaging rate (10 Hz). This result means that precise localization can be realized at a slow imaging rate, which is important for the application of kV x-ray imaging systems and EPID-based systems in image-guided radiotherapy. In conclusion, an adaptive predictor model can successfully predict irregular respiratory motion, and the adaptive prediction of respiration motion can effectively improve the delivery precision of real-time motion compensation radiotherapy.

Respiratory hysteresis complicates the external fiducial marker and internal tumor position correspondence because two distinct tumor positions during different breathing phases can yield the same external observation. Previous attempts to resolve this ambiguity have often subdivided the data into inhale/exhale stages and restricted the estimation to only one of these directions. Ruan et al. proposed a new approach to infer the internal tumor motion from the external surrogate signal using the method of *state augmentation* (Ruan et al. 2008). This method resolves the hysteresis ambiguity by incorporating higher-order system dynamics. It circumvents the segmentation of the internal/external trajectory into different phases, and estimates the inference map based on all the available external/internal correspondence pairs.

Internal organ motion analysis has revealed many unknown facts about human dynamic anatomy in normal as well as diseased conditions. New radiological or optical technologies for diagnosis or other applications will benefit from the real-time tracking technologies that have been developed for radiotherapy and discussed in this chapter and others herein.

7.11.2 Combination of RTRT System and External Surrogate Marker for Respiratory-Gating System

It would be possible to reduce the diagnostic fluoroscopic dose associated with RTRT procedures if one could predict the relationship between the external surface markers and the internal fiducial markers and use the external surface markers for pursuing or intercepting irradiation. In 2000, at NTT Hospital in Sapporo, Japan, Mitsubishi Electronics, and Hokkaido University staffs have developed an IGRT system with two fluoroscopy units for RTRT and also a respiratory-gating system.

The original type of RTRT system was not able to be installed in the small treatment room and the new system was designed to compensate for any inadequacies. The unique combination of the RTRT system and the respiratory-gating system has resulted in important findings, published in collaboration with international investigators (Berbeco et al. 2005, 2006). Assumptions about the correlation between external surface markers and internal fiducial markers have been used in some commercially available radiotherapy systems in clinical practice, and the reliability of external surface marker was examined as a focus of the research.

Berbeco et al. collaborated with NTT Hospital researchers and measured the residual tumor motion within a gating window to assess the validity of the correlation assumption for external surface based gated radiotherapy (Berbeco et al. 2005). Eight lung patients with implanted fiducial markers were studied. Synchronized internal marker positions and external abdominal surface positions were measured during the entire course of treatment. Stereoscopic imaging was used to find the internal markers in four dimensions (position and time). The data were used retrospectively to assess conventional external surrogate respiratory-gated treatment. Both amplitude- and phase-based gating methods were investigated. For each method, three gating windows were investigated, each giving 40%, 30%, and 20% duty cycle, respectively. The residual motion of the internal marker within these six gating windows was calculated. The beam-to-beam variation and day-to-day variation in the residual motion were calculated for both gating modalities. They found that the residual motion (95th percentile) was between 0.7 and 5.8 mm, 0.8 and 6.0 mm, and 0.9 and 6.2 mm for 20%, 30%, and 40% duty cycle windows, respectively. Five of the eight patients showed less residual motion with amplitude-based gating than with phase-based gating. Large fluctuations (>300%) were seen in the residual motion between some beams. Overall, the mean beam-to-beam variation was 37% and 42% from the previous treatment beam for amplitude- and phase-based gating, respectively. The day-to-day variation was 29% and 34% from the previous day for amplitude- and phase-based gating, respectively. Although gating reduced the total tumor motion, the residual motion behaved unpredictably. Residual motion during treatment could exceed that which might have been considered in the treatment plan. With this study, it was found that prediction based on external surface markers is not accurate enough to substitute for real-time tumor-tracking of internal fiducial markers, although its clinical relevance is another subject to be investigated.

In another real-time approach, Ionascu et al. have developed a dynamic data analysis technique to study the internal–external correlation and quantitatively estimate its underlying time behavior (Ionascu et al. 2007). The work quantifies the time-dependent behavior of the correlation between external respiratory signals and lung-implanted fiducial motion. For the ten patients in this study, the SI internal–external motion is well correlated but the AP internal–external motion reveals larger time shifts than for the SI direction.

It has been observed by several institutions that the end-of-exhale (EOE) tumor position is more reproducible than other phases of the breathing cycle; therefore, the gating window is often set at this phase as is our practice at Hokkaido University Hospital. From a treatment planning perspective, however, the end-of-inhale (EOI) phase might be preferred for gating because the expanded lungs will further decrease the healthy tissue within the treatment field. Berbeco et al. simulated gated treatment at the EOI phase, using a set of the data taken from NTT Hospital (Berbeco et al. 2006). This study attempted to answer the question on the amount of tumor residual motion with use of an external surrogate gating window at EOI phase. It was found that under free breathing conditions the residual motion of the tumors is much larger for the EOI phase compared to the EOE phase. The mean values of residual motion at EOI were found to be 2.2 and 2.7 mm for amplitude- and phase-based gating, respectively, and, at EOE, 1.0 and 1.2 mm for amplitude- and phase-based gating, respectively, about a factor of two difference.

Nishioka et al., also at NTT Hospital, have reported that even at the EOE phase, the external surface marker position is often inaccurate because of a baseline shift of the internal tumor motion (Nishioka et al. 2008). Synchronized internal/external position data were collected during the entire course of treatments for 12 lung patients with 24 fiducials. Baseline was determined in the exhale phase during pretreatment observation time, and a gating level of external waves was set in each treatment session in a simulation of respiratory-gated radiotherapy. In the simulation, external gating windows were defined as those below the 30% amplitude level (i.e., imaginary beams would be triggered when part of the respiratory wave falls into this window). Exhale fluctuation (EF) was defined as the phenomenon (a deviation beyond the norm) in which the lowest point of the external wave crossed downward past the predetermined baseline. Gating efficiency (GE) was defined as the ratio between the amount of gate-ON time and the total treatment time. EF occurred in 18.4% of total measurements. EF varied depending on the patient, fiducial sites, and treatment session. The mean incidence of EF for each patient varied from 2.9% to 37.5% (18.4 ± 9.9). The EF magnitude was 0.2–12.2 mm in the left–right direction, 0.7–12.7 mm in the craniocaudal direction, and 0.4–9.7 mm in the anterior–posterior direction. Total fiducial movement was 0.5–28.7 mm. GE was 36.1–69.2% (55.4 ± 11.0). EF magnitude correlated with total fiducial movement. This study showed that EF is not a rare phenomenon and needs to be taken into consideration for individualized precise 4D radiotherapy.

Wu et al. (2008) proposed to investigate an approach based on hybrid gating with dynamic internal/external correlation updates. In this approach, the external signal is acquired at high frequency (such as 30 Hz) while the internal signal is sparsely acquired (such as 0.5 Hz or less). The internal signal is used to validate and update the internal/external correlation during treatment. Tumor positions are derived from the external signal based on the newly updated correlation. Two dynamic correlation updating algorithms are introduced. One is based on the motion amplitude and the other is based on the motion phase. Nine patients with synchronized internal/external motion signals are simulated retrospectively to evaluate the effectiveness of hybrid gating. The results demonstrate that dynamically updating the internal/external correlation in or around the gating window will reduce false positive gates with relatively small diminished treatment efficiency. This improvement will benefit patients with mobile tumors, and is especially favorable for early stage lung cancers, for which the tumors are less attached or freely floating in the lung.

It is not certain whether prediction of internal organ motion with external surface marker would be accurate enough or not for guiding high-precision RTRT interventions at this moment (Kanoulas et al. 2007; McMahon et al. 2008; Seppenwolde et al. 2007). Elimination of fiducial markers is one of the dreams in RTRT and several investigators are attempting to perform real-time tracking of the tumor without fiducial markers (Cui et al. 2007; Lin et al. 2009). There is no final answer at this moment and this next horizon in radiotherapy is the research pursuit for a number of investigators.

7.12 Conclusions

Real-time tumor tracking radiotherapy systems have been developed for image-guided radiation treatments using multiple and dual kV x-ray fluoroscopy systems that are geometrically aligned with the radiation treatment device, usually a linear accelerator, to detect and monitor both patient and target position. The RTRT approach uses reference fiducial markers, placed externally, internally, or both, and real-time marker detection to guide motion-gated 3D CRT. For step-and-shoot IMRT, the RTRT system is used to deliver intensity synchronized radiation treatment that coordinates the delivery of each IMRT segment via fluoroscopic imaging. Future research directions for the RTRT system include higher fidelity motion tracking and prediction models, and IGRT approaches that do not require the use of surrogate and/or implanted fiducial markers.

Acknowledgments

We thank the many international and domestic collaborators who have contributed to the development of kilovoltage x-ray and IMRT-IGRT and who are not listed as the co-authors of this chapter. Hokkaido University has patents for real-time tumor-tracking radiotherapy and transbronchial marker-insertion techniques.

References

Ahn YC, Shimizu S, Shirato H, et al. 2004. Application of real-time tumor-tracking and gated radiotherapy system for unresectable pancreatic cancer. *Yonsei Med* 45: 584–90.

Berbeco RI, Nishioka S, Shirato H, Chen GT, and Jiang SB. 2005. Residual motion of lung tumors in gated radiotherapy with external respiratory surrogates. *Phys Med Biol* 50: 3655–67.

Berbeco RI, Nishioka S, Shirato H, and Jiang SB. 2006. Residual motion of lung tumors in end-of-inhale respiratory gated radiotherapy based on external surrogates. *Med Phys* 33: 4149–56.

Bortfeld T, Jokivarsi K, Goitein M, Kung J, and Jiang SB. 2002. Effects of intra-fraction motion on IMRT dose delivery: statistical analysis and simulation. *Phys Med Biol* 47: 2203–20.

Cui Y, Dy JG, Sharp GC, Alexander B, and Jiang SB. 2007. Multiple template-based fluoroscopic tracking of lung tumor mass without implanted fiducial markers. *Phys Med Biol* 52: 6229–42.

Hashimoto T, Shirato H, Kato M, et al. 2005. Real-time monitoring of a digestive tract marker to reduce adverse effects of moving organs at risk (OAR) in radiotherapy for thoracic and abdominal tumors. *Int J Radiat Oncol Biol Phys* 61: 1559–64.

Imura M, Yamazaki K, Shirato H, et al. 2005. Insertion and fixation of fiducial markers for setup and tracking of lung tumors in radiotherapy. *Int J Radiat Oncol Biol Phys* 63: 1442–7.

Imura M, Yamazaki K, Kubota KC, et al. 2008. Histopathologic consideration of fiducial gold markers inserted for real-time tumor-tracking radiotherapy against lung cancer. *Int J Radiat Oncol Biol Phys* 70: 382–4.

Ionascu D, Jiang SB, Nishioka S, Shirato H, and Berbeco RI. 2007. Internal-external correlation investigations of respiratory induced motion of lung tumors. *Med Phys* 34: 3893–903.

Jiang SB. 2006. Technical aspects of image-guided respiration-gated radiation therapy. *Med Dosim* 31: 141–51.

Kanoulas E, Aslam JA, Sharp GC, et al. 2007. Derivation of the tumor position from external respiratory surrogates with periodical updating of the internal/external correlation. *Phys Med Biol* 52: 5443–56.

Katoh N, Onimaru R, Sakuhara Y, et al. 2008. Real-time tumor-tracking radiotherapy for adrenal tumors. *Radiother Oncol* 87: 418–24.

Kinoshita R, Shimizu S, Taguchi H, et al. 2008. Three-dimensional intrafractional motion of breast during tangential breast irradiation monitored with high-sampling frequency using a real-time tumor-tracking radiotherapy system. *Int J Radiat Oncol Biol Phys* 70: 931–4.

Kitamura K, Shirato H, Seppenwoolde Y, et al. 2003a. Tumor location, cirrhosis, and surgical history contribute to tumor movement in the liver, as measured during stereotactic irradiation using a real-time tumor-tracking radiotherapy system. *Int J Radiat Oncol Biol Phys* 56: 221–8.

Kitamura K, Shirato H, Shinohara N, et al. 2003b. Reduction in acute morbidity using hypofractionated intensity-modulated radiation therapy assisted with a fluoroscopic real-time tumor-tracking system for prostate cancer: preliminary results of a phase I/II study. *Cancer J* 9:268–76.

Kothary N, Heit JJ, Louie JD, et al. 2009. Safety and efficacy of percutaneous fiducial marker implantation for image-guided radiation therapy. *J Vasc Interv Radiol* 20: 235–9.

Lin T, Cervino LT, Tang X, Vasconcelos N, and Jiang SB. 2009. Fluoroscopic tumor tracking for image-guided lung cancer radiotherapy. *Phys Med Biol* 54:981–92.

McMahon R, Berbeco R, Nishioka S, et al. 2008. A real-time dynamic-MLC control algorithm for delivering IMRT to targets undergoing 2D rigid motion in the beam's eye view. *Med Phys* 35: 3875–88.

Murphy MJ, Balter J, Balter S, et al. 2007. The management of imaging dose during image-guided radiotherapy: report of the AAPM Task Group 75. *Med Phys* 34:4041–63.

Nishioka S, Nishiota T, Kawahara M, et al. 2008. Exhale fluctuation in respiratory-gated radiotherapy of the lung: a pitfall of respiratory gating shown in a synchronized internal/external marker recording study. *Radiother Oncol* 86:69–76.

Oita M, Ohmori K, Obinata K, et al. 2006. Uncertainty in treatment of head-and-neck tumors by use of intraoral mouthpiece and embedded fiducials. *Int J Radiat Oncol Biol Phys* 64: 1581–8.

Onimaru R, Shirato H, Aoyama H, et al. 2002. Calculation of rotational setup error using the real-time tracking radiation therapy (RTRT) system and its application to the treatment of spinal schwannoma. *Int J Radiat Oncol Biol Phys* 54: 939–47.

Onimaru R, Fujino M, Yamazaki K, et al. 2008. Steep dose-response relationship for stage I non-small-cell lung cancer using hypofractionated high-dose irradiation by real-time tumor-tracking radiotherapy. *Int J Radiat Oncol Biol Phys* 70: 374–81.

Ren Q, Nishioka S, Shirato H, and Berbeco RI. 2007. Adaptive prediction of respiratory motion for motion compensation radiotherapy. *Phys Med Biol* 52: 6651–61.

Ruan D, Fessler JA, Balter JM, Berbeco RI, Nishioka S, and Shirato H. 2008. Inference of hysteretic respiratory tumor motion from external surrogates : a state augmentation approach. *Phys Med Biol* 53: 2923–36.

Seppenwoolde Y, Shirato H, Kitamura K, et al. 2002. Precise and real-time measurement of 3D tumor motion in lung due to breathing and heartbeat, measured during radiotherapy. *Int J Radiat Oncol Biol Phys* 53(4): 822–34.

Seppenwoolde Y, Berbeco RI, Nishioka S, Shirato H, and Heijmen B. 2007. Accuracy of tumor motion compensation algorithm from a robotic respiratory tracking system: a simulation study. *Med Phys* 34: 2774–84.

Sharp GC, Jiang SB, Shimizu S, and Shirato H. 2004a. Prediction of respiratory tumor motion for real-time image-guided radiotherapy. *Phys Med Biol* 49: 425–40.

Sharp GC, Jiang SB, Shimizu S, and Shirato H. 2004b. Tracking errors in a prototype real-time tumor tracking system. *Phys Med Biol* 49: 5347–56.

Shimizu S, Shirato H, Xo B, et al. 1999. Three-dimensional movement of a liver tumor detected by high-speed magnetic resonance imaging. *Radiother Oncol* 50: 367–70.

Shimizu S, Shirato H, Kagei K, et al. 2000. Impact of respiratory movement on the computed tomographic images of small lung tumors in three-dimensional (3D) radiotherapy. *Int J Radiat Oncol Biol Phys* 46:1127–33.

Shimizu S, Shirato H, Kitamura K, et al. 2000. Use of an implanted marker and real-time tracking of the marker for the positioning of prostate and bladder cancers. *Int J Radiat Oncol Biol Phys* 48: 1591–7.

Shimizu S, Shirato H, Ogura S, et al. 2001. Detection of lung tumor movement in real-time tumor-tracking radiotherapy. *Int J Radiat Oncol Biol Phys* 51: 304–10.

Shirato H, Shimizu S, Shimizu T, Nishioka T, and Miyasaka K. 1999. Real-time tumor-tracking radiotherapy. *Lancet* 353: 1331–2.

Shirato H, Shimizu S, Kitamura K, et al. 2000a. Four-dimensional treatment planning and fluoroscopic real-time tumor tracking radiotherapy for moving tumor. *Int J Radiat Oncol Biol Phys* 48 : 435–42.

Shirato H, Shimizu S, Kunieda T, et al. 2000b. Physical aspects of a real-time tumor-tracking system for gated radiotherapy. *Int J Radiat Oncol Biol Phys* 48: 1187–95.

Shirato H, Harada T, Harabayashi T, et al. 2003. Feasibility of insertion/implantation of 2.0-mm-diameter gold internal fiducial markers for precise setup and real-time tumor tracking in radiotherapy. *Int J Radiat Oncol Biol Phys* 56: 240–7.

Shirato H, Seppenwoolde Y, Kitamura K, Onimaru R, and Shimizu S. 2004a. Intrafractional tumor motion: lung and liver. *Semin Radiat Oncol* 14: 10–8.

Shirato H, Oita M, Fujita K, Watanabe Y, and Miyasaka K. 2004b. Feasibility of synchronization of real-time tumor-tracking radiotherapy and intensity-modulated radiotherapy from viewpoint of excessive dose from fluoroscopy. *Int J Radiat Oncol Biol Phys* 60:335–41.

Shirato H, Imura M, Fujino M, et al. 2005. Intensity synchronized radiotherapy (ISRT) with conventional fractionation schedule using fiducial markers and real-time tumor-tracking radiotherapy (RTRT) system for locally advanced lung cancer. *Int J Radiat Oncol Biol Phys* 63 (Suppl. 1): s221–s222.

Shirato H, Suzuki K, Sharp GC, et al. 2006. Speed and amplitude of lung tumor motion precisely detected in four-dimensional setup and in real-time tumor-tracking radiotherapy. *Int J Radiat Oncol Biol Phys* 64:1229–36.

Shirato H, Shimizu S, Kitamura K, and Onimaru S. 2007. Organ motion in image-guided radiotherapy: lessons from real-time tumor-tracking radiotherapy. *Int J Clin Oncol* 12: 8–16.

Taguchi H, Sakuhara Y, Hige S, et al. 2007. Intercepting radiotherapy using a real-time tumor-tracking radiotherapy system for highly selected patients with hepatocellular carcinoma unresectable with other modalities. *Int J Radiat Oncol Biol Phys* 69: 376–80.

Yamamoto R, Yonesaka A, Nishioka S, et al. 2004. High dose three-dimensional conformal boost (3DCB) using an orthogonal diagnostic X-ray set-up for patients with gynecological malignancy: a new application of real-time tumor-tracking system. *Radiother Oncol* 73: 219–22.

Yousefi S, Collins BT, Reichner CA, et al. 2007. Complications of thoracic computed tomography-guided fiducial placement for the purpose of stereotactic body radiation therapy. *Clin Lung Cancer* 8:252–6.

Wang J, Zhu L, and Xing L. 2009. Noise reduction in low-dose x-ray fluoroscopy for image-guided radiation therapy. *Int J Radiat Oncol Biol Phys* 74: 637–43.

Wu H, Zhao Q, Berbeco RI, et al. 2008. Gating based on internal/external signals with dynamic correlation updates. *Phys Med Biol* 53: 7137–50.

8

Kilovoltage Radiography for Robotic Linac IGRT

Martin J. Murphy
Virginia Commonwealth University

8.1 Introduction

Intrafraction movement by the patient and the tumor during external-beam radiotherapy remains a significant and challenging problem. Several strategies for automated interventional response to the motion are presently being pursued: (1) temporal gating of the beam; (2) realignment of the beam aperture or linear accelerator for x-ray therapy; (3) realignment of the patient; (4) electromagnetic steering of a charged particle beam. Each method requires online knowledge of changes in target position. This knowledge can presently be gained directly using fluoroscopic (Shirato et al. 2000), radiographic (Murphy and Cox 1996), or electromagnetic (Kupelian et al. 2007) methods. In addition, there is the future prospect of intrafraction magnetic resonance imaging for motion detection (Dempsey et al. 2005; Raaymakers et al. 2004).

All of these four interventional technologies require a target localization system capable of triggering the adaptive alignment response via a real-time control loop. *Real time* refers to actions that are made in response to movement in time intervals that are short compared to the characteristic time period of the motion. Different movement scenarios thus have different timing requirements.

Because target detection and adaptive alignment response are basically independent problems, one can configure a motion-adaptive image-guided radiation therapy (IGRT) system in a variety of ways. This chapter reviews the integration of a kV radiographic imaging system with a robotic manipulator that can adaptively position an x-ray linear accelerator (linac) for IGRT of intra- and extracranial targets. This system can perform real-time motion compensation in response to intrafraction patient and/or target movement.

8.2 Background and History of the CyberKnife®

The use of intrafraction kV radiography in conjunction with a robotically manipulated linac is exemplified by the CyberKnife® (Accuray Inc., Sunnyvale, CA). This device was developed by Dr. John Adler and colleagues (Adler 1999) at Stanford in the early 1990s as a frameless image-guided radiosurgery system. Unlike conventional hyperfractionated radiotherapy, radiosurgery delivers an ablative radiation dose to the target in a single fraction. The intensity of the dose, and its usual application to neurosurgical targets, requires millimeter-level precision to avoid damage to critical neurological structures. At the time, stereotactic radiosurgery could achieve this level of precision only with the attachment of a rigid frame to the patient's skeleton to immobilize the patient and to provide a system of stereotactic coordinates for aligning radiation beams with the treatment site. Although a limited amount of experimental work was being done with stereotactic body frames for extracranial applications (Hamilton et al. 1995), the requirement of rigid fixation effectively limited radiosurgery to the cranium.

It was recognized at the time that a rigid stereotactic frame severely limited the practice of radiosurgery. The conventional frame was invasive and required fixation to bony structures. This requirement ruled out all soft-tissue sites for treatment. To maintain the stereotactic coordinate system, the frame had to remain in place from the time of treatment planning to the completion of the treatment fraction. This limitation compressed the treatment experience into a single, demanding day and did not allow for fractionation even when it might have had a therapeutic advantage. In short, conventional radiosurgery practice was driven more by its technical requirements and limitations than by basic therapeutic principles.

The concept behind the CyberKnife was to eliminate the frame and use the skeletal features themselves, via stereotactic projection imaging techniques, to define the stereotactic coordinates for planning and treatment. Without the frame, though, the patient could move. Maintaining beam alignment required two things—an imaging system to continually observe the position of the treatment site and a maneuverable linear accelerator that could continually adjust its position with respect to the patient. Essentially, the CyberKnife reversed the existing radiosurgery (and conventional radiation therapy) paradigm—to bring the patient to the beam—and instead brought the beam to the patient.

Although its individual components have evolved through several generations, the basic design and operation of the CyberKnife remains as follows (Figure 8.1):

1. A lightweight X-band 6 MV electron linear accelerator (linac) is mounted to an industrial robotic manipulator that can position and orient the treatment x-ray beam with complete freedom. The linac is configured without a beam flattening filter. The beam is cylindrically collimated to produce pencil beams ranging from 5 to 60 mm in diameter at a nominal source-to-target-distance (STD) of 80 cm. The beam diameter is set either by fixed collimator inserts

or, in the most recent CyberKnife® model, by a continuously variable mechanical iris collimator. Unlike a conventional gantry-mounted linac, the axis of the treatment beam is not constrained to a mechanical isocenter.

2. A kilovoltage radiographic imaging system comprising two orthogonal sources and opposed detectors takes x-ray images at programmable intervals during the treatment fraction to monitor the target position. The target's pose (position and orientation) in the workspace of the robot is defined via radiographic landmarks relative to its pose in the treatment planning study. If the target pose changes, the imaging system detects and measures the change and signals the robot to alter the position and/or direction of the treatment beam to compensate. The robot moves to the compensating new position in approximately 250 ms. In this manner, the planned configuration of beams is maintained even when the patient moves during treatment.

Although the CyberKnife concept and design was driven by the requirements of frameless radiosurgery, it is immediately obvious that it incorporates all of the basic principles of IGRT. The imaging system can establish beam alignment with any treatment site that can be located directly via anatomical landmarks or via implanted radio-opaque fiducials in x-ray images. These capabilities extended the use of radiosurgery to extracranial sites. Without the constraint of an invasive frame, the treatments can be divided into whatever fractionation scheme best suites the therapeutic problem and applied to soft tissue as well as skeletally fixed lesions. This introduced the option of hypofractionated radiation therapy as a mid course between conventional radiotherapy and single-fraction radiosurgery.

A complete technical description of robotic radiosurgery and IGRT, as performed via the CyberKnife, includes treatment planning, treatment delivery, and quality assurance. The focus of this chapter is on the image-guidance aspects, as they continue to represent the state of the art in radiographic imaging for IGRT. The essential feature of robotic IGRT is the acquisition of near-continuous intrafraction target position information from radiographic images. This performance requirement has driven all of the design elements in the CyberKnife image-guidance system. Other forms of IGRT address more limited subcategories of this general problem.

8.3 System Description

The CyberKnife comprises an X-band 6 MV linear accelerator mounted to an industrial robotic arm (KUKA Robotics, Augsberg, Germany) with 6 degrees of positioning freedom, a patient couch, a dual kV radiographic imaging system, and computer and electronic components to support treatment planning, image processing and display, performance monitoring and fault detection, and quality assurance. The imaging system acquires pairs of 2D kilovoltage projection images, determines from them the position of the treatment site within the robotic workspace, and reports the target coordinates

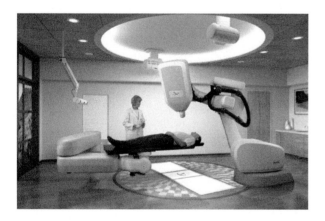

FIGURE 8.1 CyberKnife image-guided radiosurgery system with robot-mounted linac, patient couch, dual orthogonal imaging detectors in the floor, dual x-ray imaging sources mounted at the ceiling within the circular soffit, and the optical camera for the Synchrony respiratory tracking system depending from the ceiling mount at the upper left.

via a real-time control loop to the robot, which then moves to the necessary position to aim the planned beams at the target. If the target moves, the robot makes a compensating movement. This section will focus on the system design details that are relevant to intrafraction kV radiography.

8.3.1 Robotic Manipulator

In robotic IGRT, there is no mechanical isocenter—the treatment beam can be directed along any axis through any point in the vicinity of the treatment target. The significance of this from an imaging standpoint is that in principle the patient can be treated in any position from which the targeting landmarks can be seen in the imaging field of view. It is not necessary to place and hold the treatment site at a precise location (as is required for IGRT with gantry-mounted linacs). In practice, though, the patient must remain within one or two centimeters of a nominal reference setup position in order to have a practical working range for image registration and target tracking. For the purposes of coalignment of the imaging and beam delivery systems, the role of the mechanical isocenter is replaced by the concept of a *virtual isocenter*, which is nominally the origin of the imaging coordinate system and is related via a calibration procedure to the origin and orientation of the coordinate frame within which the robot defines the beam directions. In particular, it is not necessary that the linac, imaging, and treatment isocenters coincide. This has important implications for the accurate targeting of treatment sites that might be rotated relative to the treatment planning image. This topic will be elaborated upon in a later section.

The complete freedom of movement for the robotic arm supporting the linac means that the imaging and linac workspaces are not fixed and independent—it is possible for the robot to intrude into the line of sight of one or both imagers. This introduces imaging line-of-sight constraints into the beam planning procedure. From a quality assurance standpoint, the image processing and analysis software must be able to detect and accommodate unexpected obstructions or foreign objects in the radiographs.

8.3.2 Orthogonal Radiographic Imaging System

As seen in Figure 8.1, the present-generation G4 CyberKnife has two kV radiographic x-ray sources mounted at the ceiling and two 40×40 cm² amorphous silicon flat-panel digital imagers embedded in the floor on either side of the patient. The two source-to-image-receptor axes are orthogonal (for optimal 3D target position determination), while the projection of the patient's anatomy onto the floor receptors is at a 45-degree angle. The floor imagers are nominally 140 cm from the imaging center near the treatment site; source-to-image-receptor distance (SID) depends on the ceiling height (Antypas and Pantelis 2008). A nominal SID of 400 cm is typical for most model G4 installations. This geometry results in an imaging field of view of approximately 17×17 cm² at the nominal position of the treatment target.

Historically, patient setup via orthogonal planar projection images has relied upon the manual or semiautomatic 2D/2D registration of AP and lateral portal images to corresponding digitally reconstructed radiographs (DRRs) that define the ideal setup position. In this approach, accurate stereotactic 3D target position and pose measurement is problematic, partly because the two viewpoints are registered independently and partly because out-of-plane rotations are essentially undetectable. Furthermore, it constrains the imaging geometry to normal incidence projections in order to make reconstruction of the 3D position of the target tractable.

All of the image-guidance operations in a robotic IGRT system are based on automatic 2D/3D rigid registration of paired projection images to a 3D CT image. This approach uses a calibrated model of the actual kilovoltage imaging system geometry (whatever it might be) to match DRRs to the orthogonal projection images. This frees the system configuration from the conventional AP/lateral pair of views used for portal imaging, which has its origin in the visual interpretation of x-rays. From an automatic registration standpoint, the AP/lateral pair of views is in fact not optimal, as it is well known that the lateral view provides much poorer landmark visibility than the AP view. The CyberKnife and the BrainLAB ExacTrac X-ray system (BrainLAB AG, Feldkirchen, Germany) both employ symmetric oblique imaging viewpoints for the two x-ray imaging systems in order to provide balanced information to the registration process and to optimize the positioning of the imaging system elements in the treatment room. The oblique projection plane is fully accommodated in the camera model used for 2D/3D rigid registration. As observed above, both of these systems arrange the dual imaging axes to be approximately orthogonal in order to gain the best depth sensitivity, although in principle the two cameras can have an arbitrary separation angle.

Automatic 2D/3D rigid registration can completely determine the 6 degrees of freedom in the target's position and pose to within an uncertainty of a few tenths of a millimeter in translation and less than ½ of a degree in rotation (Fu and Kuduvalli 2008a; Murphy 1997). This level of precision meets the requirements of stereotactic radiosurgery. The 2D/3D rigid registration process will be discussed in more detail in a later section.

8.3.3 Synchrony Respiratory Tracking System

The ability of a kV radiography system to track targets that move with breathing will be limited by its imaging frame rate and by imaging dose considerations. It is possible, though, to combine the imaging system with a nonradiographic respiration monitor to provide a continuous surrogate measure of the target position that is periodically verified by images. This is the basis of the CyberKnife Synchrony system, which uses optical chest markers to provide a real-time respiration monitor, correlated to the tumor motion via periodic x-ray imaging (Schweikard et al. 2004). The frequency with which the imaging system updates the tumor/surrogate correlation is patient-specific and can range from once every few seconds to once per minute or longer. This will be described below in more detail.

8.4 Image Processing, Registration, and Alignment for System Guidance

The use of a dual kV radiography system in IGRT poses a problem in 2D/3D rigid image registration. The two images in the treatment room capture the patient's pose at a particular moment of time. The registration problem is to determine how that pose differs from the pose in the treatment planning image and also how it changes from one moment to the next. If there is a change, then the registration process computes the translation and rotation needed to describe the change, which is then used to either alter the beam alignment to conform to the new position or shift the patient back to the planning pose.

In the CyberKnife imaging system (as well as most other kV radiographic IGRT systems), the primary planning image that defines patient position is a CT study. This allows the most direct registration using radiographic landmarks. Much of the following discussion applies in general terms to any 2D radiographic patient positioning system.

For IGRT patient positioning systems that rely on 2D imaging devices, one conceptualizes the problem in the following way: (1) one imagines that the coordinate system of the planning CT has been transplanted to the treatment room, where it becomes the imaging coordinate frame; (2) the imaging frame is aligned with some physical reference in the treatment room; (3) the positions of the radiographic imaging system components (sources and detectors) within the imaging frame are measured with high precision (this is, the so-called camera model); (4) the camera model is used to calculate DRRs from the planning CT that emulate exactly what the imaging system would see if it were looking at the patient in the CT study; (5) one acquires alignment images and compares them to the DRRs via rigid image registration as if one were looking through the same imaging system at both the patient's CT and treatment room poses; (6) if the patient's position appears to differ in the two sets of images, the patient's CT pose is computationally altered via 2D/3D image registration until a new set of DRRs matches the alignment images, at which point one has determined the patient's shift within the imaging frame in going from the planning study to the treatment position. One then corrects either the patient or beam position.

Rigid 2D/3D registration requires an accurate measurement of the configuration of the dual imaging systems within the imaging coordinate frame. This is typically referred to as the *camera model*. The measurement is typically done using an imaging calibration phantom. A typical phantom has a number of point-like fiducials arranged in a 2D or 3D array. The phantom is imaged via CT as if it were a patient and then placed at a precise position in the treatment room, near the actual or virtual treatment beam isocenter. The position and orientation of the phantom defines the imaging coordinate system. Two projection images are acquired and registered to the phantom CT while allowing the registration process to adjust the camera model to achieve an optimal match between the phantom radiographs and the computed phantom DRRs. This calibration process is capable of determining the imaging geometry with submillimeter and subdegree accuracy.

To determine the patient's setup pose, one can do the 2D/3D registration two different ways: (1) by calculating a sequence of DRRs while iteratively adjusting the CT pose in real time, stopping when the newest set of DRRs best matches the alignment images (Murphy 1997); or (2) by precalculating a large sample of prospective patient poses, storing them in a lookup database, and then searching for the best match each time a new alignment image is taken. These two approaches represent competing tradeoffs between speed and accuracy of the registration. The most time-consuming part of 2D/3D registration has historically been the computation of the comparison DRRs, which made it difficult to do rapid repeat registrations for intrafraction movement tracking using real-time DRR iteration. Consequently, the commercially available CyberKnife employs a version of the lookup table strategy (Fu and Kuduvalli 2008a). Fast iterative 2D/3D registration was successfully used on the prototype CyberKnife at Stanford University (Murphy 1997) and has since become the basis of the BrainLAB ExacTrac x-ray system. Recently, the adaptation of graphics processing units to the image registration problem has dramatically increased the speed of DRR calculation and it is now feasible to do iterative 2D/3D DRR matching in near real time (Wu et al. 2007).

In image-guided patient setup, the patient's pose is represented entirely within the context of the imaging coordinate frame. Image registration simply emulates the effect of the patient moving around as if they were in the CT image. If the imaging system is separate from the treatment beam delivery system (as it is with the CyberKnife), a second geometrical problem enters—namely, the spatial relationship between the imaging frame and the frame of the beam delivery system. In an ideal world, the two frames would be exactly congruent and beam coordinates in the planning study would be exactly reproduced in the treatment room imaging frame; however, nothing is ever built with perfect precision. It is easiest to approach this problem by treating the imaging system as the world coordinate frame and positioning everything else (including the robotic linac) within it. It then suffices to measure the actual delivery position of the beams within the imaging frame. Any relative displacement of the two frames is a fixed, measurable offset by which one shifts either the patient or the beam positioning coordinates. However, the precision requirements for this measurement are crucial because it represents a source of systematic alignment error that affects all patients in exactly the same way.

One way to verify the imaging camera model, determine the accuracy of the registration process, and measure the offset for the beam directions in the imaging frame all at once is with a combination imaging/dosimetry phantom that can be used to completely emulate the planning and delivery process. Figure 8.2 illustrates one such phantom developed to calibrate the original

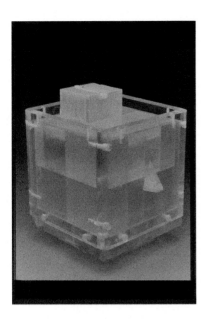

FIGURE 8.2 A dosimetric and imaging phantom that can be used to verify dose placement precision in an automated radiographic patient positioning system. The cube extending from the top has 12 layers of radiochromic film to form a 3D record of the dose position and density.

CyberKnife at Stanford (Murphy and Cox 1996). The body of the phantom itself is registered in the alignment images, but it also has four small radio-opaque fiducials attached to it to provide precise radiographic landmarks to validate the registration accuracy. Inside the phantom is a removable cube with 10 to 15 layers of radiochromic film spaced a few millimeters apart. The film cube, when exposed to a treatment dose, provides a 3D record of dose position and density relative to precisely defined landmarks that can be seen in a CT image.

The phantom is run through exactly the same end-to-end treatment procedure as a real patient. First, a CT scan is acquired and used to plan a spherical dose distribution at the precise center of the film cube. Then, the phantom is placed on the treatment couch and exposed to the planned dose using the same treatment imaging and position correction procedures as one would use for an actual patient (e.g., beam realignment for the CyberKnife; phantom repositioning for gantry linac systems).

After exposure, the center of the delivered dose distribution is measured. Any shift from the intended position of the dose can be attributed to a combination of image registration errors, robotic pointing errors, and the mechanical offset between the beam delivery system and the imaging coordinate frame. By repeating this test multiple times, the random registration and pointing errors average out. The remaining systematic errors and the coordinate frame offset can then be measured to high precision and compensated in the image alignment software. Once this calibration has been made, all subsequent tests will put the dose distribution at or very near the targeted isocenter. In the first applications of this procedure, the CyberKnife was found to have overall dose placement precision of 1.7 mm

(Murphy and Cox 1996). After numerous refinements (Chang et al. 2003), the test now shows 0.3–0.5 mm precision, depending on the imaged landmarks (Antypas and Pantelis 2008). This measurement determines the overall dose placement precision for image-guided stereotactic radiosurgery and radiotherapy, incorporating all of the uncertainties associated with target localization in the treatment planning CT study, mechanical coalignment of the imaging and linac coordinate frames, image registration precision, and mechanical positioning accuracy of the linac by the robot.

8.5 Image-Guidance Scenarios

8.5.1 Target Sites

There are two broad categories of treatment site that can be directly monitored radiographically for IGRT—those that are rigidly associated with bony landmarks and those in soft tissue. In both categories, localization can be enhanced by implanting radio-opaque fiducials in or near the target. Generally speaking, most soft-tissue sites can only be localized with confidence in kV radiographs via fiducials. In addition, some moving soft-tissue sites can be located and tracked indirectly by observing surrogate landmarks that are highly correlated with the tumor motion and inferring from them the position of the target. In this chapter, indirect localization and tracking will be considered only insofar as it involves radiographic imaging of the surrogate or a combination of target imaging and surrogate tracking.

The first applications of robotic IGRT targeted intracranial lesions using the conventional radiosurgical assumption that everything within the skull moves rigidly with it. It was therefore sufficient to use the bony outline of the skull in the 2D/3D rigid image registration process. It should be noted, though, that rotation of the skull can displace treatment sites more or less substantially according to their distance from the axes of rotation. This prompted early attention to rigid registration for all 6 degrees of freedom (Murphy 1997).

The first extracranial applications of the CyberKnife tracking system were for lesions that could be assumed to be rigidly connected to the spinal column (Chang et al. 1998; Murphy et al. 2000; Ryu et al. 2001). These treatments divided themselves into cervical, thoracic, and lumbar sites according to the clarity of the radiographic images. The cervical vertebrae can be clearly resolved in oblique kV radiographic images and consequently the neck treatments used skeletal landmarks from the outset. Vertebral bodies elsewhere are more difficult to resolve and were first targeted with the assistance of fiducial screws implanted close to the lesion (Murphy et al. 2000). This approach remained the standard of practice for spine treatments for a considerable time. It has recently been demonstrated that skeletal landmarks along the entire spine can be used for fast, robust, fully automatic 2D/3D registration and targeting (Muacevic et al. 2006).

Figure 8.3 is a screenshot of the CyberKnife image registration software for a spinal target setup using the vertebral bodies of the neck as the rigid anatomical targeting landmarks. The

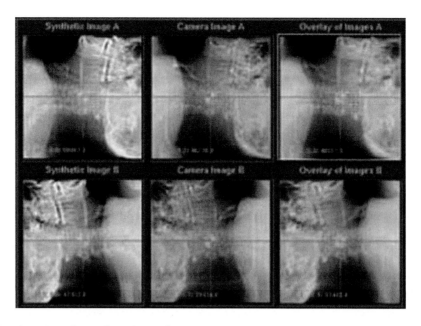

FIGURE 8.3 A screenshot from the CyberKnife tracking software, showing two orthogonal radiographs of the cervical spine (center images, top and bottom), together with the digitally reconstructed radiographs matched to them via 2D/3D rigid image registration (left images, top and bottom).

figure shows the orthogonal projection radiographs side by side with the DRRs generated by the 2D/3D rigid registration process to match the radiographs. The quality of the match can be verified by overlaying the DRRs with the radiographs to check bony landmark alignment. A visual verification of the registration is typically done before enabling the robot to shift the linear accelerator to the new position.

The first extracranial soft-tissue sites to be treated with intrafraction image guidance were pancreatic tumors (Murphy et al. 2000). To make these targets radiographically visible, small gold fiducials were sutured to the tumor during exploratory laparotomy. Although it is now sometimes feasible to locate certain thoracic tumors directly in a kV radiographic imaging system (Fu et al. 2008b), most soft-tissue lesions still require fiducial localization. (Figure 8.4 shows an instance in which fiducials have been implanted in a thoracic tumor that is itself clearly visible in outline.)

When using robotic beam targeting, it is important to recognize the interplay between translations and rotations in determining the target location via rigid registration. Unlike kV radiographic systems integrated with gantry-mounted linacs, CyberKnife-type image-guided alignment does not require that the lesion or the targeting landmark be at the imaging/treatment isocenter. If the lesion is offset from the isocenter, then the robot's translational alignment correction calculated from a rigid registration with only translational degrees of freedom will be different than the correction calculated when the registration includes rotational degrees of freedom. Consequently, the degrees of freedom allowed in the image registration should match the degrees of freedom that will be corrected (Murphy 2007).

The use of implanted fiducial markers to locate soft-tissue targets is well established but not without uncertainty. Any

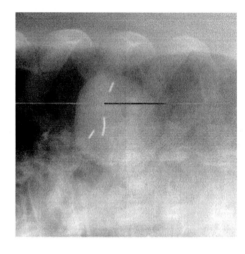

FIGURE 8.4 A radiographic image of a lung tumor containing four gold fiducials, taken with a real-time amorphous silicon imaging system during a CyberKnife lung radiosurgery treatment.

fiducial can potentially migrate within the lesion and even become lost. If only a single fiducial is implanted, there is no reliable way to tell if it has remained in the same place from treatment planning through delivery. A single point-like fiducial also does not give any indication of target rotation. Three or more fiducials are required to measure rotations; additionally, any changes in their relative spacing can be used as a signal for migration. More fiducials provide better targeting accuracy, but it has been shown that increasing the number beyond six provides little additional improvement (Murphy 2002).

Soft-tissue target sites near the diaphragm (e.g., pancreas and liver) might be expected to move in close synchrony with the diaphragm during free breathing. In this case, the diaphragm could be used as the radiographic landmark for targeting. However, it has been observed that the pancreas motion is also highly correlated with external abdominal motion (Murphy 2004), which would allow for external surrogate tracking without the added imaging dose.

8.5.2 Imaging Frequency

From the earliest development of the CyberKnife, it was recognized that, although continuous fluoroscopic imaging would provide the most complete and unambiguous target position information, the concomitant dose would be unacceptably high. For example, using the CyberKnife dose rate of 0.05–0.1 cGy per image frame for lumbar and sacral spine imaging (Table 8.1), the local dose for continuous imaging (assuming 100 ms exposure per frame) during a typical 20-min fraction would be 600–1,200 cGy. Consequently, the system was developed for periodic radiographic imaging at rates that could be adjusted to balance targeting accuracy with cumulative imaging dose. This approach introduced the problem of optimizing the imaging frequency based on how the patient/lesion moves and on how uncorrected movements would influence dose coverage.

There are three types of intrafraction target motion that can be encountered in IGRT—random, systematic, and periodic. Each requires a different approach to determining the imaging frequency.

The practical realities of tumor tracking preclude the possibility of continuous real time tracking of rapid random movements. The strategy for tracking random movements therefore assumes that most movements are small and will average out while large movements are infrequent. Rather than spend time and diagnostic imaging dose continuously observing the target position when it is not making consequential movements, the patient is instead imaged at intervals that are timed to detect and correct for the occasional large movement before a significant amount of dose has been misdirected. The frequency of imaging is related to the frequency of large movements. Imaging at regular intervals yields a random sample of the movements, which when collected into a frequency distribution can be used to estimate the optimum imaging frequency.

Generally, observations show that intrafraction movement of most sites (excepting breathing motion) does in fact consist of many small random fluctuations, together with a few large shifts, around a mean position that can drift over time (Hoogeman et al. 2008; Murphy et al. 2003). Analysis of several hundred patient position tracking records from CyberKnife treatments has shown that position sampling at approximately one minute intervals is usually sufficient to maintain one millimeter tolerance in the known target position over extended (e.g., 20–30 min) radiosurgery fractions (Murphy et al. 2003). However, the distinctive effect of systematic drift (which causes dose offset) leads to a significantly larger target coverage error compared to the effect of random motion (which results in dose blurring). This larger error is demonstrated via the population-based margin formulae developed by Stroom et al. (1999) and Van Herk

et al. (2002), which weight systematic setup errors as 3–4 times more significant than random errors. By again looking at a large body of tracking data from intrafraction radiographic imaging of cranial and spine sites and interpreting it in terms of the margins needed to maintain the prescribed intrafraction target coverage, one can show that periodic intrafraction imaging at 1–2 minute intervals is necessary to maintain 1 mm targeting tolerance in the face of the kind of systematic movement that patients actually exhibit (Murphy 2009).

If the motion is periodic, as with respiration, one can exploit a combination of radiographic imaging of the target and surrogate tracking of the breathing (Schweikard et al. 2000). This approach is developed in the CyberKnife Synchrony system. To combine tumor and surrogate tracking, it is assumed that some correlation exists between the respiratory movement of the tumor and breathing motion observed, e.g., at the surface of the chest. Rather than image the tumor continuously via fluoroscopy (Shirato et al. 2000), one can monitor it at intervals while using the correlated surrogate motion to interpolate the tumor position between images. Periodic imaging allows one to adapt the surrogate correlation function to changes that are well known to occur in respiratory tumor motion (Hosiak et al. 2004; Ozhasoglu and Murphy 2002; Tsunashima et al. 2004). The frequency of imaging is then determined mainly by the anticipated rate of change of the correlation function (Schweikard et al. 2004).

8.6 Real-Time Tumor-Tracking

When an IGRT system attempts to perform synchronous tracking of a continuously moving target, the translation of position information into a corrective beam response takes a finite amount of time that must be allowed for in the control loop; otherwise the beam will lag behind the target and be systematically out of alignment. One corrects for lag time by predicting the future position of the target (Murphy 2008; Murphy et al. 2002; Sharp et al. 2004) so as to "lead" the target with the beam. Obviously, it is possible to predict the target's future position only if the target motion is in some way deterministic. Perfectly synchronous tracking of random motion is not possible.

If image guidance is used exclusively to observe the tumor position, then all of the image acquisition, processing, and registration time is added into the system lag time. Because control loop prediction algorithms become progressively less accurate as the lag time increases, this presents a design tradeoff between longer imaging times for increased measurement accuracy versus shorter lag times for increased response accuracy. If one wishes to track tumors directly via fluoroscopy, this places severe time constraints on the image processing and analysis algorithms that can be used (see for example Cui et al. 2007).

In a system like Synchrony that combines radiography and surrogate tracking, the radiographic corrections to the surrogate correlation function are made asynchronously and consequently the image acquisition and processing time does not enter into the control loop delay. System lag is set by the response time of the optical tracking system (e.g., 30 ms) in series with the robot response. This allows one to spend more time processing the images for high accuracy than would be possible if the imaging system had direct real-time control of the robot.

8.7 Imaging Dose Considerations

Repetitive imaging during IGRT gives a non-negligible concomitant dose to the patient (Murphy et al. 2007). The clinician should take all reasonable measures to minimize this dose while maintaining adequate imaging information for treatment. When kilovoltage radiography is used for intrafraction tracking, the radiographic imaging technique, frequency, field of view, spectral hardness, and other parameters can (and should) be adjusted to optimize the cost/benefit of the imaging dose. As discussed earlier, imaging frequency should be tailored to the timescale of anticipated movement. Even continuous movement, as with respiration, does not require continuous fluoroscopic imaging. The Nyquist theorem shows that data sampling at rates higher than twice the highest frequency in the signal spectrum adds no additional information. If breathing is reasonably regular and has a period of 2–4 s, then acquiring an image every second is nominally sufficient. This has encouraged those who use intrafraction imaging to develop pulsed fluoroscopy to reduce unnecessary dose (Shirato et al. 2004).

The imaging field of view should likewise be minimized. Although this does not reduce local dose and its deterministic risk for skin and eye injury, it does reduce effective dose, which is the quantity of significance when estimating stochastic risk of radiation-induced cancer.

In the CyberKnife imaging system, the x-ray source/patient entrance distance is nominally 250 cm for cranial radiosurgery and 240 cm for body radiosurgery. The source operates at between 100 and 120 kV, has 2 mm of aluminum filtration, and is collimated to a square field that is nominally 17×17 cm^2 at the patient (Murphy et al. 2007). The source collimator is telescopic, which allows the field size to be adjusted. Table 8.1 summarizes the ranges of technique and approximate entrance dose per image for targets at various body locations (data provided by Accuray Inc., Sunnyvale, CA). For the abdominal and pelvic sites, the patient's body weight strongly influences the technique required to get good images. As previously described, the Synchrony technique refers to a special function of the CyberKnife system that tracks thoracic and abdominal treatment sites that move

with breathing; the x-ray imaging technique for these sites uses a shortened exposure period to reduce motion blurring. The total exposure for each target position determination has contributions from two orthogonal imaging projections, with a doubling of dose wherever the collimated source fields overlap at the patient. These dose levels are typical for fixed kV radiographic imaging systems in the treatment room (e.g., the BrainLAB ExacTrac system).

8.8 Summary

This chapter reviews technical elements of intrafraction kV radiographic imaging as it is employed for target tracking by the CyberKnife image-guided radiosurgery system. This particular system incorporates all of the essential elements of 2D radiographic imaging for beam alignment, and it is the only commercially available system that couples the image-guidance process directly to the beam delivery system via robotic principles. However, much of this review is generally applicable to the use of 2D radiography for patient/beam alignment in IGRT.

The use of kilovoltage projection imaging provides improved image quality and a reduction in imaging dose compared to megavoltage portal images (Murphy et al. 2007). Experience with the CyberKnife has demonstrated that frame-based radiosurgical dose placement precision can be maintained in a frameless system that can detect and adapt to patient movement via intrafraction kV imaging. It has further demonstrated that, for treatment sites rigidly connected to radiographic landmarks such as bony anatomy or implanted fiducials, it is sufficient to acquire a pair of orthogonal projection images and register them via 2D/3D rigid registration techniques to the planning CT study. The use of automatic 2D/3D registration furthermore allows complete freedom in placing and orienting the imaging components to optimize the workspace configuration in the treatment room.

8.9 Disclosure

The author discloses a financial interest in Accuray Incorporated, manufacturers of the CyberKnife.

References

Adler JR, Murphy MJ, Chang S, and Hancock S. 1999. Image-guided Robotic Radiosurgery, *Neurosurgery* 44: 1299–1307.

Antypas C and Pantelis E. 2008. Performance evaluation of a CyberKnife G4 image-guided robotic stereotactic radiosurgery system, *Phys Med Biol* 53: 4697–4718.

Chang SD, Murphy MJ, Geis P, et al. 1998. Clinical experience with image-guided robotic radiosurgery in the treatment of brain and spinal cord tumors, *Neurologia Medico-Chirurgica* 38(11): 780–783.

Chang SD, Main W, Martin DP, Gibbs IC, and Heilbrun MP. 2003. An analysis of the accuracy of the CyberKnife: a robotic frameless stereotactic radiosurgical system, *Neurosurgery* 52(1): 140–147.

TABLE 8.1 Measured planar radiographic entrance dose levels per image for the CyberKnife image-guided radiosurgery system

Site	Kv	mA	Ms	mAs	mGy
Cranium and C-spine	105–125	100	100	10	0.25
T-spine	120–125	100–150	100–125	10–20	0.25–0.50
L-spine	120–125	100–200	100–150	10–30	0.25–0.75
Sacrum	120–125	100–300	100–300	10–90	0.25–2.00
Synchrony	120–125	100–300	50–75	5–22.5	0.10–0.50

Cui Y, Dy JG, Sharp GC, Alexander B, and Jiang SB. 2007. Multiple template-based fluoroscopic tracking of lung tumor mass without implanted fiducial markers, *Phys Med Biol* 52(20): 6229–6242.

Dempsey J, Benoit D, Fitzsimmons J, et al. 2005. A device for real time 3D image-guided IMRT, *Int J Radiat Onc Biol Phys* 63: S202–S202.

Fu D and Kuduvalli G. 2008a. A fast, accurate, and automatic 2D-3D image registration for image-guided cranial radiosurgery, *Med Phys* 35(5): 2180–2194.

Fu D, Kahn R, Wang B, et al. 2008b. Fiducial-free lung tumor tracking for CyberKnife radiosurgery, *Int J Radiat Oncol Biol Phys* 72(1): S608–S609.

Hamilton AJ, Lulu BA, and Fosmire H. 1995. Preliminary clinical experience with linear accelerator-based spinal stereotactic radiosurgery, *Neurosurgery* 36: 311–319.

Hoogeman MS, Nuyttens JJ, Levendag PC, and Heijmen BJM. 2008. Time dependence of intrafraction patient motion assessed by repeated stereoscopic imaging, *Int J Radiat Oncol Biol Phys* 70(2): 609–618.

Hosiak JDP, Sixel KE, Tirona R, Cheung PCF, and Pignol JP 2004. Correlation of lung tumor motion with external surrogate indicators of respiration, *Int J Radiat Oncol Biol Phys* 50(4): 1298–1306.

Kupelian P, Willoughby T, Mahadevan A, et al. 2007. Multi-institutional clinical experience with the Calypso System in localization and continuous, real-time monitoring of the prostate gland during external radiotherapy, *Int J Radiat Oncol Biol Phys* 67(4), 1088–1098.

Muacevic A, Staehler M, Drexler C, Wowra B, Reiser M, and Tonn JC. 2006. Technical description, phantom accuracy, and clinical feasibility for fiducial-free frameless real-time image-guided spinal radiosurgery, *J Neurosurg Spine* 5(4): 303–312.

Murphy MJ and Cox RS. 1996. Accuracy of Dose Localization for an Image-guided Frameless Radiosurgery System, *Med Phys* 23: 2043–2049.

Murphy MJ 1997, An automatic six-degree-of-freedom image registration algorithm for image-guided frameless stereotaxic radiosurgery, *Med Phys* 24: 857–866.

Murphy MJ, Adler JR, Bodduluri M, et al. 2000. Image-guided radiosurgery for the spine and pancreas, *Comput Aided Surg* 5: 278–288.

Murphy MJ. 2002. Fiducial-based targeting accuracy for external-beam radiotherapy, *Med Phys* 29: 334–344.

Murphy MJ, Jalden J, and Isaksson M. 2002. Adaptive filtering to predict lung tumor breathing motion during image-guided radiation therapy, Proceedings of the 16th International Congress on Computer-Assisted Radiology and Surgery, Paris, pp. 539–544.

Murphy MJ, Chang S, Gibbs I, et al. 2003. Patterns of patient movement during image-guided frameless radiosurgery, *Int J Radiat Oncol Biol Phys* 55(5): 1400–1408.

Murphy MJ. 2004. *Tracking moving organs in real time*, Seminars in Radiation Oncology, Chen and Bortfield, Editors, Vol. 14, no. 1, pp. 91–100.

Murphy MJ. 2007. Image-guided patient positioning: if one cannot correct for rotational errors in external-beam radiotherapy setup, should the rotations be measured? *Med Phys* 34(6): 1880–1883.

Murphy MJ, Balter J, Balter S, et al. 2007. The management of imaging dose during image-guided radiotherapy, Report of the AAPM Task Group 75, *Med Phys* 34(10): 4041–4063.

Murphy MJ. 2008. Intra-fraction geometric uncertainties in frameless image-guided radiosurgery, *Int J Rad Onc Biol Phys* 73(5): 1364–1368.

Ozhasoglu C and Murphy MJ. 2002. Issues in respiratory motion compensation during external-beam radiotherapy, *Int J Radiat Oncol Biol Phys* 52:1389–1399.

Raaymakers BW, Lagendijk JJW, Van der Heide UA, et al. 2004. Integrating a MRI scanner with a radiotherapy accelerator: a new concept of precise on line radiotherapy guidance and treatment monitoring, 14th Proceedings of the International Conference on the Use of Computers in Radiation Therapy (Seoul, South Korea), pp. 89–92.

Ryu S, Kim D, Murphy MJ, et al. 2001. Image-guided frameless robotic stereotactic radiosurgery to spinal lesions, *Neurosurgery* 49: 838–847.

Schweikard A, Glosser G, Bodduluri M, Murphy MJ, and Adler JR. 2000. Robotic motion compensation for respiratory movement during radiosurgery, *Comput Aided Surg* 5: 263–277.

Schweikard A, Shiomi H, and Adler J. 2004. Respiration tracking in radiosurgery, *Med Phys* 31: 2738–2741.

Sharp GC, Jiang SB, Shimizu S, and Shirato H. 2004. Prediction of respiratory tumour motion for real-time image-guided radiotherapy, *Phys Med Biol* 49: 425–440.

Shirato H, Shimizu S, Kunieda T, et al. 2000. Physical aspects of a real-time tumor-tracking system for gated radiotherapy, *Int J Radiat Oncol Biol Phys* 48: 1187–1195.

Shirato H, Oita M, Fujita K, Watanabe Y, and Miyasaka K. 2004. Feasibility of synchronization of real-time tumor-tracking radiotherapy and intensity-modulated radiotherapy from viewpoint of excessive dose from fluoroscopy, *Int J Radiat Oncol Biol Phys*, 60: 335–341.

Stroom JC, DeBoer HCJ, Huizenga H, and Visser AG. 1999. Inclusion of geometrical uncertainties in radiotherapy treatment planning by means of coverage probability, *Int J Radiat Oncol Biol Phys* 43(4): 905–919.

Tsunashima Y, Sakae T, Shioyama Y, et al. 2004. Correlation between the respiratory waveform measured using a respiratory sensor and 3D tumor motion in gated radiotherapy, *Int J Radiat Oncol Biol Phys* 60(3): 951–958.

Van Herk M, Bemeijer P, Lebesque JV. 2002. Inclusion of geometric uncertainties in treatment plan evaluation, *Int J Radiat Oncol Biol Phys* 52(5): 1407–1422.

Wu J, Kim M, Peters C, Liu J, Palta J, Li S, and Samant S. 2007. Patient positioning using a fast robust 2D-3D registration strategy with a registration quality evaluator, *Int J Radiat Oncol Biol Phys* 69(3) S43–S43.

9

Respiratory-Correlated CT

Carnell J. Hampton
Wake Forest University

9.1 Introduction: Challenges of Respiratory Motion in Radiotherapy

Effective management of intrafraction organ motion during radiotherapy has historically been considered a "holy grail" that, when viewed in the context of improvements in image-guided radiotherapy (IGRT), may now be achievable in the common practice of clinical radiation therapy (Shirato et al. 2007). Intrafraction motion has many physiological sources, including the motion of organs associated with cardiac, gastrointestinal, and respiratory function. Even before the introduction of advanced, computer-aided diagnostic-quality imaging as the basis for 3D treatment planning, clinicians and physicists were well aware of and considered the consequences of organ motion for the placement and planning of radiotherapy portals. For much of the modern history of external beam radiotherapy, the delivery of radiation to targets in the thoracic cavity involved the planning of relatively simple, large treatment portals because of a lack of quality methods for assessing and quantifying disease *in situ* over the course of therapy. This method of delivering radiation prescriptions attempted to balance the need to deliver therapeutic doses of radiation to cancer cells while acknowledging the tradeoff of limiting doses to the critical structures. The resulting suboptimal delivery associated with this still recent era of radiotherapy is evident in the historically low local control rates for certain cancers of the lung and abdomen associated with convention fractionated radiotherapy when compared with dramatically improved local control provided by new, highly focused hypofractionated dose schemes (Fakiris et al. 2009). The

opportunity for hypofractionated radiotherapy and other delivery schemes that leverage favorable radiobiology, however, have only been possible because of a technological evolution in imaging and image-guided interventions. While improvements in diagnostic imaging have increased the ability of clinicians to detect disease, the targeting of tumor targets remains fraught with uncertainties including target delineation variability, daily setup uncertainty and, to a lesser degree, intrafraction motion, that greatly influence the optimal dosimetric delivery of radiotherapy. The common usage of PET/CT imaging has paid dividends toward the addressing the challenge of improving target delineation variability (Greco et al. 2007; Senan et al. 2005). With IGRT rapidly becoming the standard of care in radiotherapy, many of the challenges related to daily setup uncertainty are also being addressed (Bissonnette et al. 2009a, 2009b; Dawson and Jaffray 2007; Xing et al. 2006). Intrafraction motion assessment has benefited in many ways from the advances and investment in IGRT technology, thus making the attempt to manage the uncertainties desirable as well as feasible (Sonke et al. 2009).

The complex physiological and pathological processes involved in the voluntary and involuntary motion of muscles during respiration have been difficult to model, much less account for in a practical manner when performing routine clinical delivery. Then there is the matter of correlating visible external anatomic motion associated with respiration with the actual motion of the internal target. Uncertainty abounds from the complexities related to the mechanics of imaging moving targets to the task of reliably predicting the stability of a patient's respiratory pattern for a particular treatment or even a treatment course (Balter et al. 1996; Redmond et al. 2009; Spoelstra 2009).

TABLE 9.1 A sample of published lung motion data

	Lower Lobe			Middle Lobe			Upper Lobe		
Observer	SI	AP	LR	SI	AP	LR	SI	AP	LR
Barnes	18.5 (9–32)			7.5 (2–11)					
Erridge	12.5 (6–34)	9.4 (5–22)	7.3 (3–12)						
Plathow	9.5 (4.5–16.4)	6.1 (2.5–9.8)	6.0 (2.9–9.8)	7.2 (4.3–10.2)	4.3 (1.9–7.5)	4.3 (1.5–7.1)	4.3 (2.6–7.1)	2.8 (1.2–5.1)	3.4 (1.3–5.3)

Source: The mean range of motion and minimum–maximum ranges in millimeters. Adapted from AAPM Report #76
SI = superior/inferior direction; AP = anterior/posterior direction; LR = left/right direction.

9.1.1 Organ Motion and Dynamic Imaging

An important aspect in quantifying the uncertainty of target motion is the use of an appropriate imaging technique that captures the desired information with sufficient spatial and temporal resolutions. Fluoroscopy, because of its once widespread use in radiotherapy simulation, has traditionally been used to assess the motion of tumors of the thoracic and abdominal cavities, either imaging the target directly or relying on some surrogate for the target (Ekberg et al. 1998). Direct target observation using fluoroscopy is difficult for most soft-tissue targets without the presence of a radiographic fiducial marker such as surgical clips, bony landmarks, or an indwelling catheter imbedded in or near the tumor. The 2D nature of fluoroscopy also yields limited information regarding the true 3D motion of targets. More recently, 3D imaging modalities have been used to provide improved visualization of anatomy in motion. Dynamic fast MRI has been used to visualize respiratory motion and quantify tumor motion in three dimensions and even to assess the correlation between internal targets and external surrogates (Plathow et al. 2005). Published studies using a number of imaging methods have demonstrated that both the lung and the liver demonstrate widely varying magnitudes of motion (Tables 9.1 and 9.2). Lung tumor motion has been shown to exceed 2 cm while some liver tumors can exhibit motion in excess of 4 cm even with shallow breathing (Barnes et al. 2001; Suramo et al. 1984).

9.1.2 CT Imaging Artifacts for Dynamic Targets

The primary imaging modality useful in the calculation of dose deposition in radiotherapy is computed tomography. Modern computed tomography imaging uses a rotating single collimated x-ray source and multiple coplanar and noncoplanar mounted detectors to acquire projection data that can be reconstructed into a "slice" of tomographic data. When coupled with patient translation, multiple slices can be acquired and "stacked" into a 3D dataset. The electron densities derived from Hounsfield units captured in CT image voxels are useful in calculating the deposition of dose for radiation beams traversing the patient contour (Xing et al. 2007). The earliest implementation of CT imaging involved the rather slow acquisition of data, providing temporally averaged data that blurred the effects of intrafraction motion and presenting a case not unlike that of the free-breathing

TABLE 9.2 A sample of published liver motion in SI direction in millimeters

Observer	Shallow Breathing	Deep Breathing
Weiss	13 ± 5	
Suramo	25 (10–40)	55 (30–80)
Davies	10 (5–17)	37 (21–57)

Source: Adapted from AAPM Report #76

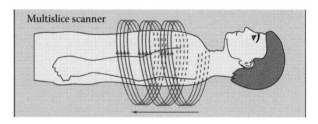

FIGURE 9.1 An illustration of modern multislice computed tomography image acquisition. Adapted from BMJ 2002; 322: 1078.

radiotherapy patient during the course of therapy. The evolution of CT imaging includes the transition from the acquisition of a single slice of significant thickness to multiple submillimetric slices simultaneously (Figure 9.1). With this evolution, data acquisition times are now relatively rapid, resulting in the acquisition of data randomly distributed throughout the breathing cycle. The limitations of CT imaging are apparent as unwanted imaging features result from the miscorrelation of the temporal patterns of highly mobile anatomy and image acquisition.

These artifacts within an image slice are evidence of the violation of assumptions made by common projection reconstruction algorithms regarding anatomic invariability during CT data acquisition. The result of temporal miscorrelation is somewhat unpredictable and potentially significant especially when viewed in the context of targeting small, mobile lesions with small-field radiotherapy portals and highly focused radioablative doses (Shimizu et al. 2001). Errors in target delineation can adversely affect dose-calculation accuracy. Phantom studies can demonstrate some of the potentially significant imaging effects, but the not unsubtle and tell-tale artifacts, including skips, volume averaging, and mislocations when imaging the diaphragm of patients can often be seen on CT treatment planning patient datasets (Figure 9.2).

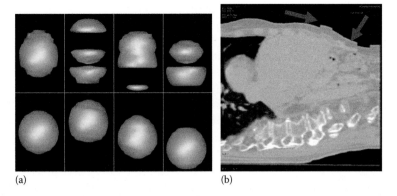

FIGURE 9.2 (a) CT images of a spherical object in motion (top row) along with 4DCT images of the object imaged in varying states of the motion cycle (bottom row). (Reproduced from Rietzel et al., *Med. Phys.*, 32: 874–889, 2005b. With permission.) (b) Artifacts captured on a sagittal view from a helical CT acquisition for a clinical patient.

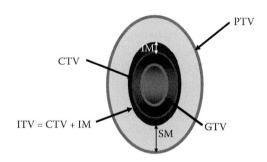

FIGURE 9.3 ICRU 62 descriptions of radiation therapy target constructs.

While margins can play an important role in overcoming the uncertainty in target delineation when imaging mobile targets, there is little consensus on the appropriate selection of margins nor the method by which they are applied, when the international standards and practices of ICRU 62 are used as a guide (ICRU). The international consensus nomenclature addresses intra- and interfraction uncertainties but fails to explicitly address uncertainty in target delineation, although the effects—while difficult to quantify practically—have been demonstrated academically (Steenbakkers et al. 2005).

9.1.3 Dosimetric Effect of Respiratory Motion

The ICRU 62 nomenclature specifies the internal tumor volume (ITV) as an expansion of the margin of the clinical tumor volume (CTV), to account for uncertainty with respect to target size, shape, and position variability relative to anatomy (ICRU). The ITV reflects patient-specific measurements or perhaps, patient-population based observations derived from temporally correlated studies or empirical margin calculators (Figure 9.3). In the absence of respiratory-correlated CT-based treatment planning, it is difficult to know the magnitude of margin needed to accurately reflect uncertainties resulting in the needless exposure of nontarget tissue to high doses of radiation or inadequate coverage of the clinical target. While covering the limits of target motion with the ITV may ensure coverage, the

increased likelihood of exposing healthy tissue in the radiation field to high doses may make the development of an acceptable treatment plan more challenging. Deleterious effects resulting from temporal miscorrelations have been simulated, predicting negative consequences to optimal clinical outcomes (Mechalakos et al. 2004) in patients with large respiration-induced motion. While normal breathing and conventional (1–2 cm) 2D GTV-PTV margin expansion are typically adequate to prevent consequential deviations from desired coverage, individual patients with large breathing excursions and/or irregularly shaped and large tumors are at some risk for decreases in tumor control probability (Bissonnette et al. 2009a, 2009b; Hughes et al. 2008). The same study revealed similar limitations for the coverage of lung tumors using GTV/CTV-to-PTV margin expansions (0.5–1 cm longitudinally, 0.5 cm axially) typically found in stereotactic body radiotherapy (SBRT). Target coverage as evaluated by DVH analysis indicated that mobility-related factors were negatively correlated with a loss of coverage for lung tumors (Wulf et al. 2003). Others have suggested that the use of "standard" or population-based margins not based on respiratory-correlated imaging may unnecessarily irradiate normal tissue when tumor motion estimated with time-averaged imaging is less than predicted (van Sornsen de Koste et al. 2001). The conclusion of many investigators is that dose delivery to targets with margins optimized based on respiratory-correlated imaging is a requirement for dose escalation.

9.1.4 Reproducibility of the Breathing Cycle

It is entirely feasible that methods to accurately quantify respiratory motion can be found given advances in imaging. A fundamental consideration, however, for methods mitigating the consequences of respiratory motion in radiotherapy is the realistic observation that the respiratory cycle may not behave predictably for imaging and treatment sessions nor for the duration of therapy. This uncertainty can make the class of solutions based on the observation of a single or few respiratory imaging sessions risky and can lead to flawed radiation delivery if assumptions are made incorrectly. Clinical studies involving the use of imaging prior to daily radiotherapy and later, other in-room, real-time imaging modalities (Section 9.1.5), point to the importance of measuring patient-specific breathing variations to minimize the uncertainty associated with breathing cycle variability (Bissonnette et al. 2009a, 2009b; Purdie et al. 2006). Published clinical experiences promote, for some, the importance of tracking and gating technologies that link precision therapy to knowledge of the location of the tumor at all times (Smith et al. 2009; Underberg et al. 2005).

9.1.5 Real-time Assessment of Motion

Real-time imaging in or near the treatment room is integral to closing the loop between uncertainties associated with the simulation and treatment of patients in general, and the localization of mobile targets specifically. While conventional 4D CT systems in the simulation suite or CT-on-rail systems within the treatment delivery room can provide assessments of the reproducibility of target motion on the day of treatment (Purdie et al. 2006, Slotman et al. 2006, Juhler-Nottrup et al. 2008), they cannot provide real-time imaging of the mobile target along with synchronous delivery of therapy. Table 9.3 describes many of the commercial systems available for real-time imaging and delivery. Real-time tracking technologies can be grouped by their ability to directly or indirectly track tumor motion. A drawback of many direct imaging systems is the requirement that patients endure an invasive implantation procedure. A related consideration is the ability to correlate external surrogates to internal targets when indirect tumor tracking is used. Another important factor when weighing real-time technologies is an evaluation of whether a particular target tracking technology involves the delivery of additional nontherapeutic ionizing radiation and whether the imaging dose is justified. One limitation of real-time motion assessment and therapy is the potential for inefficient dose delivery.

So-called low duty cycle techniques are ultimately a tradeoff between efficiency and treatment precision that must be considered when evaluating the appropriateness of a real-time technique for a particular patient and treatment delivery method. The limitations of real-time imaging and gating will be discussed in more detail in Section 9.1.6.3).

Beyond initial real-time imaging for tumor localization, real-time imaging also plays a significant role throughout the delivery process, providing feedback for adaptation of the therapy delivery system. Real-time assessment of the respiratory signal contributes to predictive algorithms that can theoretically be used to account for time delays in data processing and mechanical repositioning of the delivery system (Keall et al. 2001, Seppenwoolde et al. 2002; Sharp et al. 2004).

9.1.6 Motion-Management Techniques

9.1.6.1 Physiological Management

While various technologies for real-time assessments and therapy have been commercialized, there are a few practical, low-tech methods for respiratory motion management that have been used clinically. Deep-inspiration breath-hold methods seek to delivery therapy during a reproducible state of maximum breath-hold while using a spirometry system that monitors the air-flow associated with respiration (Rosenzweig et al. 2000). By coaching the patient during simulation, the point of maximum lung inflation can be determined and used for CT-simulation image acquisition. The acquired deep-inspiration CT dataset is subsequently used for treatment planning and reference images are created for delivery. Therapy is delivered by turning the beam on only during a period where the patient maintains a target breath-hold level. Variations on this technique have been used clinically, including allowing the patient to direct self-held breath-holds with the ability to interlock the beam when the breath-hold is relinquished (Kim et al. 2001). A key indication for this method is the ability of a patient to maintain a reproducible breath-hold. A training session used to monitor and coach patients prior to a simulation session has been suggested as a possible method of increasing the chances of obtaining a reproducible breathing signal. Such a session, however, typically requires increased personnel and technical resources relative to normal simulation sessions.

TABLE 9.3   Commercial real-time motion assessment technologies

Technology	Target Imaging Method	Uses Ionizing Radiation	Correlation Method	Comments/References
BrainLab Adaptive Gating	Direct	Yes	Fiducials	Figure 9.4c; Willoughby et al. 2006; Jin 2008
Mitsubishi/RTRT	Direct	Yes	None	Shirato 2007
Anzai AZ-733V	Indirect	No	Electronic feedback	Li et al. 2006
Accuray Synchrony	Indirect	Yes	Infrared fiducials	Figure 9.4d; Ozhasoglu et al. 2008
Varian RPM	Indirect	No	Infrared fiducials	Figure 9.4a; Vedam et al. 2003
Vision/Gate RT	Indirect	No	3D surface	Figure 9.4b; Hughes et al. 2009

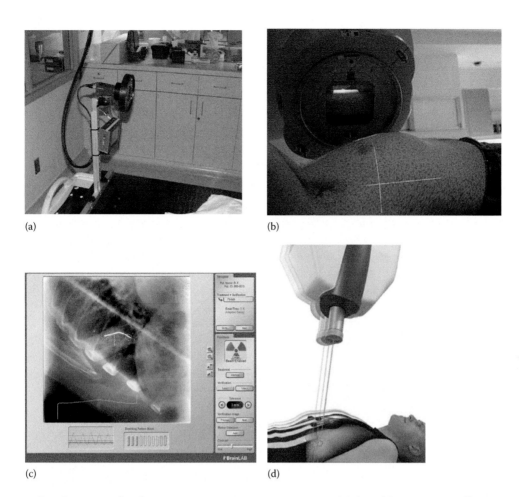

FIGURE 9.4 Examples of commercial real-time motion assessment/management technology. (a) Varian RPM, (b) Vision RT, (c) BrainLab Adaptive Gating, (d) Accuray Synchrony. (Images used with permission from Accuray Incorporated: Darren J. Milliken, Counsel; Vision RT permission granted by Norman Smith, CEO, Vision RT Ltd.)

9.1.6.2 Physical Management

An active-breathing control (ABC) technique has been used to improve the reproducibility of a patient's breath-hold (McNair et al. 2009; Remouchamps et al. 2003; Wong et al. 1999). A spirometry-like device uses a balloon valve to force a breath-hold at a specified lung volume for a predefined and patient dependent duration of time. Like all breath-hold techniques, a patient's pulmonary function status and comfort with the technique is a key factor that limits applicability to patients with undiminished respiratory status. These techniques are therefore better suited for therapy to patients with abdominal malignancies. Another method of forcing a desired respiratory state involves the use of an abdominal compression device to control diaphragmatic motion (Heinzerling et al. 2008; Lax et al. 1994). Typically, shallow breathing can be forced by applying pressure to the abdomen using a compression "paddle" during simulation and treatment. On-board fluoroscopic treatment available on some IGRT-capable linear accelerators allow for the monitoring of the reproducibility of motion range.

9.1.6.3 Respiratory Gating/Synchronization

The technique of synchronizing the delivery of radiation during a particular portion of the respiratory cycle has come to be widely known as gating. A gating technique can be used during both imaging and treatment to reduce the uncertainty related to the position of mobile tumors (Vedam et al. 2003). The potential for margin reduction becomes feasible with gating since radiation is only delivered during a set window of the respiratory cycle. The width of this window influences the level of residual motion captured during beam-on. For simulation and treatment, a respiratory signal must be acquired using either an internal fiducial marker or an external signal as a surrogate for internal targets. Commercial systems have typically used a detector system capable of directly or indirectly capturing anterior–posterior abdominal movement associated with respiration. During imaging, the detected respiratory signal can be used to trigger CT acquisition once per breathing cycle over several cycles (Figure 9.5a). This approach is called *prospective 4D CT*. The detected respiratory signal is used to automatically enable the radiation beam for image acquisition or treatment. Systems that detect internal fiducial markers utilize multidimensional fluoroscopic or similar imaging modalities to track markers, triggering the delivery of radiation when the target is in the desired position. Gated delivery is complex, requiring rigorous patient-related quality assurance (Huntzinger et al. 2006; Jiang et al. 2008). Sources of error include the potential for the use of an inadequate surrogate for tumor motion, resulting in misalignment of the position of the gate with respect to the motion of anatomy during respiration.

Irregular breathing can affect the initial gated imaging session causing the capture of unintended portions of the breathing cycle (Figure 9.5b). The duty cycle—a measure of treatment efficiency—for gated therapy has been measured to be about 30–50% of an ungated therapy for 3D conformal radiotherapy (Jiang 2006a,b). Gated IMRT delivery is even more inefficient because of the time needed to account for the beam-off time associated with step-and-shoot MLC motion. Even when delivery efficiency is increased by favoring a larger gating window, a tradeoff is made with respect to residual tumor motion that implies dosimetric consequences for the target. The choice of the proper

gating window customized for each patient to maximize the tradeoff is evidence of the effort that must be invested in proper implementation of gated therapy. The target/anatomy within the gating window becomes the focus of the treatment planning process and the associated generation of reference imaging for proper treatment setup. Consistency is required between the gating window used for treatment planning and the daily patient setup requiring image-guidance techniques to minimize the inter- and intrafractional miscorrelations that can occur between the internal target, the bony anatomy, and any external gating device. Simulation studies (Juhler-Nottrup et al. 2008a, 2008b) have showed that even when an IGRT-like bony anatomy matching setup strategy is used for lung radiotherapy, the center of volume variance for targets over the course of therapy can measure up to 5 mm. It was theorized by the authors that some of this variation could have been the result of systematic changes in baseline position due to miscorrelation of the external/internal motion. The benefits of gated delivery at end-exhalation were explored for SBRT by a group of researchers (Guckenberger et al. 2009) who computed the relationship between tumor-motion

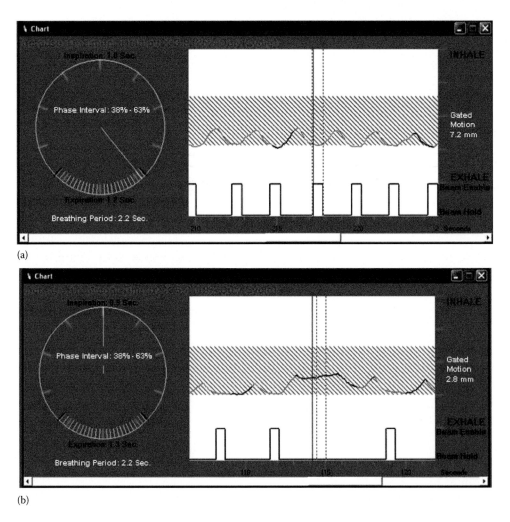

(a)

(b)

FIGURE 9.5 Respiratory traces of patients used for 4D CT simulation. (a) Regular breathing trace; (b) breathing trace of a patient affected by an interruption in the regular breathing cycle.

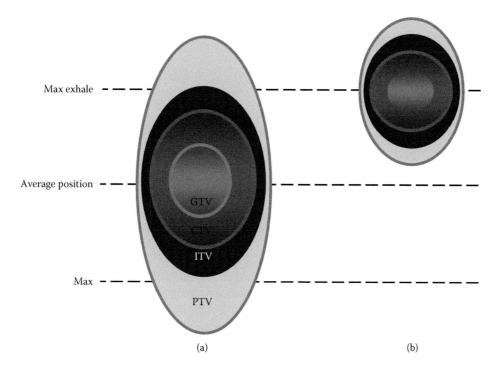

Max exhale

Average position

GTV

CTV

ITV

Max

PTV

(a)   (b)

FIGURE 9.6 An illustration of target structures created using 4-D CT data. (a) A target expansion reflecting the encompassing volume of all breathing phases plus setup margin. (b) The target expansion covers motion during a portion of the breathing cycle, near maximum exhalation, typical of that used for gated treatment delivery.

amplitudes and the magnitude of safety-margins needed to provide adequate dosimetric coverage of the CTV (Figure 9.6). When compared with free-breathing techniques, the reduction in treatment margins achieved by gating techniques (37.5% gating window) was 5 mm when compensating for cranial–caudal motions of less than 15 mm. The role of gating for targets with respiratory-induced motion >15 mm may be better justified when the expense of complex gated techniques provides confidence of significant target margin reduction.

9.1.6.4 Motion Compensation

In contrast to the complexity of gated or synchronized therapy, the simplicity of motion compensation techniques make them most likely to be implemented in the largest number of radiotherapy clinics. While gating of the therapy process with the respiratory cycle possesses numerous uncertainties and tradeoffs, motion compensation techniques can be uncoupled from the radiation delivery process if the appropriate measures are taken during treatment simulation, planning, and daily setup to minimize or eliminate systematic uncertainties while compensating for suspected random uncertainties. In fact, motion compensation techniques make only minimal assumptions about reproducibility of a patient's breathing pattern from simulation to the end of therapy and rely on the systematic application of target margins. The technological requirements for motion compensation present few barriers for many modern radiotherapy departments. The independence of the simulation and treatment delivery allow even those

radiotherapy departments without modern CT equipment but with access to diagnostic imaging departments with modern CT scanners the opportunity for motion compensation.

At minimum, motion compensation requires data that provide measures of the mean tumor position and the range of tumor motion. These data must be gathered at the time of CT acquisition such that many of the effects of target motion affecting radiotherapy treatment planning (Section 9.1.2) can be mitigated. One method of obtaining the necessary data is to acquire CT data in a slow-scanning mode, mimicking the early era CT acquisition techniques described in Section 9.1.2. During this procedure, patients continue free-breathing during the scan. With the treatment couch also slowed such that the time of a full respiratory cycle is longer than data acquisition, the slow-CT scan provides for the extent of target motion anatomy during the acquisition. The result is a blurred image reflecting the target motion at the time of simulation. Slow-CT works only in high-contrast areas of anatomy such as lung tumors since the motion blurring can obscure targets in close proximity to normal density (e.g., water-equivalent) anatomy. Another limitation is the increased dose associated with the longer acquisition time for slow-scanning techniques.

A directed breath-hold CT acquisition can be thought of as a form of manually gated data acquisition, capturing only the anatomy associated with a distinct portion of the breathing cycle. By acquiring imaging data in two separate scans while a patient holds their breath during maximum exhale followed by inhale, distinct data sets capturing the extent of tumor motion are available for image fusion (Hughes et al. 2008). The combined datasets provide a target for treatment planning without the blur associated with slow-CT imaging. Breath-hold CT acquisition accomplishes the goal of determining tumor motion extent but does so without collecting organ motion information. The simulation paradigm suffers from being dissimilar to the treatment delivery paradigm, which is most likely performed during free-breathing or light respiration, creating the possibility that the tumor excursion measured in the two scans may be inconsistent with the normal range of motion. Breath-hold scans also suffer from motion artifacts that can effect the delineation of targets (Rietzel et al. 2005b).

9.2 4D CT Image Formation

Many of the motion management techniques described in the previous sections have found limited usefulness in radiotherapy clinics for many reasons. The use of generous margins for both setup and intrafraction uncertainty based on experience and practice is a typical solution. There has been a general lack of understanding of how the absence of patient-specific motion management has a disparate impact on the population of patients undergoing thoracic or abdominal radiotherapy. Even relatively basic motion encompassing methods such as slow-CT and breath-hold CT have not been widely implemented because of the initial unavailability of even low-tech imaging technology like commercial image-fusion software. These methods also possessed some well-described limitations (Section 9.1.6.4).

Four-dimensional computed tomography (4D CT), also known as respiratory correlated CT, is a technique that presents an opportunity to collect comprehensive temporal information as well as 3D spatial information useful for treatment planning and delivery (Rietzel et al. 2005a, 2005b). In fact, both the blurred "average" image of a slow-CT and the separate gates of the breath-hold methods can be thought of as subsets of a 4D CT dataset. 4D CT technology, as deployed commercially within radiotherapy clinics, uses similar hardware to that described for gated image acquisition, including technology that uses external surrogates to correlate the respiratory cycle with the acquisition of CT slice data. 4D CT simulation can use either a prospective or retrospective protocol to reconcile the captured temporal and spatial information. A prospective protocol (previously described in Section 1.6.3) results in the collection of a single dataset, reflecting spatial information during a single selected phase of the respiratory cycle. Prospective, gated-CT acquisition is indeed a time-resolved 3D CT imaging and is classified by some as 4D CT, but falls short of providing optimal information about the totality of organ or target, given that it captures data from one preselected breathing cycle window. A retrospective acquisition method, in contrast, produces multiple 3D datasets capturing spatial imaging at several phases of the breathing cycle (Section 9.2.2). Retrospective acquisition acquires data nearly continuously during periodic motion using an axial cine scanning mode or a very-low pitch helical scanning mode. The retrospective acquisition method is described in literature most

often associated with 4D simulation with applicability to motion compensation techniques as well as gated treatment delivery.

9.2.1 Simulation

4D CT simulation becomes an option for any patient for whom there is a concern that respiratory motion may complicate or compromise the creation of a deliverable treatment plan that meets the prescribed parameters. Data from studies attempting to correlate the position of tumors within the lung with an expected magnitude and trajectory have generally been conflicting, suggesting that perhaps any patient with targets in the thorax or abdomen may be a candidate for 4D CT simulation (Seppenwoolde et al. 2002). 4D CT, in fact, provides a method of "triage" because of the ease with which it can be incorporated into the simulation workflow. While a reproducible breathing pattern is desirable, especially for gated treatment delivery, retrospective 4D CT is generally robust enough to yield useful information for motion compensation even when the measured breathing cycle is less than optimal (Riboldi et al. 2009).

9.2.2 Image Acquisition

4D CT simulation typically begins by positioning the patient on the CT table using conventional simulation techniques and appropriate immobilization. Prior to image acquisition, a device capable of monitoring the anterior–posterior motion of an external surrogate of the respiratory cycle is placed in contact with the patient. Alternately, a device that directly measures respiratory volume can also be use to provide respiratory cycle data. Using either method, information about the length of a breathing period can be determined typically with commercial software and provided as input to the CT scan parameters. For retrospective sorting of 4D CT images, a cine CT scan is initiated during free-breathing such that multiple rotations of the CT for image acquisition are performed at a single couch location for a time equivalent to the maximum observed respiratory cycle plus the time needed for one full CT tube rotation. By acquiring data by this method, multiple images of a particular portion of the anatomy at different times throughout the breathing cycle are acquired before moving to another "slice" of anatomy and repeating the process until the desired longitudinal section of anatomy is covered. In between table positions, the x-ray source is turned off. While image acquisition is being performed, the marker measuring the respiratory signal is continuously collecting phase and amplitude information and correlating respiration with a temporal stamp from the CT scanner marking whether an image is actively being acquired (x-ray beam is "on") or not ("off").

The CT acquisition should use a slice thickness appropriate for the site being imaged with awareness that the amount of scan data, as well as dose, generated by the cine CT technique increases as the slice width decreases. Once the desired longitudinal range is covered, the respiratory signal tagged with the x-ray on/off information is typically processed offline by taking the temporally and sequentially acquired reconstructed

CT slice data and matching each slice data with the nearest corresponding phase of the respiratory cycle during which it was acquired. The slice data are then resorted such that for each phase of the respiratory cycle, a complete, sorted set of images covering the complete longitudinal range is available, i.e., there is a set of slices all at end expiration, another set at end inspiration, and others for a number of phases in between (Figure 9.7). The number of phases represented in the final sorting is prescribed by directing the frequency with which the respiratory cycle is sampled. Ten phases are typically used covering a complete breathing cycle by dividing the total breathing period by 1/10th, e.g., a 6-s breathing cycle sampled every 0.6 s. If end inspiration is 0% of the breathing cycle, end expiration is typically around 50–60% of the breathing period after inspiration (Rietzel et al. 2005b). Multiple options are available for treatment planning using the resulting multiple sorted datasets (Section 9.2.4).

9.2.3 Respiratory Coaching

Practically, 4D CT data acquisition can be accomplished with the patient performing reproducible, free breathing. Irregularities in a patient's breathing cycle can impact the retrospective resorting algorithm. Since the number of discrete phases is preselected, phase selection during the resorting process chooses the nearest appropriate phase within a range or phase tolerance. Incorrectly sorted slices can either be incorporated into the dataset, resulting in artifacts, or they can be excluded from the individual phase datasets—a choice that has consequences for treatment planning when the individual phase datasets are used for determining optimal gating phases (Rietzel et al. 2006a). Partial volume-like effects due to the velocity of moving objects during CT scanner rotation can be seen in reconstructed images with the effect pronounced for spherical geometries (Rietzel et al. 2005b).

Respiratory coaching at the time of simulation and treatment has been used by some to regularize patient's respiratory cycles during 4D CT acquisition, especially if gated treatment delivery is the goal. Regular breathing helps to maximize the benefit of gated delivery by improving selection of peak inhale and exhale phases during which residual motion of a target can be minimized. Audio, visual, and combined audiovisual biofeedback techniques have been used to investigate improvements in breathing reproducibility for 4D CT simulation and treatment (George et al. 2006). While these techniques have shown some reduction in variability for a given duty cycle, gains have to be placed in context with the presence of other limitations including cycle to cycle reproducibility that are not specifically addressed by the described methods.

9.2.4 4D CT Treatment Planning

Once 4D CT data are acquired and processed, it is available in the form of multiple 3D datasets available for use in the treatment planning process. In some treatment planning/ virtual simulation software packages, processed 4D CT data can be viewed along side other multimodality datasets for side-by-side assessment and incorporation into the planned target design. In this environment, the impact of potential temporal miscorrelation associated with temporally uncorrelated datasets is readily apparent. In Figure 9.8, target volumes associated with temporal imaging (ITV_{4D} and ITV_{Gating}) of a highly mobile target are dramatically different than the gross tumor visualized with a lung window on a helical CT dataset (Figure 9.8b), which appears to be affected by CT reconstruction errors.

4D CT data presents the possibility to incorporate patient-specific motion details for both targets and organs of interest. One of the most comprehensive methods of incorporating temporal information into the treatment planning process

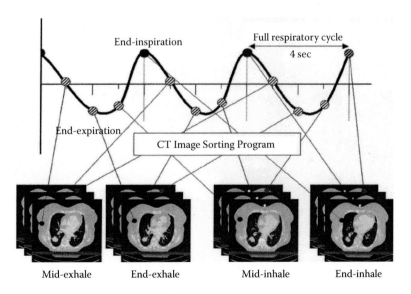

FIGURE 9.7 A diagram depicting the process of retrospectively sorting 4D CT data. (From Underberg, RWM, et al., *Int. J. Radiat. Oncol. Biol. Phys.*, 60: 1283–1290, 2004.)

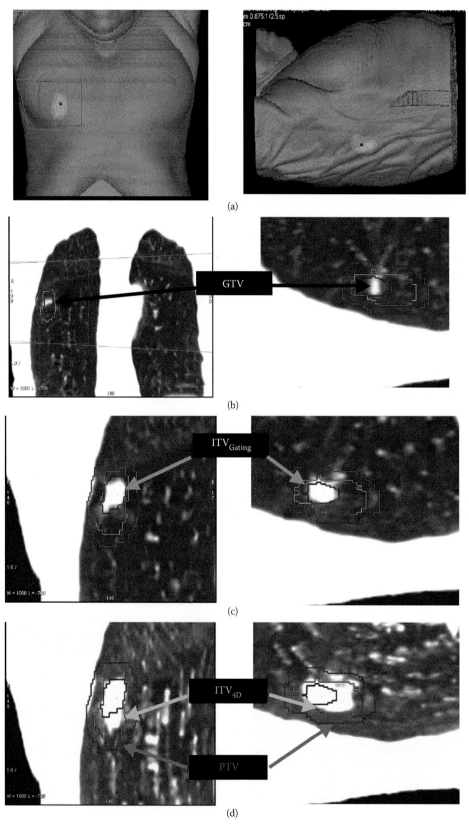

FIGURE 9.8 Target volumes derived from 4D CT data. 3D representation of a patient with a lung lesion from coronal and sagittal viewpoints (a). 2D views of the patient with contours overlaid atop (b) a conventional helical CT scan, (c) a 30% phase dataset, chosen as the gating window, and (d) a MIP dataset. The blue contour (ITV$_{Gating}$) represents the target within a chosen gating window. The yellow contour (ITV$_{4D}$) was created by contouring the target on the phase datasets. The red contour represents a PTV expanded from ITV$_{4D}$ contour.

is to import the multiple 3D phase datasets into the virtual simulation or treatment planning software where contours can be drawn on each phase images (Rietzel et al. 2006a, 2006b). Given the raw phase datasets, targets can be contoured on each dataset—a time-consuming process that ultimately leads to the examination of maximal excursions of motion as well as other parameters associated with the contour centroids. Manual contouring on multiple respiratory phase images is challenging to implement clinically, given the time- and personnel-related constraints common in most clinics (Cover et al. 2006). Animated cine loop visualization of organ and target motion displayed in axial, sagittal, and coronal planes, in combination with the ability to contour on those visualizations, provides users with a more robust and elegant method of defining targets.

Approaches seeking to create composite volumes have been created from the union of phase contours. Breath-hold-type targeting can be derived from 4D data by choosing to create a composite volume based on contours derived from the fusion of exhale and inhale phase datasets. Care must be taken to choose the extrema phases by visual inspection since there are potential phase shifts between internal target motion and external surrogates (Rietzel et al. 2005b). The approximated composite contour can be easily verified by displaying the overlaid contour on each of the phase images. This retrospective 4D CT technique addresses one of the inadequacies of estimating an accurate motion envelope based on extrema contours since the data were acquired under a free-breathing protocol instead of as separate fused breath-hold scans. Other potential sources of error remain, including the potential of hysteresis effects that are not captured with extrema imaging techniques (Seppenwolde 2002). If gated treatment delivery is a goal, then the phase data can be also observed to determine the optimal phases for which the target exhibits minimal residual motion (Figure 9.8c). Planning target volumes for gated therapy derived from phase bins near end expiration have been shown to provide a reduction in planning target volume versus targets created using population-derived margins or motion-encompassing derived margins (Underberg et al. 2005).

Beyond time-saving methods such as 4D CT-derived extrema imaging, other methods have been described that produce composite image datasets approximating tumor excursion. The maximum intensity projection (MIP) or maximum intensity volume (MIV) is created by projecting the maximum Houndsfield unit value for corresponding voxels from each phase dataset onto a new synthetic CT volume (Rietzel 2008) (Figure 9.8d). For lung tumors, significant density differences between tumor tissue voxels involved in breathing and surrounding tissues will indicate the GTV extent. Care must be used in relying solely on MIP or MIV display for target delineation because of target boundary uncertainties resulting from the possible occlusion of targets adjacent to or abutting high-density structures (Underberg et al. 2005). Differences between MIP or MIV contours and the composite contours created from the union of contours on multiple datasets may also be subject to the same intra- and interuser variability observed for manual contouring. A motion-similar technique similar to the MIP or MIV approach

makes use of a time-weighted mean or midventilation projection image (Smith et al. 2009; Wolthaus et al. 2006).

To minimize the time-consuming process of contouring on multiple phase datasets, automatic deformable image registration has been used to create motion envelopes based on contours originally defined on one phase dataset (Zhang et al. 2005). Deformable image registration uses nonrigid techniques to track voxel changes due to the deformation of organs and targets caused by respiration. The union of the original contour and the contours deformed through the remaining phase datasets ideally captures the tumor excursion although, practically, the analytical solution to the optimization problem that is the basis of deformable image registration dose not necessarily give an exact answer. Motion envelopes derived from deformable registration must be validated to ensure that they are not compromised. Deformable image registration requires a separate segmentation step to minimize complications that arrive from applying the registration algorithm to stationary and moving anatomy found within the region of the thoracic cavity.

9.2.5 4D Dose Calculation

4D dose calculation approaches have been described that also make use of deformable image registration to assess dose on a per voxel basis. The use of 4D treatment planning allows for the creation and evaluation of 4D DVHs for both targets and normal lung (Rietzel et al. 2005a). It is generally accepted that the motion of lung tissue within a "static" dose distribution results in the blurring of deposited dose (Lujan et al. 1999). 4D dose calculation has been used to derive information on the relationship between motion amplitude of targets and the corresponding increase in field size needed to compensate dosimetrically when compared to free-breathing treatment. Dosimetric optimization seeks to minimize the overcompensation of margins when target motion due to respiration is large (Mutaf and Brinkmann 2008). High-accuracy treatments such as SBRT require optimization of margins while balancing target coverage, normal organ dosing, and respiratory motion compensation. It has been shown that geometrical optimization using a motion encompassing ITV construct can lead to overcompensation for breathing motion and increased doses to normal lung tissue when motion due to respiration is less than 2 cm (Gukenberger 2009). A related treatment planning approach that has been described aims to incorporate the effects of tumor motion on dose calculation by blurring a static dose distribution in response to quantitative data on an individual patient's tumor-temporal derived probability density function (van Herk et al. 2003; Yan et al. 1997).

9.2.6 PTV Generation

4D CT provides a means of reducing some of the uncertainties common to the delineation of thoracic and abdominal targets and improves the process by which gross tumor volumes are created when compared with helical scanning only. Interobserver contour variation must still be explicitly accounted for (Stroom and Heijmen 2002). Consensus on appropriate clinical target volume (CTV) expansion accounting for microscopic disease is generally absent in the literature, reflecting limited correlation research with pathological data (Grills et al. 2007; Stroom et al. 2007). Composite target volumes, generated by manual contouring on multiple phase datasets, extrema segmentation, or rapid segmentation using MIP, MIV, or midventilation synthetic targets, generally capture an approximation of internal motion and can be classified as representative of the encompassing internal tumor volume (ITV) concept described in ICRU 62 formulation (Hughes et al. 2008). Many of the approaches described in literature for the generation of planning target volumes (PTV) add safety margins to the GTV or CTV, reflecting internal and setup uncertainty margins added in quadrature (Rietzel et al. 2006b). Others have simply expanded the ITV isotropically with a margin reflecting measured setup data for a population of relevant patients for a given immobilization/treatment system (Nelson et al. 2006; Slotman et al. 2006). On-board IGRT imaging is most appropriate for the gathering of interfrational as well as intrafractional uncertainty data (Bissonnette et al. 2009a, 2009b; Grills et al. 2008). Beyond the ITV concept, 4D CT provides quantitative, individualized data about internal tissues useful in the determination of systematic and random uncertainties associated with the treatment planning of targets affected by physiological motion. When 4D CT is combined with IGRT, treatment planning margin recipes may be employed using appropriate uncertainty data to calculate geometrically or dosimetrically optimized dose distributions for the common clinical situation of treatment for a free-breathing patient (McKenzie et al. 2000; Stroom and Heijmen 2002). The potential for dose escalation for an individual patient highlights the importance of appropriate margin determination and the role that 4D CT and IGRT play in properly accounting for uncertainties both during treatment planning as well as throughout the treatment process through adaptive techniques. The addition of 4D cone-beam computed tomography (4D CBCT) technology and the potential for margin reduction and adaptive treatment planning are addressed in Sections 9.3.1 and 9.3.2.

9.2.7 Temporal Imaging and Multimodality Imaging

The use of physiological imaging in modern radiotherapy treatment planning has become typical for a number of anatomical sites. The presence of combination PET/CT scanners has streamlined the acquisition of anatomical and physiological imaging in the treatment position while minimizing the limitations inherent in the registration of datasets acquired on separate scanners (Jarritt et al. 2006; Nehmeh et al. 2004; Erdi et al. 2004). Respiratory motion impacts the accurate acquisition of PET images. 4D PET will be discussed further in Chapter 14.

9.3 Image-Guided and Gated Treatment Delivery

Many of the choices available to the planner for 4D treatment planning have been described in previous sections. While many methods preserve delivery time by including temporal information in the treatment planning process, their application to a particular patient's course of therapy may not be appropriate especially if nonoptimal treatment plans are required to compensate for intra- and interfractional motion. Despite the increased treatment time and the additional workload associated with assuring the quality of a dynamic process, consideration of motion-compensating tracking/gated treatment delivery options may be most appropriate especially for large motion amplitudes in the range of >15 mm (Gukenberger 2009). When coupled with image-guidance, gating techniques allow for the use of minimal safety margins around target tissues since setup and localization uncertainties are effectively minimized (Underberg et al. 2005).

Gated treatment delivery typically utilizes much of the same hardware used during the simulation process. A detected stable signal correlated either directly or indirectly to the internal target motion due to respiration is used to enable the radiation beam, delivering dose during a prespecified phase (Brandner et al. 2006; Smith et al. 2009). Most commercial systems allow for manual intervention in the event of a loss of respiratory signal stability. Breathing coaching, if used during simulation, is also used for gated treatment. If detected, variations in residual motion during the gating window can be resolved by narrowing the window at a cost of longer delivery times. When gating is used for intensity-modulated radiotherapy (IMRT), care must be taken to consider the effect of interplay between leaf motion and target motion as well as the potential for a significant increase in treatment time relative to conventional and non-gated IMRT (Jiang 2006a, 2006b).

Gated treatment delivery has been discussed most frequently as a solution in radiotherapy for thoracic tumors including nonsmall-cell lung cancer (NSCLC) and metastatic lung tumors. With lower lobe tumor motion measured up to 1.85 cm in published studies (Barnes et al. 2001), and varying greatly from patient to patient, gated delivery provides margin reduction, minimization of unnecessary dose to normal tissues, and improved dose coverage relative to radiotherapy delivered during free breathing. Much of the published literature has described theoretical benefits of gated therapy for dose escalation (Nelson et al. 2006) and SBRT. The efficacy of gated delivery in concert with image guidance for correction of setup errors, and methods accounting for delineation uncertainties and baseline drifts has been demonstrated (Guckenberger et al. 2009).

Gated treatment for abdominal cancers such as those involving the liver has been studied as an optimal solution for an organ with a mean displacement measured up to 2.5 cm (Suramo et al. 1984). Since the liver is poorly imaged when using planar imaging techniques, it is common for gated therapy to utilize planar IGRT of an internal surrogate, stereoscopic fluoroscopy, or respiratory-correlated CBCT to provide visualization of a target. While there is the potential for complications when fiducial implantations are performed (Murphy 2004), imaging of internal surrogates provides the validation of respiratory signal tracking necessary when external fiducials are used (Jin et al. 2008; Willoughby et al. 2006). Given an accurate patient setup and a stable respiratory trace, a megavoltage beam can be gated to the requested phase. In one published study, gated SBRT has been described with excellent clinical results (Wurm et al. 2006). Comparisons between expected setup based on markers placed on the skin and gated localization based on internal markers within the liver demonstrated the potential for setup errors if gated localization is not used.

While gating is most often described as a solution for the problem of respiratory motion in radiotherapy for lung and liver tumors, the technique has also played a role in the treatment of other cancers. For breast cancer, one published simulation study evaluated the effects of CTV-PTV margin expansions needed to compensate for intrafraction respiratory motion states ranging from respiratory gated (symbolically negligible motion) to heavy breathing (George et al. 2003). DVH analysis of contoured target and normal structures indicated increases in heterogeneity for the PTV, decreases in CTV heterogeneity and increased doses to normal structures with increased respiratory motion. As in the case of other clinical sites, the dosimetric improvements derived from gating techniques must be weighed against the increased effort needed for implementation.

9.3.1 4D/gated Treatment Delivery Quality Assurance

At each step in the process of 4D radiotherapy, from simulation to treatment delivery, technical, patient- and process-related quality assurance procedures must be employed to prevent systematic errors that can compromise patient care. All applicable linac and CT imaging quality assurance tests described in guidance documents should be performed with the specified tolerances and frequencies. AAPM Task Group 142's report on quality assurance of medical accelerators list monthly and annual tests related to respiratory gated accelerator operation that should be performed by a qualified medical physicist (QMP) (Klein et al. 2009) (Table 9.4).

Dynamic phantoms capable of producing simple cyclical motion or more complex human respiratory simulations are particularly useful in evaluating the feedback processes involved in image acquisition and treatment delivery. General as well as technology-specific quality assurance parameters are described in the report of AAPM Task Group 76 (Keall et al. 2006). A necessary measure in assuring the quality of temporal imaging and/or delivery is to confirm the synchronization of the radiation beam with the patient's respiratory cycle. External respiration monitors must accurately predict internal tumor position to prevent the consequences described in Section 9.1.6.3. Training, competence, and vigilance by the radiation oncology staff involved in respiratory management are highly recommended.

For some commercial 4D CT acquisition methods, the analysis of peak inhalation and exhalation data for retrospective

TABLE 9.4 A summary of quality assurance recommendations for respiratory gating as described in AAPM Report # 142

Procedure	Tolerance	
	Monthly	Annual
Beam output constancy	2%	
Beam energy constancy		2%
Phase, amplitude beam control	Functional	
In-room respiratory monitoring system	Functional	
Temporal accuracy of phase/ amplitude gate on		100 ms of expected
Calibration of surrogate for respiratory phase/amplitude		100 ms of expected
Gating interlock	Functional	Functional

4D CT reconstruction includes the automatic assignment of motion phases based on the rise and fall of an abdominal surrogate. The automated routines used in this process, however, may be subject to incorrect phase assignments as well as the invalidation of some phase segments when processing irregular breathing cycles. This deficiency suggests that a quality assurance process is needed to insure the correct determination of respiratory phase and to minimize the image artifacts caused by inaccurate phase assignments. Rietzel et al. (2006a) have proposed manual postprocessing that has been demonstrated to improve the resorting process and minimize motion artifacts (Figure 9.9).

With the increased interest in highly conformal, hypofractionated treatment routines, the localization process involved in the delivery of therapy for highly mobile tumors takes on added significance. For gated delxivery, verification of setup typically makes use of gated or cine 2D radiographs (Jiang 2006a,b), fluoroscopy (Hugo et al. 2007), or perhaps gated or respiratory-correlated 3D images. Care must also be taken when targets are localized for treatment with portals designed based on motion encompassing target volumes derived from 4D. Underberg et al. (2006) used repeat CT scanning during a 5-week course of radiotherapy to show the potential for interfractional shifts of center of mass ITV position, which was surmised to be caused by radiation-induced changes in the surrounding normal tissues. The reported findings strengthen the case for the need for daily IGRT as a means of mitigating the potential for mislocalization of therapy portals and assuring the quality of the prescribed stereotactic therapy (Figure 9.10). Haasbeek et al. (2007) further explored the necessity for adaptive therapy using repeat 4D CT to demonstrate minimal dosimetric impact due to the time trends of mobile targets over a short hypofractionated treatment course.

9.3.2 IGRT for Treatment Quality Assurance

For mobile targets that can be directly and easily visualized using 3D imaging, IGRT has proven to be an important tool for localization for therapy (Bissonnettee et al. 2009a, 2009b,

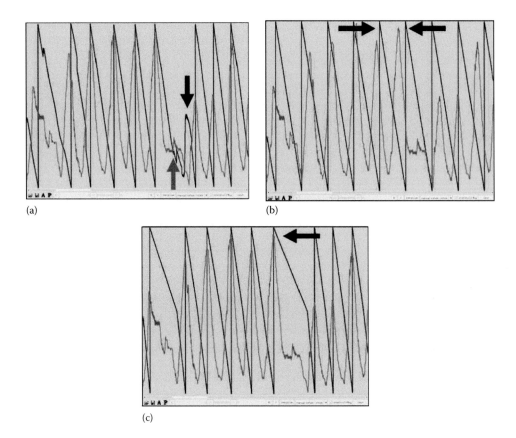

FIGURE 9.9 Mischaracterization of phase assignments. Irregularities in the detected breathing trace (gray line) have the potential to create incorrect phase assignments (black line) when automatic routines are used. Manual intervention can be used to properly assign the peak inhalation and expiration phases. (Adapted from Rietzal E, Chen GTY., *Med. Phys.*, 33: 377–379, 2006a. With permission.)

Wang et al. 2009). 3D CBCT of free-breathing patients typically encompasses multiple breathing cycles, blurring visualization of the tumor in the direction of respiratory motion. It is assumed that the 3D CBCT image of the tumor resembles the geometry and positioning of the temporally constructed ITV derived from 4D simulation imaging. Online techniques that align the CBCT to the ITV have been demonstrated to overcome challenges presented by baseline variations in tumor position and significantly reduce the potential for interfractional setup errors when compared with techniques that perform matching of bony anatomy only (Guckenberger et al. 2006; Purdie et al. 2006) (Figure 9.10).

A technique described by Masi et al. (2008) has proven effective for mitigating interfractional differences in tumor position caused by respiratory motion by using the active breathing control (ABC) device to train patients. Respiratory-correlated cone-beam computed tomography (RC-CBCT) has also been shown to be an effective method of verifying the mean position, trajectory, and shape of moving tumors (Sonke et al. 2005, 2009). The technique relies on the detection of an internal surrogate in the 2D x-ray projections acquired while rotating about the patient. After processing, the acquired data are used to produce binned datasets corresponding to phases of the breathing cycle and allowing for quantification of breathing

motion prior to therapy. Comparison of RC-CBCT with 4D CT datasets have confirmed that target motion is relatively stable from initial simulation through the course of treatment (Purdie et al. 2006) while also demonstrating intrafractional stability (Bissonnette et al. 2009a, 2009b). The potential for large intrapatient changes in tumor motion between fractions was noted for select patients. With the selective application of gating techniques for those patients who will receive the most benefit, it is expected that image-guided techniques such as RC-CBCT will continue to be the subject of study, especially as this functionality is commercialized and implemented.

9.4 Summary and Recommendations

More information, provided by 4D CT imaging technologies and placed in the hands of planners and clinicians, potentially increases the probability of improving clinical outcomes. IGRT and real-time imaging in the treatment suite is integral to closing the loop by reducing uncertainties associated with the simulation and treatment of patients in general and the quantification of mobile targets specifically. Many techniques are now available for both assessing intrafraction motion due to respiration and, given that *a priori* information, intervening and directing in the clinical radiation

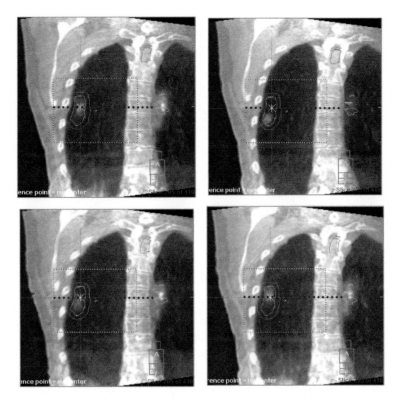

FIGURE 9.10 (See color insert) IGRT of a lung lesion. Coronal views of reconstructed CBCT data acquired on four different fractions. Baseline shift of the target relative to the bony anatomy.

delivery. Tradeoffs exist for each 4D approach that influence a range of parameters from the accuracy of the intervention to the length of a therapy session. Care must be taken to consider how shifts in the baseline position of targets at the initiation of therapy, during therapy, and throughout the treatment course affect localization and targeting. Adherence to guidance provided by vendors, as well as users and professional societies, must be considered when implementing a particular 4D CT approach.

References

Balter JM, Ten Haken RK, Lawrence TS, et al. Uncertainties in CT-based radiation therapy treatment planning associated with patient breathing. *Int. J. Radiat. Oncol. Biol. Phys.* 1996; 36: 167–174.

Barnes EA, Murray BR, Robinson DM, et al. Dosimetric evaluation of lung tumor immobilization using breath hold at deep inspiration. *Int. J. Radiat. Oncol. Biol. Phys.* 2001; 50: 1091–1098.

Bissonnette J, Franks KN, Purdie TG, et al. Quantifying interfraction and intrafraction tumor motion in lung stereotactic body radiotherapy using respiration-correlated cone beam computed tomography. *Int. J. Radiat. Oncol. Biol. Phys.* 2009a; 75: 688–695.

Bissonnette J, Purdie TG, Higgins JA, et al. Cone-beam computed tomography image guidance for lung cancer radiation therapy. *Int. J. Radiat. Oncol. Biol. Phys.* 2009b; 73: 927–934.

Brandner ED, Heron D, Wu, A, et al. Localizing moving targets and organs using motion-managed CTs. *Med. Dosim.* 2006; 31: 134–140.

Cover KS, Lagerwaard FJ, Senan S. Color intensity projections: A rapid approach for evaluating four-dimensional CT scans in treatment planning. *Int. J. Radiat. Oncol. Biol. Phys.* 2006; 64: 954–961.

Dawson LA, Jaffray DA. Advances in image-guided radiation therapy. *J. Clin. Oncol.* 2007; 8: 938–947.

Ekberg L, Holmberg O, Wittgren L, et al. What margins should be added to the clinical target volume in radiotherapy treatment for lung cancer? *Radither. Oncol.* 1998; 48: 71–77.

Erdi YE, Nehmeh SA, Pan T, et al. The CT motion quantitation of lung lesions and its impact on PET-measured SUVs. *J. Nucl. Med.* 2004; 45: 1287–1292.

Fakiris AJ, McGarry RC, Yiannoutsos CT, et al. Stereotactic body radiotherapy for early-stage non-small-cell lung carcinoma: Four-year results of a prospective phase II study. *Int. J. Radiat. Oncol. Biol. Phys.* 2009; 75: 677–682.

George R, Keall PJ, Kini VR, et al. Quantifying the effect of intrafraction motion during breast IMRT planning and dose delivery. *Med. Phys.* 2003; 30: 552–562.

George R, Vedam SS, Ramakrishnan V, et al. Audio-visual biofeedback for respiratory-gated radiotherapy: Impact of audio instruction and audio-visual biofeedback on respiratory-gated radiotherapy. *J. Radiother. Oncol. Phys.* 2006; 65: 924–933.

Greco C, Rosenzweig K, Cascini GL, et al. Current status of PET/ CT for tumor volume definition in radiotherapy treatment planning for non-small cell lung cancer (NSCLC). *Lung Can.* 2007; 57: 125–134.

Grills IS, Fitch DL, Goldstein NS, et al. Clinicopathologic analysis of microscopic extension in lung adenocarcinoma: Defining clinical target volume for radiotherapy. *Int. J. Radiat. Oncol. Biol. Phys.* 2007; 69: 334–341.

Grills I, Hugo G, Kestin LL, et al. Image-guided radiotherapy via daily online cone-beam CT substantially reduces margin requirements for stereotactic lung radiotherapy. *Int. J. Radiat. Oncol. Biol. Phys.* 2008; 70: 1045–1056.

Guckenberger M, Krieger T, Richter A, et al. Potential of image-guidance, gating and real-time tracking to improve accuracy in pulmonary stereotactic body radiothearpy. *Radiother. Oncol.* 2009; 91: 288–295.

Gukenberger M, Meyer J, Vordermark D, et al. Magnitude and clinical relevance of translational and rotational patient setup errors: A cone-beam CT study. *Int. J. Radiat. Oncol. Biol. Phys.* 2006; 65: 934–942.

Haasbeek CJA, Lagerwaard FJ, Cuijpers JP, et al. Is adaptive treatment planning required for stereotactic radiotherapy of stage I non-small cell lung cancer? *Int. J. Radiat. Oncol. Biol. Phys.* 2007; 67: 1370–1374.

Heinzerling JH, Anderson JF, Papiez L, et al. Four-dimensional computed tomography scan analysis of tumor and organ motion at varying levels of abdominal compression during stereotactic treatment of lung and liver. *Int. J. Radiat. Oncol. Biol. Phys.* 2008; 70: 1571–1578.

Hughes S, McClelland J, Chandler A, et al. A comparison of internal target volume definition by limited four-dimensional computed tomography, the addition of patient-specific margins, or the addition of generic margins when planning radical radiotherapy for lymph node-positive non-small cell lung cancer. *Clin. Oncol.* 2008; 20: 293–300.

Hughes S, McClelland J, Tarte S, et al. Assessment of two novel ventilatory surrogates for use in the delivery of gated/ tracked radiotherapy for non-small cell lung cancer. *Radiother. Oncol.* 2009; 91: 336–341.

Hugo GD, Yan D, Liang J. Population and patient-specific target margins for 4D adaptive radiotherapy to account for intra- and inter-fraction variation in lung tumour position. *Phys. Med. Biol.* 2007; 52: 257–274.

Huntzinger C, Munro P, Johnson S, et al. Dynamic targeting image-guided radiotherapy. *Med. Dosim.* 2006; 31: 113–125.

International Commission on Radiation Units and Measurements. ICRU Report 62. Prescribing, recording, and reporting photon beam therapy (Supplement to ICRT Report 50). *Bethesda,* MD: ICRU, 1999.

Jarritt PH, Carson KJ, Hounsell AR, et al. The role of PET/CT scanning gin radiotherapy planning. *Br. J. Radiat.* 2006; 79: S27–S35.

Jiang SB, Wolfgang JI, Mageras GS. Quality assurance challenges for motion-adaptive radiation therapy: Gating, breath-holding, and four-dimensional computed tomography. *Int. J. Radiat. Oncol. Biol. Phys.* 2008; 71: S103–S107.

Jiang SB. Radiotherapy of mobile tumors. *Semin. Radiat. Oncol.* 2006a; 38: 239–248.

Jiang SB. Technical aspects of image-guided respiration-gated radiation therapy. *Med. Dosim.* 2006b; 31: 141–151.

Jin J-Y, Yin F-F, Tenn SE, et al. Use of the brainlab exactrac x-ray 6D system in image-guided radiotherapy. *Med. Dosim.* 2008; 33: 1124–1134.

Juhler-Nottrup T, Korreman SS, Pedersen AN, et al. Interfractional changes in tumour volume and position during entire radiotherapy courses for lung cancer with respiratory gating and image guidance. *Acta Oncol.* 2008a; 47: 1406–1413.

Keall PJ, Kini VR, Vedam SS, et al. Motion adaptive x-ray therapy: A feasibility study. *Phys. Med. Biol.* 2001; 46: 1–10.

Keall PJ, Mageras GS, Balter JM, et al. The management of respiratory motion in radiation oncology report of AAPM task group 76. *Med. Phys.* 2006; 33: 3874–3900.

Kim DJW, Murray BR, Halperin R, et al. Held-breath self-gating technique for radiotherapy of non-small-cell lung cancer. Int. *J. Radiat. Oncol. Biol. Phys.* 2001; 49: 43–49.

Klein EE, Hanley J, Bayouth J, et al. Task Group 142: Quality assurance of medical accelerators. *Med. Phys.* 2009; 36: 4197–4212.

Lax I, Blomgren H, Naslund I, et al. Stereotactic radiotherapy of malignancies in the abdomen: Methodological aspects. *Acta Oncol.* 1994; 33: 677–683.

Li XA, Stepaniak C, Gore E. Technical and dosimetric aspects of respiratory gating using a pressure-sensor motion monitoring system. *Med. Phys.* 2006; 33: 145–154.

Lujan AE, Larsen, EW, Balter JM, et al. A method for incorporating organ motion due to breathing into 3D dose calculations. *Med. Phys.* 1999; 26: 715–720.

Masi l, Casamassima F, Menichelli C, et al. On-line image guidance for frameless stereotactic radiotherapy of lung malignancies by cone-beam CT: Comparison between target localization and alignment on bony anatomy. *Acta Oncol.* 2008; 47: 1422–1431.

McKenzie AL, van Herk M, Mijnheer B. The width of margins in radiotherapy treatment plans. *Phys. Med. Biol.* 2000; 45: 3331–3342.

McNair HA, Brock J, Symonds-Taylor JRN, et al. Feasibility of the use of the active breathing coordinator (ABC) in patients receiving radical radiotherapy for non-small cell lung cancer (NSCLC). *Radiother. Oncol.* 2009; 93: 434–429.

Mechalakos J, Yorke E, Mageras GS, et al. Dosimetric effect of respiratory motion in external beam radiotherapy of the lung. *Radiother. Oncol.* 2004; 71: 191–200.

Murphy MJ. Tracking moving organs in real time. *Semin. Radiat. Oncol.* 2004; 14: 91–100.

Mutaf YD, Brinkmann DH. Optimization of internal margin to account for dosimetric effects of respiratory motion. *Int. J. Radiat. Oncol. Biol. Phys.* 2008; 70: 1561–1570.

Nehmeh SA, Erdi YE, Pan T, et al. Four-dimensional (4D) PET/CT imaging of the thorax. *Med. Phys.* 2004; 31: 3179–3186.

Nelson C, Starkschall G, Chang JY. The potential for dose escalation in lung cancer as a result of systematically reducing margins used to generate planning target volume. *Int. J. Radiat. Oncol. Biol. Phys.* 2006; 65: 573–586.

Ozhasoglu C, Saw CB, Chen HC. Synchrony-CyberKnife respiratory compensation technology. *Med. Dosim.* 2008; 33: 117–123.

Plathow C, Zimmermann H, Fink C, et al. Influence of different breathing maneuvers on internal and external organ motion: Use of fiducial markers in dynamic MRI. *Int. J. Radiat. Oncol. Biol. Phys.* 2005; 62: 238–245.

Purdie TG, Moseley DJ, Bissonnette J, et al. Respiration correlated cone-beam computed tomography and 4DCT for evaluating target motion in stereotactic lung radiation therapy. *Acta Oncol.* 2006; 45: 915–922.

Redmond KJ, Song DY, Fox JL, et al. Respiratory motion changes of lung tumors over the course of radiation therapy based on respiration-correlated four-dimensional computed tomography scans. *Int. J. Radiat. Oncol. Biol. Phys.* 2009; 75: 1605–1612.

Remouchamps VM, Letts N, Vicini FA, et al. Initial clinical experience with moderate deep-inspiration breath hold using an active breathing control device in the treatment of patients with left-sided breast cancer using external beam radiation therapy. *Int. J. Radiat. Oncol. Biol. Phys.* 2003; 56: 704–715.

Riboldi M, Sharp GC, Baroni G, Chen GTY. Four-dimensional targeting error analysis in image-guided radiotherapy. *Phys. Med. Biol.* 2009; 54: 5995–6009.

Rietzel E, Chen GTY, Choi NC, et al. Four-dimensional image-based treatment planning: Target volume segmentation and dose calculation in the presence of respiratory motion. *Int. J. Radiat. Oncol. Biol. Phys.* 2005a; 61: 1535–1550.

Rietzel E, Pan T, Chen GTY. Four-dimensional computed tomography: Image formation and clinical protocol. *Med. Phys.* 2005b; 32: 874–889.

Rietzel E, Chen GTY. Improving retrospective sorting of 4D computed tomography data. *Med. Phys.* 2006a; 33: 377–379.

Rietzel E, Liu AK, Doppke KP, et al. Design of 4D treatment planning target volumes. *Int. J. Radiat. Oncol. Phys.* 2006b; 66: 287–295.

Rietzel E, Liu AK, Chen GTY, et al. Maximum-intensity volumes for fast contouring of lung tumors including respiratory motion in 4D CT planning. *Int. J. Radiat. Oncol. Biol. Phys.* 2008; 71: 1245–1252.

Rosenzweig KE, Hanley J, Mah D, et al. The deep inspiration breath-hold technique in the treatment of inoperable non-small-cell lung cancer. *Int. J. Radiat. Oncol. Biol. Phys.* 2000; 48: 81–87.

Senan S, De Ruysscher E. Critical review of PET-CT for radiotherapy planning in lung cancer. *Crit. Rev. Oncol. Hemotol.* 2005; 56: 345–351.

Seppenwoolde Y, Shirato H, Kitamura K, et al. Precise and real-time measurement of 3D tumor motion in lung due to breathing and heartbeat measured during radiotherapy. *Int. J. Radiat. Oncol. Biol. Phys.* 2002; 53: 822–834.

Sharp GC, Jiang SB, Shimizu S, et al. Prediction of respiratory tumour motion for real-time image-guided radiotherapy. *Phys. Med. Biol.* 2004; 49: 425–440.

Shimizu S, Shirato H, Ogura S, et al. Detection of lung tumor movement in real-time tumor-tracking radiotherapy. *Int. J. Radiat. Oncol. Biol. Phys.* 2002; 51: 304–310.

Shirato H, Shimizu S, Kitamura K, et al. Organ motion in image-guided radiotherapy: Lessons from real-time tumor-tracking radiotherapy. *Int. J. Clin. Oncol.* 2007; 12: 8–16.

Slotman BJ, Lagerwaard FJ, Senan S. 4D imaging for target definition in stereotactic radiotherapy for lung cancer. *Acta Oncol.* 2006; 45: 966–972.

Smith RL, Lechleiter K, Malinowski K, et al. Evaluation of linear accelerator gating with real-time electromagnetic tracking. *Int. J. Radiat. Oncol. Biol. Phys.* 2009; 74: 920–927.

Sonke J, Rossi M, Wolthaus J, et al. Frameless stereotactic body radiotherapy for lung cancer using four-dimensional cone beam CT guidance. *Int. J. Radiat. Oncol. Biol. Phys.* 2009; 74: 567–574.

Sonke J-J, Zijp L, Remeijer P, et al. Respiratory correlated cone-beam CT. *Med. Phys.* 2005; 47: 1422–1431.

Spoelstra FOB, Pantarotto JR, Sornsen de Koste JR, et al. Role of adaptive radiotherapy during concomitant chemoradiotherapy for lung cancer: Analysis of data from a prospective clinical trial. *Int. J. Radiat. Oncol. Biol. Phys.* 2009; 75: 1092–1097.

Steenbakkers RJHM, Duppen JC, Fitton I, et al. Observer variation in target volume delineation of lung cancer related to radiation oncologist-computer interaction: A "Big Brother" evaluation. *Radiother. Oncol.* 2005; 77: 182–190.

Stroom JC, Heijmen BJM. Geometrical uncertainties, radiotherapy planning margins, and the ICRU-62 report. *Radiother. Oncol.* 2002; 64: 75–83.

Stroom J, Blaauwgeers H, van Baardwijk A, et al. Feasibility of pathology-correlated lung imaging for accurate target definition of lung tumors. *Int. J. Radiat. Oncol. Biol. Phys.* 2007; 69: 267–275.

Suramo I, Paivansalo M, Myllyla V. Cranio-caudal movements of the liver, pancreas and kidneys in respiration. *Acta Radiol. Diagn.* 1984; 25: 129–131.

Underberg RWM, Lagerwaard FJ, Cuijpers JP, et al. Four-dimensional CT scans for treament planning in stereotactic radiotherapy for stage I lung cancer. *Int. J. Radiat. Oncol. Biol. Phys.* 2004; 60: 1283–1290.

Underberg RWM, Lagerwaard FJ, Slotman BJ, et al. Benefit of respiration-gated stereotactic radiotherapy for stage I lung cancer: An analysis of 4DCT datasets. *Int. J. Radiat. Oncol. Biol. Phys.* 2005; 62: 554–560.

Underberg RWM, Lagerwaard FJ, van Tinteren H, et al. Time trends in target volumes for stage I non-small-cell lung cancer after stereotactic radiotherapy. *Int. J. Radiat. Oncol. Biol. Phys.* 2006; 64: 1221–1228.

van Herk M, Witte M, van der Geer J, et al. Biologic and physical fractionation effects of random geometric errors. Int. J. *Radiat. Oncol. Biol. Phys.* 2003; 57: 1460–1471.

van Sornsen de Koste JR, Lagerwaard FJ, Schuchhard-Schipper RH, et al. Dosimetric consequences of tumor mobility in radiotherapy of stage I non-small cell lung cancer – an analysis of data generated using 'slow' CT scans. *Radiother. Oncol.* 2001; 61: 93–99.

Vedam SS, Keall PJ, Docef A, et al. Predicting respiratory motion for four-dimensional radiotherapy. *Med. Phys.* 2004; 31: 2274–2283.

Vedam SS, Kini VR, Keall PJ, et al. Quantifying the predictability of diaphragm motion during respiration with a noninvasive external marker. *Med. Phys.* 2003; 30: 505–513.

Wang ZH, Nelson JW, Yoo S, et al. Refinement of treatment setup and target localization accuracy using three-dimensional cone-beam computed tomography for stereotactic body radiotherapy. *Int. J. Radiat. Oncol. Biol. Phys.* 2009; 73: 571–577.

Willoughby TR, Forbes AR, Buchholz D, et al. Evaluation of an infrared camera and X-ray system using implanted fiducials in patients with lung tumors for gated radiation therapy. *Int. J. Radiat. Oncol. Biol. Phys.* 2006; 66: 568–575.

Wolthaus JWH, Schneider C, Sonke JJ, et al. Mid-ventilation CT scan constructed from four-dimensional respiration-correlated CT scans for radiotherapy planning of lung cancer patients. *Int. J. Radiat. Oncol. Biol. Phys.* 2006; 65: 1560–1571.

Wong JW, Sharpe MB, Jaffray DA, et al. The use of active breathing control (ABC) to reduce margin for breathing motion. *Int. J. Radiat. Oncol. Biol. Phys.* 1999; 44: 911–919.

Wulf J, Hadinger U, Oppitz U, et al. Impact of target reproducibility on tumor dose in stereotactic radiotherapy of targets in the lung and liver. *Radiother. Oncol.* 2003: 66; 141–150.

Wurm RE, Gum F, Erbel S, et al. Image guided respiratory gated hypofractionated stereotactic body radiotherapy (H-SBRT) for liver and lung tumors: Initial experience. *Acta Oncol.* 2006; 45: 881–889.

Xing L, Siebers J, Keall P. Computational challenges for image-guided radiation therapy: Framework and current research. *Semin. Radiat. Oncol.* 2007;17: 245–257.

Xing L. Overview of image-guided radiation therapy. *Med. Dosim.* 2006; 31: 91.

Yan D, Vicini F, Wong J, et al. Adaptive radiation therapy. Phys. *Med. Biol.* 1997; 42: 123–132.

Zhang TZ, Orton NP, Tome WA, et al. On the automated definition of mobile target volumes from 4D-CT images for stereotactic body radiotherapy. *Med. Phys.* 2005; 32: 3493–3502.

10

4D PET/CT in Radiotherapy

Sadek A. Nehmeh
Memorial Sloan-Kettering
Cancer Center

Yusuf E. Erdi
Memorial Sloan-Kettering
Cancer Center

Recent progress in combined modality treatments, incorporating radiochemotherapy, and the technical advances in radiation delivery and medical imaging, in particular PET, have yielded significant improvements in treatment outcomes in NSCLC. In radiotherapy, accurate tumor delineation is crucial for preventing geographical misses, and consequently for improving local tumor control.[1] 18F-Fluorodyoxydoglucose (18FDG) PET imaging has been shown to add significantly to the accuracy of conventional anatomic imaging (CT and MRI) in defining the extents of lung disease[2,3] and to have higher sensitivity and specificity than CT. The superiority of PET over conventional imaging in detecting distant disease may also result in modifying patient disease management.[4] Moreover, the newly developed PET radiotracers capable of targeting tumor growth, hypoxia, and tumor perfusion, enable the definition of new biological subvolumes within the gross target volume (GTV), known as biological target volumes (BTVs).[5,6] Recent studies have proposed that escalating the dose to these targeted subvolumes (BTVs) within the GTV can improve local control, thus radiotherapy outcome. With the advances in radiation delivery techniques, in particular intensity-modulated radiotherapy (IMRT), as well as image-guided radiation therapy (IGRT), and with PET assisting in delineating subtarget BTVs, it has become plausible to escalate the dose to these radiation resistant regions (e.g., hypoxic subvolumes), while sparing normal tissues from high doses.[7]

Early assessment of tumor response to therapy, including both chemo- and radiotherapies, is critical for optimizing patient management, and consequently treatment outcome and survival. One method to assess tumor response to therapy is by measuring the decrease in anatomical tumor volume. Another method is to quantify the decrease of tumor cell metabolism along the course of therapy.[8] Assessment of tumor response, using 18FDG-PET, following radiotherapy, has been widely explored.[9] 18FDG-PET has been shown to predict an early response to radiotherapy. IMRT treatment outcome, with the integration of PET/CT, showed an overall survival rate of 97% and 91% at 1 and 2 years, respectively, compared to 74% and 54% without the integration of PET/CT.[10]

One prerequisite to benefit from combined PET/CT modality in the areas of tumor delineation, radiation dose escalation, and tumor response assessment is the accurate coregistration of CT and PET images, both for external surfaces and anatomy and internal anatomy. External PET-to-CT coregistration has become trivial with both image sets acquired with the patient in the same position on a now-widely available hybrid PET/CT scanner. However, due to respiratory motion and the differences in PET and CT image acquisition times to image the thorax (PET is an integrated image over tens of minutes, and CT is a rapidly acquired image over approximately one minute), misregistration of internal organs between the two modalities is common.[11–14] Breathing-induced image artifacts, in both PET and CT, have also been reported.[4,15–18] For example, in CT, breathing motion may cause the exclusion of some anatomic structures or repeated scanning of others, resulting in image artifacts, thus affecting the accuracy of diagnosis and target volume definition in radiotherapy.[19] In PET, breathing may result in blurring the lesion, thus providing inaccurate lesion location as well as inaccurate quantification of the specific uptake value (SUV), which is an indicator of the amount of radioligand uptake and, thus, the amount of disease present.[14,19] Also, because of differences in time resolution between the two modalities, CT may not spatially match the PET images, thus resulting in an inaccurate attenuation correction

(AC) in the PET images. Consequently, the target may be mis-localized,[12,17,20] and the SUV may again be erroneous. When not accounted for in radiotherapy, breathing-induced artifacts can result in unnecessarily exposing normal tissues to high radiation doses, and/or partially missing the target volume, thus reducing local control. Moreover, because of SUV inaccuracies due to motion blurring and misregistered CT AC, the change in SUV values between pre- and post-PET scans may not be reliable for assessing tumor response to therapy, unless SUV values have been accounted for respiratory motion in both PET and CT images.

Many methods have been developed to address respiratory motion in PET/CT imaging. In the balance of this review, these will be discussed together with the different respiratory tracking techniques. The role of 4D PET/CT in delineating the GTV, staging the disease, and monitoring tumor response will also be discussed.

10.1 Respiratory Motion Tracking Systems

Although respiratory gating is not yet standard in the context of PET imaging, several related techniques have been developed to account for respiratory motion artifacts. For this purpose, a large number of respiration monitoring systems to track the breathing motion and assist in performing four-dimensional (4D) radiotherapy, 4D-CT, 4D cone beam CT, and 4D-PET have been investigated. Such breathing motion tracking systems are described herein.

10.1.1 Visual Tracking

Recently, a novel in-house system, the 3D respiratory tracking system (3DRTS), has been developed and reported for 4D PET/CT applications.[21] 3DRTS uses miniature wireless cameras (DynaSpy, Inc., Model# RC211) and an edge detection technique to track, simultaneously and in real-time, the 3D motion of a set of fiducial markers (FMs) placed on the thorax. The small, concise size, and wireless transmission features of the camera selected for this application enable its installation inside the PET/CT gantry. Figure 10.1 shows the 3DRTS setup for respiratory-gated PET/CT. With one camera, it is possible to deduce the two-dimensional (2D) information of the FM motions. With two cameras, using a stereocamera technique, it is possible to deduce the third dimension of the motion. The user first identifies the positions of the FMs, using a graphical user interface (GUI) developed for this purpose. Then, the 2D motion of each FM is displayed by the 3DRTS graphical interface at rate of 30 fps. At an user-defined breathing amplitude, a trigger can be delivered to the PET/CT scanner for a gated PET of CT image acquisition.

A major advantage of the new system is its capability to track simultaneously the 2D motion (with one camera) of multiple markers (rather than just one as is the case for the other systems). Moreover, 3DRTS can provide 3D motion information of the FMs. While the authors used the camera described previously for tracking, the 3DRTS software can support any standard digital camera, like web cameras, personal video cameras,

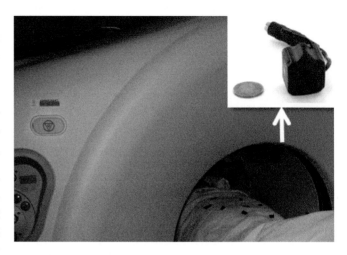

FIGURE 10.1 3DRTS setup inside the PET/CT gantry during 4D acquisition. 3DRTS uses a miniature wireless camera (top right) to simultaneously track the 2D motion of multiple FMs (black markers on the patient's thorax).

etc., making the tracking system both easy to implement as well as affordable.

10.1.2 Pressure Sensor

Pressure sensors are dedicated respiration sensors that were originally designed for use in radiation therapy and medical imaging. One such device is the AZ-733V sensor (Anzai Medical, Tokyo, Japan; http://www.anzai-med.co.jp). A pressure sensor consists of an elastic belt that can be fastened around the patient's abdomen or thorax. A load cell is placed inside the belt in order to measure the change in pressure due to the change in stress during breathing. This change in pressure is usually correlated to breathing amplitude and is displayed as a function of time. Pressure sensors have been explored in the areas of gated radiotherapy,[22,23] 4D-CT and 4D cone beam CT during radiotherapy delivery,[23,24] and gated PET.[25]

10.1.3 Spirometer

Another respiratory sensor is the spirometer. The spirometer measures air flow to and from the lungs using an air tube placed in the nose or mouth of the patient. Part of the breathed air flows to a sensor attached to the other end of the tube, and the measured air flow is converted into the volume of air in the patient's lungs. This lung volume is then displayed as a function of time. An example of such a device is the PMM spirometer (Siemens Medical Systems, Erlangen, Germany). Spirometers have also been investigated for gated radiotherapy,[22,26,27] quantitative CT,[28] and gated PET.[25]

10.1.4 Temperature Sensor

Temperature sensors are used to measure, with a high temporal resolution, the changing temperature of air respired by the patient. With the use of room temperature as a reference, the outside air passing through the sensor during inspiration is at a lower temperature than that of the air from the lungs passing through it during expiration. One example of temperature sensors is the BioVet CT1 System (Spin Systems, Brisbane, Australia). The BioVet CT1 system was initially designed for use in medical imaging research on small animals. Temperature sensors have been used in the settings of respiratory-gated radiotherapy[19] and respiratory-gated PET.[29]

10.1.5 Real-Time Position Management Respiratory Gating System

The real-time position management respiratory gating system (RPM) (Varian Medical Systems, Palo Alto, CA) was initially designed for gated radiotherapy. The RPM uses a video camera to monitor and thus track the vertical displacement of two infrared (IR) reflective markers rigidly mounted on a plastic block placed on the patient's thorax.[11] The motion of the IR markers is displayed by a graphical interface on the RPM workstation. The RPM setup for 4D PET/CT is shown in Figure 10.2. The RPM has been used in gated radiotherapy of lung,[30] respiratory-gated CT,[31,32] 4D-CT,[30,33,34] and 4D-PET imaging.[11,15–17]

With the exception of the spirometer and the temperature sensor, the aforementioned systems provide a respiratory signal through the measurement of the displacement at a particular zone of the thoracic cage. These systems provide an accurate and reproducible respiratory signal.[35] While the spirometer may reflect lung movement, or at least lung volume changes, most accurately, it is generally less well tolerated by patients than the other systems over the long duration of typical PET emission image acquisitions.

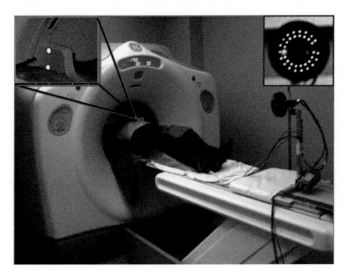

FIGURE 10.2 RPM setup during 4D PET/CT acquisition. The RPM tracks two IR reflective markers located on the anterior chest surface (top left) using an IR video camera (top right).

10.2 Respiratory Motion Artifacts in PET/CT

Respiratory motion artifacts in PET/CT imaging fall into three categories that are modality specific: (a) CT, (b) PET, and (c) PET/CT. These classes are now reviewed.

10.2.1 Respiratory Motion Artifacts in CT

Respiration-induced artifacts in CT images are mainly caused by the dynamic interaction between transaxial image acquisition, which primarily proceeds from head to foot along the long axis of the body, and the asynchronous motion of tumor and normal tissues.[19] Commonly observed artifacts include distortion of the dome of the liver at the lung–diaphragm interface, splitting of a tumor into two distinct parts, out-of-order shuffling of the transaxial slices, and creation of discontinuities in the diaphragm/lung interface.[19] These artifacts yield distortion of both the lesion shape and size and consequently an inaccurate definition of the target volume in planning of radiotherapy. Figure 10.3 illustrates the different motion artifacts of an oscillating spherical phantom for which CT images were acquired at random phases of the motion.[19]

Figure 10.4 shows an example of distortions of the dome of the liver at the lung–diaphragm interface, as may commonly appear in clinical CT images due to breathing. The most superior aspect of the dome was first imaged during full inspiration in a most superior position and then imaged multiple times again more inferiorly as the respiratory cycle proceeded to expiration during helical CT image acquisition.

10.2.2 Respiratory Motion Artifacts in PET

In PET imaging, data are usually acquired for 3–7 min per field of view (FOV). Therefore, the images are time averaged over many breathing cycles (average breathing period is 5 s), which results in blurring the target volume.[15–17] Figure 10.5 demonstrates such artifacts for an oscillating point source compared to a static point source. Because of motion, the counts are redistributed along the direction of the motion, thus resulting in an overestimation of the target volume (Figure 10.5b). Therefore, when used in radiotherapy treatment planning, blurred PET images may result in an excessively large planning target volume, and therefore, an unnecessarily large radiation dose to the normal tissues.[15] PET image intensities may be either lower (as in Figure 10.5b) or higher (not shown) than expected for a non-point source target volume experiencing motion due to breathing, depending on the target size and magnitude of motion.

10.2.3 Respiratory Motion Artifacts in PET/CT

In addition to the CT and PET breathing-induced artifacts previously discussed, respiratory motion in hybrid PET/CT can result in hybrid motion artifacts, primarily due to the temporal

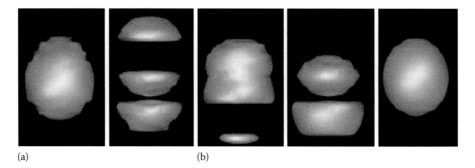

(a)   (b)

FIGURE 10.3 CT images of a sphere in sinusoidal motion along the axial direction (arrow), with the CT image plane oriented left to right and orthogonally to the plane of the figure. (a) Artifacts obtained in helical CT acquired at random phases during the motion. (b) For reference, the CT image of the stationary sphere is also shown. (From Rietzel, E., Pan, T., Chen, G.T., *Med Phys*, 32: 874–89, 2005. With permission.)

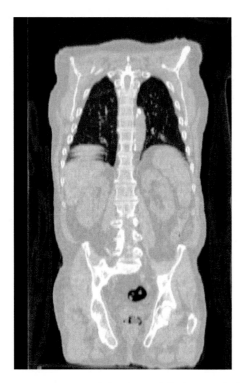

FIGURE 10.4 Distortion of the dome of the liver at the lung–diaphragm interface in helical CT due to breathing.

mismatch between PET images and the corresponding CT-based attenuation map. Previous studies have shown that this effect may result in mislocalizing the lesion.[12,17] Figure 10.6 shows an example where a lung lesion was incorrectly localized in the liver in the PET images due to a temporal mismatch between the PET and CT image sets.[12] The same lesion was confirmed to reside in the lower lung lobe for PET images reconstructed without CT-based attenuation correction.[12]

Erdi and coworkers have also shown that such mismatches may result in changes in lesion size and SUV fluctuations of up to 24%.[13] Figure 10.7 shows one PET image set reconstructed with CT attenuation maps acquired at different breathing phases. The corresponding SUVs are also reported.[13]

10.3 Correction for Breathing Artifacts in PET/CT

Two approaches have been suggested in order to incorporate PET/CT images of the thorax in the treatment planning of radiotherapy: (1) acquire PET and CT data in 4D and then match the two data sets on a respiratory phase-by-phase basis and (2) match the CT temporal resolution with that of PET by smearing the CT data. While the first method corrects for most of the breathing-induced artifacts discussed before, the second is restricted to improving the spatial matching between PET and CT images and therefore improves the accuracy of AC. Both approaches will be described herein.

10.3.1 Breathing Phase Matched PET/CT

Two techniques have been described in order to achieve phase matched PET/CT imaging.

10.3.1.1 Four-Dimensional PET/CT

4D PET was first developed for cardiac imaging to assess myocardial motion and to obtain the ejection fraction.[36] In the last decade, the cardiac-gated technique was expanded to correct for breathing-induced motion artifacts in the thorax.[15–17] In gated mode, PET data are acquired in each cycle into multiple time bins (8–10 bins), the width of which is predefined by the user. A trigger generated at a user defined phase or amplitude of the breathing cycle is usually fed into the PET scanner. This trigger initiates the data collection cycle, i.e., into the first bin. With a 10-bin gated scan setup, a respiratory-gated study is usually acquired for at least 1 min/bin, for a total of 10 min per bed position (each bed position covers about 15 cm in the Z direction), to collect relatively acceptable statistics. The resulting bins' images each correspond to one breathing phase of the respiratory motion, thus revealing the fourth dimension (time). Because of the reduced acquisition time per bin relative to the static clinical setup, which typically uses at least 3 min per bed position, 4D-PET images have poorer count rate statistics, and therefore are characterized by increased noise level and reduced

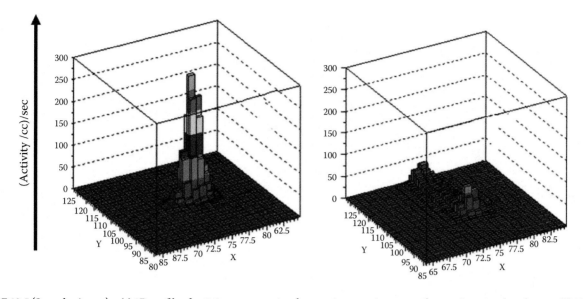

FIGURE 10.5 (See color insert) (a) 3D profile of activity concentration for a stationary point source shows a Gaussian distribution. (b) The activity concentration of the same point source is stretched due to the motion. The two peaks correspond to the end points of the oscillating motion.

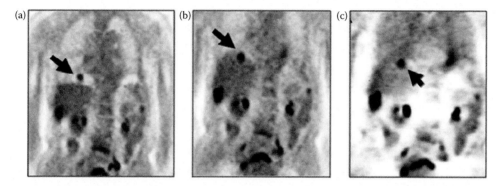

FIGURE 10.6 Mislocalization of liver lesion due to temporal mismatch between PET and CT images. (a) A focal [18]FDG uptake in the lower lobe of the right lung appears in the PET with CT attenuation corrected images. (b) The same lesion appears in the liver when PET images were corrected for attenuation using [68]Ge transmission rod sources. (c) The finding in (b) was confirmed in the nonattenuation corrected PET images. (Sarikaya I, Yeung HW, Erdi Y, et al., Respiratory artefact causing malpositioning of liver dome lesion in right lower lung, *Clin Nucl Med*, 28: 943–44, 2003).

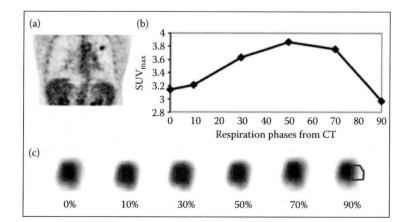

FIGURE 10.7 (a) Coronal image with an upper-left lung lesion. (b) Variation in SUV_{max} due to correcting for attenuation in the PET images using CT data acquired at different phases within the breathing cycle. (c) Cross sections of PET lesion reconstructed with different phase CTAC. The same threshold window is used for all PET images. The lesion boundary is drawn on the 0% phase and copied onto other phases. At the 90% phase, 9-mm displacement of the region of interest can clearly be seen. (From Erdi, Y.E., et al. *J Nucl Med*, 45: 1287–92, 2004.)

(a)   (b)

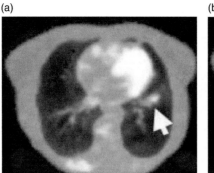
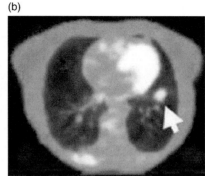

FIGURE 10.8   A transaxial fused PET/CT slice through a patient's lesion as it appears (a) in the nongated acquisition and (b) in the 4D PET/CT study. (From Nehmeh, S.A., et al., *Med Phys*, 31: 3179–86, 2004. With permission.)

signal-to-noise ratio (SNR). Also, if the 4D-PET was acquired separately, at least an additional 15 min (including setup) would be required. All of these effects, together with the lengthy procedure to process the 4D-PET data, especially matching each PET bin with the corresponding CT one for AC, have resulted in limiting the regular application of 4D-PET for daily clinical practice.

PET/CT scanners have recently been equipped with list mode data acquisition whereby events from each coincidence pair of 511 keV photons are stored in a list stream with a time stamp for later reconstruction. It has been demonstrated that the list-mode data acquisition can be performed with either cardiac or respiratory triggering during a normal static image acquisition.[37] List-mode data may be retrospectively sorted into multiple bins, according to the breathing amplitude and/or phase, thus resulting into 4D-PET images.

For accurate AC in 4D-PET images, 4D-CT becomes a requirement in order to spatially match between the corresponding two image sets on a bin-by-bin basis.[11,13] Pan et al. introduced a novel method, the 4D-CT imaging, to acquire CT images of all phases of the breathing cycle.[31] Their 4D-CT protocol uses cine mode acquisition, a "step-and-shoot" technique, to acquire repeated axial CT images for a specified period of time at each table position. The scan time per axial position is usually set equal to the average breathing cycle period plus the duration of the image reconstruction. The reconstruction time for two consecutive CT images at each axial position is on the order of 0.1–0.5 s.[31] Nehmeh et al. adopted this technique where they used a "shoot" period (cine duration) equivalent to one breathing period plus one second and a table increment (cine CT axial field of view) of 10 mm (4 × 2.5 mm slice thickness).[11] The x-ray tube speed was set to 2 rotations/s. The cine interval between images was 0.45 s, and each image was reconstructed with 360° of data.

Finally, the 4D-PET data are corrected for attenuation using the corresponding matching 4D-CT images. In a proof of principal study that included four patients, Nehmeh and coworkers showed an improvement in the coregistration of PET and CT lesions' centroids of up to 41%, reductions in PET target volume of up to 42%, and an increased lesion SUV of up to 16%,

as a result of breathing motion correction using 4D PET/CT Figure 10.8.

Although, it is still cumbersome to acquire 4D-PET data due to its prolonged acquisition and processing time, it is expected that with the new acquisition and processing protocols that have been implemented on the PET scanners by manufacturers, those limitations will be minimized, and 4D PET/CT will become a clinically feasible solution to improve the accuracy of tumor delineation and quantification that are affected by internal organ motion, especially due to breathing.

10.3.1.2   Deep Inspiration Breath-Hold PET/CT

Breath-hold CT (BH-CT) is well-established in clinical practice for CT image acquisition for diagnostic and radiation treatment planning purposes. However, breath-hold PET (BH-PET) appears to be clinically impossible because of the requirement to collect at least 3 min of data per FOV, unless PET data from multiple BH periods can be selected into a single data set.[17,20] Deep inspiration breath-hold (DIBH) PET/CT has been used as an alternative to 4D PET/CT using the RPM system in its amplitude-gating mode to monitor the patient respiratory motion.[17] In the DIBH PET/CT protocol proposed by Nehmeh et al.,[17] the patient is instructed to breathe deeply and then hold their breath for 20 s for a series of repeated cycles. First, CT data are acquired for the whole axial length of the thorax (approximately 16 seconds on average). PET data for one FOV are then acquired over nine 20-s frames for a total of 3 min. In case the patient fails to hold their breath in any of the frames, additional frames may be acquired. After each BH period, the patient is instructed to breathe normally. Even though in the study of Nehmeh et al.[17] PET data were acquired for only one FOV (~15.2 cm), which corresponds to more than half the axial length of the lungs, the DIBH procedure may be extended to cover the whole thorax. To ensure the accuracy of AC, PET data must be acquired at the same breathing amplitude as that during which CT data were acquired. Therefore, the amplitude threshold (a user-adjustable RPM option for defining the amplitude at which a trigger should be delivered) is set at the same breath-hold level used during the CT study.[17] Nehmeh and coworkers[16,17] showed an increase in lesion SUV by as much as 83% and an improved spatial matching between PET and CT by as much as 50% using DIBH PET/CT versus standard free-breathing PET/CT. In a prospective study, Meirelles and coworkers[20] showed that DIBH CT resulted in detection of 2.2 additional nodules per patient on average, especially nodules smaller than 0.5 cm. DIBH CT also allowed more precise localization and characterization of pulmonary lesions than free-breathing CT.[20] DIBH PET/CT also reduced misregistration between PET and CT caused by internal motion.[20,38] In one case, focal ^{18}F-FDG uptake apparently localized to the lung on conventional PET/CT was shown to actually represent a rib metastasis on BH PET/CT (Figure 10.9).[39] This finding was confirmed in CT images.

DIBH data acquisition has significant advantages over 4D protocols. First, unlike 4D acquisitions, DIBH does not require the patient to follow verbal instructions (breathe in, breathe out) to maintain a regular breathing motion. Second, image acquisition of 3 min per bed, equivalent to the standard clinical acquisition time per bed, can be acquired in DIBH. This would correspond to at least 30 min of acquisition time in 4D-PET for a total of 10 bins, as in the protocol suggested by Nehmeh et al.[15–17] Third, in case of sudden breathing irregularities, the corresponding data may be disregarded for inclusion in the final DIBH dataset. This exclusion of data, however, is not possible in 4D-PET. Finally, DIBH-PET and DIBH-CT are acquired according to the standard clinical PET/CT protocol. Consequently, no further rebinning of the CT data to spatially match the PET slices is required, which minimizes the postprocessing time.[17]

10.3.2 PET-Matched CT

PET-matched CT techniques do not account for breathing motion in the PET images but rather blur the CT images to spatially match the PET ones. Two techniques have been suggested to attain this goal; maximum intensity projection CT, and average CT.

10.3.2.1 Maximum Intensity Projection CT: MIP-CT

Maximum intensity projection (MIP) CT images are formed by identifying and assigning the maximum pixel value from all the 4D-CT phases for each pixel in a CT image.[31] All image phases are collapsed to a single static CT image that displays the maximum intensity of each pixel. With MIP-CT images, the extent of tumor motion is represented as a region of pixels (voxels) having high intensities[40]; therefore, MIP-CT images should spatially match PET images that inherently include motion through image blurring due to the required acquisition times. Consequently, use of MIP-CT images should result in a more accurate AC in PET images, since image blurring due to motion is not corrected for and is essentially equivalent for each imaging modality. One major advantage of this technique is that MIP-CT images can be generated without the need for gating[33] or respiratory motion tracking. Figure 10.10 shows an example of the use of MIP-CT to better determine the extent of a PET-defined GTV.

10.3.2.2 Average CT: ACT

Similar to the use of MIP-CT, the average CT (ACT) technique attempts to match PET temporal resolution in order to improve the PET-to-CT registration.[41] In ACT, each slice location is

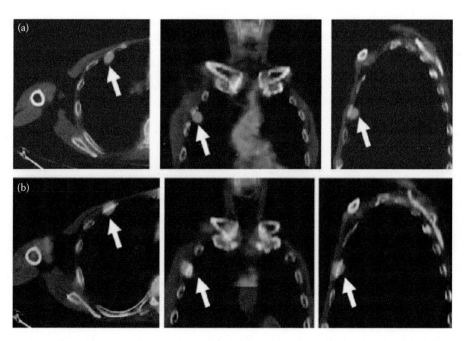

FIGURE 10.9 Transaxial, coronal, and sagittal views of (a) standard- and (b) DIBH-fused PET and CT images. Arrows point to a lesion in a rib, based on CT images. The PET lesion appears partially in lung in the free-breathing images, and only marginally matching the CT lesion because of respiratory motion. DIBH resulted in improved coregistration between PET and CT, and improved lesion localization.

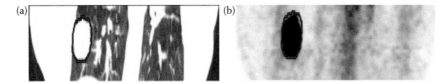

FIGURE 10.10   MIP-CT GTV (a) and the corresponding PET GTV (b). The MIP-CT GTV was contoured (red outline) and then copied to the registered PET GTV for comparison. MIP-CT accurately matches the extent of the PET GTV; therefore, the MIP-CT image set should serve as an accurate attenuation correction map for the PET image.

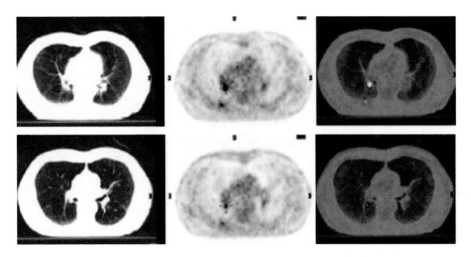

FIGURE 10.11   CT, PET, and fused PET/CT transaxial images at lesion location. Using ACT for AC in PET images (top row) resulted in improved lesion contrast, and an increase in its SUV by 63% compared to helical CT for AC (bottom row). The cross hair points to the lesion.

cine CT-scanned at a very high speed gantry rotation over one breath cycle. The cine CT images, acquired at each slice location, are then averaged to yield an ACT image that thus matches the PET temporal resolution. Pan and coworkers showed that using ACT images for PET AC resulted in improvements for the assessment of lymph node [18]FDG uptake, detectability, and the accuracy of tumor targeting for radiation treatment.[41] Figure 10.11 shows an example of improved PET-to-CT coregistration, and therefore an increased [18]FDG focal uptake, when using ACT to correct for attenuation in PET images. In this particular example, the SUV increased by 63% over that measured in the helical-CT attenuation corrected PET images.[41] As for MIP-CT, ACT does not require gating[33] or respiratory motion tracking. However, the technique still has the same drawback as MIP-CT in that it does not correct for motion artifacts in PET and CT images.

10.4 Clinical Use of 4D PET/CT in Radiation Treatment Planning

Respiratory motion management is a well-known concept for CT-based radiation treatment planning (RTP). Recently, an AAPM task group recommended that respiratory motion management technology is appropriate when target motion is greater than 5 mm, a method of respiratory motion management is available, and the patient can tolerate the procedure.[42] Incorporation

of 4D-PET data into RTP requires the accurate matching PET and CT, as described earlier. Use of 4D-PET in RTP provides information about the extent of tumor motion and improves the RTP-related processes of (1) target definition, (2) staging, and (3) therapy monitoring, as now reviewed.

10.4.1 Target Definition

Target volume delineation may be considered as the largest source of uncertainty in conformal radiation treatment and is a major step during the planning phases for IMRT and IGRT. The advent of hybrid PET/CT imaging, incorporating anatomical and metabolic information, has allowed the reduction of this uncertainty in defining the extent of the target volume.[43] Also, the use of PET/CT in radiotherapy planning enabled reduction of interobserver variability, compared to conventional CT-only contouring.[16,38] In the thorax, however, breathing motion can be a major challenge for defining the target volume, even with PET/CT. The International Commission of Radiation Units and Measurements (ICRU) recommends the clinical target volume (CTV) to be expanded to the internal target volume (ITV) with an internal margin that takes into account tissue deformations and physiologic movements due to respiration, cardiac motion, and peristalsis.[44]

The previously discussed techniques to correct for breathing-induced artifacts in hybrid PET/CT imaging[11,31,33] have facilitated delivery of 4D radiation plans. 4D PET/CT enabled smaller

FIGURE 10.12 (See color insert) Transaxial ¹⁸F-FDG PET image through a patient's lesion in nongated mode (a) and the corresponding image in gated mode acquired in the first bin (b). (c) Planning target volume in nongated (light blue) and gated (pink) modes. Note that light blue extends under whole pink area. Gating, in this particular case, has mainly spared left lung tissues from high dose regions.

target volumes and tighter corresponding margins.[15] These actions result in reduced dose to normal tissues and consequently decrease the risk of radiation-induced injury. In a proof of principal study that included four NSCLC patients, Nehmeh and coworkers showed reductions in the tumor volume by as much as 43% using 4D PET/CT images compared to standard nongated ones.[11] Figure 10.12a shows an example of the blurring of the planning target volume due to respiratory motion. The target volume with increased metabolic uptake had a range of motion shown by image intensities as delineated by the contour in Figure 10.12b. The corresponding gated 4D PET image (Figure 10.12b) shows a much smaller target volume.[15] In this particular example, the overestimation of the planning target volume resulted in a 12% increase in the normal tissue complication probability (NTCP) compared to the NTCP that would have been realized if the smaller target volume had been used from the gated PET images (personal communication with Nehmeh et al.). This yielded a higher exposure to normal lung tissues and therefore a reduction in the dose delivered to the target volume.

In another simulation study that investigated the effect of tumor motion on tumor control probability (TCP), Ling and coworkers demonstrated an average decrease of TCP of 8.1%[45] for a tumor motion amplitude of 3 cm (corresponding to diaphragm and gross-target volume excursions from end-inspiration to end-expiration). This result means that use of respiration correlated 4D-RTP will improve target under-dosing conditions, and due to exact depiction of lesion localization, irradiation of large parts of normal tissues can be omitted. In lung cancer, these improvements will emphasize the importance of the clinical concept of elective nodal irradiation of large macroscopically normal parts of the mediastinum when defining the CTV.[46]

10.4.2 Improved Staging and Disease Management

CT-based RTP has many limitations. First, the true extent of intrathoracic disease is not well delineated on CT scans. Second, CT fails to detect lesions in normal-sized lymph nodes or distinguish reactive hyperplasia from lesions. Consequently, patients are generally under-staged based on CT-only imaging. In the last decade, PET scanning has become an integral component of lung cancer staging because of its superior sensitivity and specificity over CT alone, in particular in the detection of nodal and distant metastases. Of significance, cancer staging using PET imaging usually yields important revisions in patient management.[47] The American Society of Clinical Oncology published evidence-based guidelines for the diagnostic evaluation of patients with NSCLC.[48] These recommendations include that FDG-based PET complements radiologic findings and PET imaging should be performed when there is no evidence of distant metastatic disease on CT.[49] Clinically, PET is always accompanied by CT because the relatively poor spatial resolution of PET limits its utility in the evaluation of the primary tumor and precise anatomic location of regions of focal increased uptake in nodes and metastatic lesions. Additionally, the introduction of integrated PET-CT scanners with automatic fusion of PET and CT images overcomes limitations inherent to both modalities when used separately. In fact, staging of NSCLC has been reported to be more accurate with integrated PET-CT than when using visual correlation of PET and CT images performed separately.[50] The limitations of both PET and CT data sets can further be reduced by acquiring 4D PET/CT data, using the techniques reviewed earlier in this chapter. 4D PET/CT approaches further enhance the detectability of lesions, which can be jeopardized by motion blurring in standard clinical PET images.[15,51] In addition, signal loss due to motion can only be recovered using 4D PET.[52]

10.4.3 Therapy Monitoring

The treatment responses measured by FDG-PET/CT after radiotherapy reflect the combined effects of changes in metabolism and physical size for the underlying target and normal tissues.[53] In a study that monitored tumor response during the course of radiotherapy, Erdi and coworkers showed a reduction in the measured SUV and lesion volume as a function of delivered radiation dose (Figure 10.13).[8] However, if this decrease is to be quantified in order to assess tumor response, breathing motion would need to be accommodated or otherwise lesion motion will constitute a major source of error. Clinical non-4D PET images are average images acquired over multiple respiratory cycles and SUVs are determined by searching the entire image volume for the maximum voxel intensity, which inherently is an average intensity value. The combined changes of SUV by PET, and the size measurements by non-4D CT may exaggerate, or diminish, the magnitude of response measurement errors depending on the average respiratory motion captured during the scan. Such

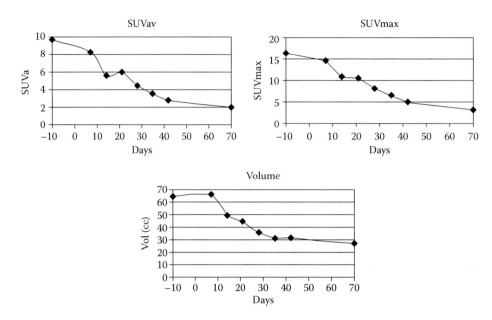

FIGURE 10.13 Therapy response parameters [SUV$_{avg}$, SUV$_{max}$, V$_{FDG}$] for one NSCLC patient. Radiation therapy started at day 0. Data points indicate actual scan days.

errors are particularly important when the size of lesion does not shrink quickly or significantly in post-treatment CT or PET scans. One also needs to consider the potential effects of postradiation inflammation on SUV measurements, which manifests as increased metabolism and thus, increased FDG uptake, and should give an ample time for the inflammation to subside for the lesion to show more accurate SUV values. At the posttherapy follow-up scan, it is important to use 4D imaging since lesion motion leads to distribution of activity into a larger volume, and will underestimate the SUV values of the lesion.[15]

10.5 Conclusion

PET/CT has provided inline fusion of anatomic and functional information. In addition to improving localization and characterization of sites of radiotracer uptake, this combined imaging modality has also increased the accuracy of diagnosis, staging, restaging, and monitoring of tumor response in different types of cancers. Moreover, PET has been shown to have a crucial role in accurately delineating the target volume, and identifying biological subvolumes within the GTV, enabling targeted dose-modulated radiotherapy techniques, and thus, better optimizing patient management. In lung, however, accuracy of any of the above described advantages of PET/CT is jeopardized due to breathing motion.

In this work, we have described the different approaches to correct for respiratory motion artifacts in PET images. Each of those techniques has its advantages and disadvantages, while the optimum clinical approach remains to be determined. The main concern with 4D-CT is the increased radiation dose. 4D-CT provides information about the extent of tumor motion, information critical for radiotherapy planning; however, during this procedure, the patient receives a dose that is at least three folds

higher in a standard PET/CT procedure, which is the main disadvantage of 4D-CT. 4D-PET images are acquired over shorter times than the standard PET acquisitions. This approach has two main disadvantages. First, it becomes clinically impractical to acquire more than one PET FOV, yielding only partial coverage of the lungs. Second, 4D-PET images have lower counts and therefore are noisier than standard PET images. Approaches to improve the statistics of 4D-PET while conserving temporal resolution include stacking of the 4D-PET image sets preceded by a nonrigid registration in image space.[54,55] However, because of the low-count issue, it is perhaps not advisable to perform any registration based on the PET images.

The average-CT technique[41] helps better spatially match PET and CT images. However, other motion artifacts (motion blurring, underestimation of SUV, etc.) will remain uncorrected.

In cases where patients can hold their breath, the DIBH PET/CT acquisition method proposed by Nehmeh and coworkers[17] may be the motion correction technique of choice. This method has the advantage of restricting the CT acquisition to the most reliable breathing phase, thus reducing the patient's dose. Moreover, previous studies showed that acquiring CT images at end inspiration increases the detectability of lung nodules.[20] Furthermore, PET data, acquired at only end inspiration, allows longer acquisition times as well as recovery of image statistics, which should improve PET/CT detectability.

Finally, motion-correction in PET/CT imaging has been shown to improve image quality and quantitation. However, whether those improvements make any difference in the final diagnosis and/or patient management compared to noncorrected images is still to be investigated. Studies aiming to evaluate the diagnostic value of motion-free PET/CT images of lung are currently being conducted.

References

1. Senan S, Ruysscher DD. Critical review of PET-CT for radiotherapy planning in lung cancer. *Crit Rev Oncol Hematol* 2005; 56:345–51.

2. Dwamena BA, Sonnad SS, Angobaldo JO, et al. Metastases from non-small cell lung cancer: mediastinal staging in the 1990's. Metaanalytic comparison of PET and CT. *Radiology* 1999; 213:530–6.

3. Bujenovic S. The role of positron emission tomography in radiation treatment planning. *Semin Nucl Med* 2004; 34:293–9.

4. Erdi YE, Rosenzweig K, Erdi AK, Macapinlac HA, Hu YC, Braban LE, Humm LE, Squire OD, Chui CS, Larson SM, Yorke, ED. Radiotherapy treatment planning for patients with non-small cell lung cancer using positron emission tomography (PET). *Radiother Oncol* 2002; 62(1):51–60.

5. Lee N, Nehmeh S, Schöder H, Fury M, Chan K, Ling CC, Humm J. Prospective trial incorporating pre-/mid-treatment [(18)F]-misonidazole positron emission tomography for head-and-neck cancer patients undergoing concurrent chemoradiotherapy. *Int J Radiat Oncol Biol Phys* 2009; 75(1):101-8.

6. Lee NY, Mechalakos JG, Nehmeh S, Lin Z, Squire OD, Cai S, Chan K, Zanzonico PB, Greco C, Ling CC, Humm JL, Schöder H. Fluorine-18-labeled fluoromisonidazole positron emission and computed tomography-guided intensity-modulated radiotherapy for head and neck cancer: a feasibility study. *Int J Radiat Oncol Biol Phys* 2008; 70(1):2–13.

7. Ling C, Hymm J, Larson S, Amols H, Fuks Z, Leibel S, et al. Towards multidimensional radiotherapy (MD-CRT): biological imaging and biological conformality. *Int J Oncol Biol Phys* 2000; 47:551–60.

8. Erdi YE, Macapinlac H, Rosenzweig KE, Humm JL, Larson SM, Erdi AK, Yorke ED. Use of PET to monitor the response of lung cancer to radiation treatment. *Eur J Nucl Med* 2000; 27(7):861–6.

9. Brock CS, Young H, O'Reilly SM, Mathews J, Osman S, Evans H, et al. Early evaluation of tumour metabolic response using [18F]fluoro-deoxyglucose and positron emission tomography: a pilot study following a phase II chemotherapy schedule for temozolomide in recurrent high-grade glioma. *Br J Cancer* 2000; 82:608–15.

10. Rothschild S, Studer G, Seifert B, Huguenin P, Glanzmann C, Davis JB, Lütolf UM, Hany TF, Ciernik IF. PET/CT staging followed by intensity-modulated radiotherapy (IMRT) improves treatment outcome of locally advanced pharyngeal carcinoma: a matched-pair comparison. *Radiat Oncol* 2007; 2:22.

11. Nehmeh SA, Erdi YE, Pan T, et al. Four-dimensional (4D) PET/CT imaging of the thorax. *Med Phys* 2004; 31:3179–86.

12. Sarikaya I, Yeung HW, Erdi Y, et al. Respiratory artefact causing malpositioning of liver dome lesion in right lower lung. *Clin Nucl Med* 2003; 28:943–44.

13. Erdi YE, Nehmeh SA, Pan T, et al. The CT motion quantitation of lung lesions and its impact on PET-measured SUVs. *J Nucl Med* 2004; 45:1287–92.

14. Beyer T, Antoch G, Muller S, et al. Acquisition protocol considerations for combined PET/CT imaging. *J Nucl Med* 2004; 45(suppl 1):25S–35S.

15. Nehmeh SA, Erdi YE, Ling CC, et al. Effect of respiratory gating on quantifying PET images of lung cancer. *J Nucl Med* 2002; 43:876–81.

16. Nehmeh SA, Erdi YE, Rosenzweig KE, et al. Reduction of respiratory motion artifacts in pet imaging of lung cancer by respiratory correlated dynamic PET: methodology and comparison with respiratory gated PET. *J Nucl Med* 2003; 44:1644–48.

17. Nehmeh SA, Erdi YE, Meirelles GSP, et al. Deep-inspiration breathhold PET/CT of the thorax. *J Nucl Med* 2006; 48:22–6.

18. Erdi YE, Nehmeh SA, Pan T, et al. The CT motion quantitation of lung lesions and its impact on PET-measured SUVs. *J Nucl Med* 2004; 45:1287–92.

19. Rietzel E, Pan T, Chen GT. Four-dimensional computed tomography: image formation and clinical protocol. *Med Phys* 2005; 32:874–89.

20. Meirelles GS, Erdi YE, Nehmeh SA, Squire OD, Larson SM, Humm JL, Schöder H. Deep-inspiration breath-hold PET/CT: clinical findings with a new technique for detection and characterization of thoracic lesions. *J Nucl Med* 2007; 48(5):712–9.

21. Amin Haj-Ali, Qing Chen, Hazim A. Jaradat, Paul Booth, Maryam Mehryar, John L. Humm, Sadek A. Nehmeh. A miniature and wireless tracking system for respiratory gated PET/CT. *J Nucl Med* 2009; 50(suppl 2):1543.

22. Kubo HD, Hill BC. Respiration gated radiotherapy treatment: a technical study. *Phys Med Biol* 1996; 41:83–91.

23. Xa L, Stepaniak C, Gore E. Technical and dosimetric aspects of respiratory gating using a pressure-sensor motion monitoring system. *Med 2009; Phys* 2006; 33:145–54.

24. Dietrich L, Jetter S, Tücking T, et al. Linac-integrated 4D cone beam CT: first experimental results. *Phys Med Biol* 2006; 51:2939–52.

25. Martínez-Möller A, Bundschuh R, Navab N, et al. Comparison of respiratory sensors and its compliance for respiratory gating in emission tomography. (Proceedings of Annual Meeting of Society of Nuclear Medicine, Washington, DC, June 2007). *J Nucl Med* 2007; 48(suppl 2):426.

26. Zhang T, Keller H, O'Brien MJ, et al. Application of the spirometer in respiratory gated radiotherapy. *Med Phys* 2003; 30:3165–71.

27. Ozhasoglu C, Murphy MJ. Issues in respiratory motion compensation during external-beam radiotherapy. *Int J Radiat Oncol Biol Phys* 2002; 52:1389–99.

28. Kalender WA, Rienmüller R, Seissler W, et al. Measurement of pulmonary parenchymal attenuation: use of spirometric gating with quantitative CT. *Radiology* 1990; 175:265–68.

29. Boucher L, Rodrigue S, Lecomte R, et al. Respiratory gating for 3-dimensional PET of the thorax: feasibility and initial results. *J Nucl Med* 2004; 45:214–19.

30. Yorke E, Rosenzweig KE, Wagman R, et al. Interfractional anatomic variation in patients treated with respiration-gated radiotherapy. *J Appl Clin Med Phys* 2005; 6:19–32.

31. Pan T, Lee TY, Rietzel E, et al. 4D-CT imaging of a volume influenced by respiratory motion on multi-slice CT. *Med Phys* 2004; 31:333–40.

32. Chang J, Sillanpaa J, Ling CC, et al. Integrating respiratory gating into a megavoltage cone-beam CT system. *Med Phys* 2006; 33:2354–61.

33. Pan T, Sun X, Luo D. Improvement of the cine-CT based 4D-CT imaging. *Med Phys* 2007; 34:4499–503.

34. Chi PC, Balter P, Luo D, et al. Relation of external surface to internal tumor motion studied with cine CT. *Med Phys* 2006; 33:3116–23.

35. Guivarc'h O, Turzo A, Visvikis D, et al. Synchronization of pulmonary scintigraphy by respiratory flow and by impedance plethysmography. *Proc SPIE Med Imaging* 2004; 5370:1166–75.

36. Hoffman EJ, Phelps ME, Wisenberg G, Schelbert HR, Kuhl DE, Electrocardiographic gating in positron emission computed tomography. *J Comput Assist Tomogr* 1979; 3, 733–39.

37. Kinahan PE, Vesselle H, MacDonald L, Alessio AM, Kohlmyer S, Lewellen T, Whole-body respiratory gated PET/CT. *J Nucl Med Meet. Abst.* 2006; 47:187P.

38. Nagel CCA, Bosmans G, Dekker ALAJ, et al. Phased attenuation correction in respiration correlated computed tomography/positron emitted tomography. *Med Phys* 2006; 33:1840–1847.

39. Duggan DM, Ding GX, Coffey CW II, et al. Deep-inspiration breath-hold kilovoltage cone-beam CT for setup of stereo-tactic body radiation therapy for lung tumors: initial experience. *Lung Cancer* 2007; 56:77–88.

40. Underberg RW, Lagerwaard FJ, Slotman BJ, Cuijpers JP, Senan S, Use of maximum intensity projections _MIP_ for target volume generation in 4DCT scans for lung cancer. *Int J Radiat Oncol Biol Phys* 2005; 63:253–60.

41. Pan T, Mawlawi O, Nehmeh SA, Erdi YE, Luo D, Liu HH, Castillo R, Mohan R, Liao Z, Macapinlac HA. Attenuation correction of PET images with respiration-averaged CT images in PET/CT. *J Nucl Med* 2005; 46:1481–7.

42. Keall PJ, Mageras GS, Balter JM, et al. The management of respiratory motion in radiation oncology report of AAPM Task Group 76. *Med Phys* 2006; 33(10):3874–900.

43. Greco C, Rosenzweig K, Cascini GL, Tamburrini O. Current status of PET/CT for tumour volume definition in radio-therapy treatment planning for non-small cell lung cancer (NSCLC). *Lung Cancer* 2007; 57(2):125-34.

44. International Commission on Radiation Units and Measurements (ICRU). Prescribing, Recording and Reporting Photon Beam Therapy. ICRU Report 50 1993.

45. Ling CC, Yorke E, Amols H, Mechalakos J, Erdi Y, Leibel S, Rosenzweig K, Jackson A. "High-tech will improve radio-therapy of NSCLC: a hypothesis waiting to be validated". *Int J Radiat Oncol Biol Phys* 2004; 60(1):3–7.

46. Nestle U, Weber W, Hentschel M, Grosu AL. Biological imaging in radiation therapy: role of positron emission tomography. *Phys Med Biol* 2009; 54(1):R1–R25.

47. Lardinois D, Weder W, Hany TF, et al. Staging of non-small-cell lung cancer with integrated positron-emission tomography and computed tomography. *N Engl J Med* 2003; 19:2500–7.

48. Pfister DG, Johnson DH, Azzoli CG, et al. American Society of Clinical Oncology treatment of unresectable non-small-cell lung cancer guideline: update 2003. *J Clin Oncol* 2004; 22:330–53.

49. Macapinlac HA. Clinical applications of positron emission tomography/computed tomography treatment planning. *Semin Nucl Med* 2008; 38(2):137–40 (Review).

50. Antoch G, Stattaus J, Nemat AT, et al. Non-small cell lung cancer: dual-modality PET/CT in preoperative staging. *Radiology* 2003; 229:526–33.

51. Park SJ, Ionascu D, Killoran J, Mamede M, Gerbaudo VH, Chin L, Berbeco R. Evaluation of the combined effects of target size, respiratory motion and background activity on 3D and 4D PET/CT images. *Phys Med Biol* 2008; 53(13):3661–79.

52. Pevsner A, Davis B, Joshi S, et al. Evaluation of an auto-mated deformable image matching method for quantifying lung motion in respiration-correlated CT images. *Med Phys* 2006; 33:369–76.

53. Pöttgen C, Levegrün S, Theegarten D, et al. Value of 18F-fluoro-2-deoxy-D-glucose-positron emission tomog-raphy/computed tomography in non-small-cell lung cancer for prediction of pathologic response and times to relapse after neoadjuvant chemoradiotherapy. *Clin Cancer Res* 2006; 12(1):97–106.

54. Klein GJ, Reutter RW, Huesman RH. Four-dimensional affine registration models for respiratory-gated PET. *IEEE Trans Nucl Sci* 2001; 48:756–60.

55. Thorndyke B, Schreibmann E, Maxim P, et al. Enhancing 4D PET through retrospective stacking. *Med Phys AAPM Meet* 2005; TU-D-J-6C-08.

11

On-Board Digital Tomosynthesis: An Emerging New Technology for Image-Guided Radiation Therapy

Q. Jackie Wu
Duke University

Devon Godfrey
Duke University

Lei Ren
Duke University

Sua Yoo
Duke University

Fang-Fang Yin
Duke University

External-beam radiation therapy is a common treatment modality for cancers. The treatment course typically consists of 30–40 daily fractions of 180–200 cGy over several weeks. On-board imaging (OBI) guidance is often designed to track shifts in patient positioning and tumor location immediately before treatment sessions. Many clinicians believe that daily imaging followed by any required adjustments to the plan or patient positioning would make radiation treatments more precise, especially if decisions for plan revisions can be based on 3D volumetric imaging of soft-tissue targets and nearby tissues.

Digital tomosynthesis (DTS) is a relatively new modality in image-guided radiation therapy (IGRT). DTS reconstructs a stack of image slices from projections obtained from a limited gantry rotation angle. Recent investigations of DTS for target localization are motivated by its advantages of shorter imaging time, increased mechanical clearance, and potential reduction of imaging dose. This chapter describes recent clinical investigations in developing and implementing the DTS technology for online image-guided patient positioning and target localization.

11.1 Introduction

IGRT represents a new era in the field of high-precision radiation therapy. Improved target localization capabilities through various (OBI) platforms, such as ultrasound, computed tomography, and magnetic resonance imaging technologies, have helped to fully realize the maximization of target dose and the minimization of normal organ/tissue spills. The recent development and wide application of OBI devices (Fox et al., 2006; Jaffray et al., 1999, 2002; Letourneau et al., 2005; Oldham et al., 2005; Pisani et al., 2000; Sharpe et al., 2003; Sorcini and Tilikidis, 2006; Yin et al., 2008) is intended to track tumor locations before, during, and after treatment to monitor inter- and intrafaction variations in patient position and anatomic locations. Figure 11.1a shows a typical OBI configuration (Varian Medical Systems, Palo Alto, CA). It consists of a kilovoltage (kV) x-ray source and an amorphous-silicon flat panel detector mounted orthogonally to the MV-beam axis. The available clinical imaging capabilities from this configuration are 2D electronic portal imaging using mega-voltage (MV) x-ray beams, 2D radiographic or fluoroscopic imaging using kV x-ray beams, and 3D kV cone beam computed tomography (3D CBCT) using kV x-ray beams.

The advantages of 3D CBCT over the 2D radiographic methods are the acquisition and reconstruction of a volumetric dataset, enabling anatomy to be displayed and analyzed throughout a contiguous set of 2D image slices, with improved soft-tissue contrast. The full 3D spatial/anatomic information from 3D CBCT improves patient positioning accuracy (Li et al., 2006; Oldham et al., 2005; Wang et al., 2007; Yin et al., 2008). The relatively high soft-tissue contrast is important for sites like the prostate and breast, where the relative position of target versus bony anatomy can potentially vary from one fraction to another, and rotational variations are

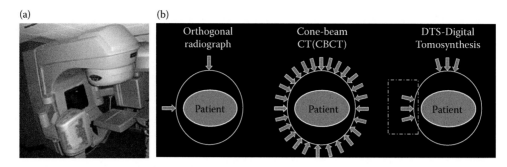

FIGURE 11.1 On-board imaging (OBI) technology. (a) Configuration of on-board imager (OBI) with a linear accelerator. (b) Illustration of imaging methods using 2D radiographs, CBCT, and DTS.

important for sites like head-and-neck where isocenter alignment alone is not sufficient. However, technical limitations (e.g., gantry rotational clearance) and imaging dose considerations may preclude the utilization of CBCT for daily positioning in many patients. For example, we have evaluated the radiation dose of several preset CBCT imaging techniques and found that the CBCT dose ranged from 5 to 9 cGy for standard CBCT scans of the head and neck and abdominal regions (Kim et al., 2008). In the study, thermoluminescence dosimeters (TLD) were placed in head and body CT phantoms, revealing that the standard head protocol was delivering a dose of 8.4 cGy and the standard body (pelvis) protocol was delivering 4.6 cGy, on average. More importantly, the radiation dose is delivered to the entire imaging volume, which is often much larger than the treatment volume. For example, use of daily CBCT imaging for IGRT of the breast will include and deliver unintended radiation dose to the contralateral breast, which is considered sensitive to secondary cancers from low-dose exposure (Hall and Brenner, 2008; Suit et al., 2007).

All forms of tomography rely on the motion of the x-ray source and/or detector during an exposure to create parallax, whereby the projected motion of objects is dependent on their distance from the detector. In traditional geometric tomography, a single long exposure is made while the acquisition system is in motion, creating an image where the anatomy at the target/focus level remains sharp (i.e., stationary), while off-plane structures are blurred by the system motion according to their distance from the focal plane. By varying the extent and path of motion, a variety of effects can be obtained, with variable depth of field and different degrees of blurring of "out-of-plane" structures. Both DTS and CT are tomographic imaging techniques (Kak and Slaney, 1999), which use a series of discrete projection images along with image processing to reconstruct a stack of user-selected focal planes in the imaged object. In CT, the source/detector makes a complete 360° rotation about the subject, obtaining a complete set of data from which images may be reconstructed. In DTS, only a small rotation angle (e.g., 40°) with a small number of discrete exposures (e.g., 10–80 projections) are used (Dobbins and Godfrey, 2003). This limited projection dataset can be digitally processed to yield a series of slices at different depths and with different thicknesses, similar to conventional tomography. However, due to the incomplete nature of the acquired projection data, tomosynthesis only generates slices in a single orientation (e.g., coronal) and is

unable to offer the extremely narrow slice widths or slice profiles that CT offers. In general, the tomosynthetic reconstruction usually suffers from "tomosynthetic noise," i.e., blurred images of off-plane structural detail, superimposed over the focused image of the reconstructed planes (Badea et al., 2001). However, DTS still allows very-high in-plane resolution, even though the out-of-plane resolution is reduced relative to CT. Methods of improving the out-of-plane resolution have been proposed and explored (Badea et al., 1998; Dobbins and Godfrey, 2003; Kolitsi et al., 1993).

Figure 11.1b illustrates the most common configuration of DTS imaging in radiation therapy: a kV OBI x-ray system mounted on a conventional linear treatment accelerator (linac). The linac machine is an isocentric system, and therefore the DTS projection images are acquired during the isocentric rotation of the x-ray tube-detector system around the patient. As discussed earlier, the resolution is very high within DTS slices reconstructed parallel to the central projection image in the scan, but the slice-to-slice resolution is low due to the limited scan angle. Thus, an excellent stack of coronal section images can be rendered from a DTS scan centered about the anterior–posterior (AP) view, but high-quality sagittal or axial views cannot be reconstructed from the same scan. Alternatively, stacks of sagittal DTS slices can be acquired from a scan centered about the right or left lateral view. Oblique DTS planes can also be reconstructed with gantry pointing at oblique angles. However, no view exists, which will allow the reconstruction of high-quality axial DTS images.

DTS has been proven to been a powerful diagnostic imaging modality for a variety of imaging sites (breast, lung, joints, etc.) (Duryea et al., 2003; Fahrig et al., 1997; Godfrey et al., 2006a; Niklason et al., 1997). DTS is an emerging OBI modality for per-fraction target localization in radiation treatment (Chang et al., 2009; Maltz et al., 2009; Yoo et al., 2009; Zhang et al., 2009). In particular, it is anticipated that DTS technology will be able to reduce imaging time, minimize mechanical clearance concerns (and thus, reduce the probability of device-patient collisions), and reduce imaging dose compared to CBCT. Figure 11.1b demonstrates the differences between 2D radiographic, CBCT, and DTS acquisitions for an existing, commercially available OBI geometry. While a 2D radiograph requires only 1 x-ray projection and an orthogonal pair requires 2 x-ray projections, CBCT imaging typically uses 600 to 700 x-ray projections acquired over 360° of rotation (~2 projections per degree) during

~1 min of continuous scanning for half-fan mode and ~200° of rotation for a full-fan mode. DTS, on the other hand, is generally implemented with only 40° of rotation (~80 x-ray projections) or less, acquired in less than 10 s.

The clinical feasibility of using DTS technology for on-board target localization is under active investigation (Godfrey et al., 2006b; Messaris et al., 1999; Pang and Rowlands, 2005; Wu et al., 2007). This chapter introduces and reviews on-board DTS for IGRT. The principles of DTS and reconstruction algorithms pertinent to isocentric systems are presented. A method for generating reference DTS (RDTS) images from a conventional planning CT is also presented. Bony and soft-tissue visibility in patients' on-board DTS images from different anatomic sites, such as breast, head and neck, prostate, and liver, are reviewed and discussed. The preliminary findings on target localization for various treatment anatomical sites are discussed. Finally, gated DTS acquisition is presented as a method for improving target visibility in anatomic regions that are prone to respiratory motion.

11.2 Isocentric DTS Reconstruction

11.2.1 On-Board DTS Reconstruction

The DTS image reconstruction is similar to CT reconstruction. Each projection image is first corrected for detector individual pixel response by flood and dark-field images, and the corrected projection data are run through a logarithmic transformation prior to tomographic reconstruction, to remove the exponential function inherent to Beer's law of attenuation (Godfrey et al., 2006b). The reconstruction geometry (using OBI system) is shown in Figure 11.2, which portrays the detector at the isocenter for simplification of the reconstruction mathematics (Godfrey et al., 2006b). The filtered back-projection reconstruction (Feldkamp et al., 1984) can be formulated as

$$f(x,z/y) = \int_{\beta=\min\beta}^{\max\beta} \frac{d^2}{(d-s)^2} \int_{-\infty}^{\infty} \frac{d}{\sqrt{d^2+p^2+\zeta^2}}$$
$$R(\beta,p,\zeta)h\left(\frac{d\cdot t}{d-s}-p\right)dpd\beta, \quad (11.1)$$

where $f(x,z/y)$ is the reconstructed plane (x, z) through a given depth y; β refers to the projection angle; d is the source-to-isocenter distance; $s = -x\sin\beta + y\cos\beta$ is the distance of a voxel from the detector plane; P and ζ are the detector axes perpendicular and parallel to the axis of rotation, respectively; $R(\beta, P, \zeta)$ is the cone-beam projection data; and $h(\cdot)$ denotes a 1 D ramp filter with a Hamming window, applied along P, with $t = x\cos\beta + y\sin\beta$. Thus, the Feldkamp DTS technique is analogous to Feldkamp CBCT (Feldkamp et al., 1984) solved only for specified depths y, with a small total scan angle of $|\beta \max - \beta \min| \ll 2\pi$.

11.2.2 Reference DTS Reconstruction

In IGRT, the patient on-board image volume is usually registered with a reference image volume for detection of patient positioning

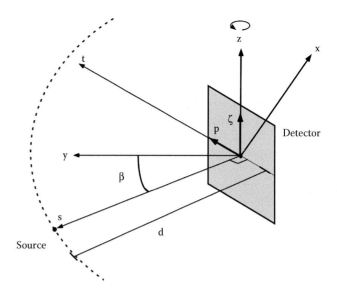

FIGURE 11.2 Digital tomosynthesis acquisition geometry with OBI configuration. (From Godfrey, DJ, et al., *Int J Radiat Oncol Biol Phys*, 68: 8–15, 2006b. With permission.)

errors. The planning CT image set is used as reference image data for registration with on-board CBCT volumes. However, due to the unique slice profile of DTS slices, anatomy is rendered differently in on-board DTS images than in corresponding planning CT slices (Godfrey et al., 2007). As a result, conventional planning CT image data do not appear to be adequate for registration with on-board DTS images (Godfrey et al., 2007).

To create a more exact reference set for DTS registration, we have pioneered a method for simulating reference DTS (RDTS) slices directly from conventional planning CT volumes (Godfrey et al., 2007). Using the ray-tracing algorithm (Siddon, 1985), forward cone-beam projections are computed through the planning CT volumes at geometries matching those of the actual projections acquired during an on-board DTS scan (Figure 11.2). DTS slices are then reconstructed from the simulated cone-beam projections, resulting in RDTS slices whose slice profile exactly matches that of the on-board DTS image data (Godfrey et al., 2007). Reconstruction of RDTS slices can be performed using the Feldkamp DTS algorithm described previously in Equation 11.1. This method permits registration of daily acquired on-board DTS images with RDTS images that share similar image information. The pairing of DTS and RDTS images is a key step in implementing the DTS technique for IGRT target verification (Godfrey et al., 2007).

11.3 Image Guidance Using DTS for Head–Neck Cancer Treatment

Head-and-neck was the first clinical site studied for DTS-based IGRT application at our institution (Wu et al., 2007). This clinical study evaluated DTS as a daily imaging technique for patient positioning based on bony anatomy and compared the results with 3D CBCT and 2D radiography. Sixty-five imaging datasets were acquired for 10 patients (ranging from 4 to 7 scans per patient, mean 6.5 scans/patient). For each treatment, the patient was initially positioned using laser marks. OBI datasets including 2D kV-radiographs, DTS, and CBCT were obtained to measure daily patient positioning variations.

Figure 11.3 shows sample DTS images of a head-and-neck case. The images were acquired using the standard CBCT imaging acquisition protocol for the head-and-neck region and were reconstructed in the coronal and sagittal orthogonal views, using a 40° scan angle for each. Consecutive DTS slices were reconstructed at 0.5 mm increment (slice spacing), but only every 20th slice is displayed in the figure. The display window and level were adjusted to provide the optimal contrast for bony anatomy as well as soft tissues. As a tomographic technique, the DTS images provide clear rendering of bony anatomy. The DTS images also appear to resolve the overlying anatomy onto distinct slices, but each slice plane contains some low-frequency shading from neighboring slices (which is characteristic of DTS imaging).

Figure 11.4 shows sample reference images, either RDTS or planning CT images, and the corresponding on-board images of DTS and CBCT, paired for patient positioning analysis. Bony anatomy is rendered differently with different imaging techniques. For example, differences in the appearance of bony edges are evident when the CBCT images are compared to the on-board DTS slices. On the other hand, reference images and corresponding on-board images from the same imaging technique (i.e., RDTS and DTS, CT, and CBCT) contain very similar image information that enables direct comparison and assessment of patient position (Godfrey et al., 2007).

Daily patient positioning variation was retrospectively measured in this study after all the image data were collected. All on-board images, 2D radiographs, CBCTs, and DTS images, as well as their corresponding reference images, were loaded into a dedicated OBI image evaluation station. On-board DTS images were registered with RDTS images to determine patient positioning corrections, and the results were compared with CT-CBCT registration to evaluate their accuracy. The image datasets of each modality were grouped and analyzed together. Four reconstructed DTS datasets (DTS with 40 and 20° projection arcs in coronal and sagittal views) were treated as four

independent modalities. Positioning variation measured by each modality was blinded to the other modalities.

For a given daily measurement, the origin $(0, 0, 0)$ was defined as the point in space marked by the initial patient setup using laser marks, not the isocenter detected using imaging guidance. The difference was defined as the daily isocenter positioning variation. Each imaging method returned a shift vector $Pi(j)$ that had a lateral (X, left–right), vertical (Y, anterior–posterior), and longitudinal (Z, superior–inferior) coordinate, where j indexed the imaging method ($j = $ 2D, 40° DTS-Coronal, 20° DTS-Coronal, 40° DTS-Sagittal, 20° DTS-Sagittal or CBCT) and i stands for the fraction number for a particular patient. The magnitude of $Pi(j)$ is $V_i(j) = \sqrt{X_i^2(j) + Y_i^2(j) + Z_i^2(j)}$. The mean and standard deviation of the daily positioning variation along each individual axis and of the vector magnitude were computed across all imaging fractions.

Table 11.1A summarizes the isocenter positioning differences (translations only) between the DTS and CBCT techniques (Wu et al., 2007). The mean differences between any of the four DTS and CBCT-based positioning methods were less than 0.1 cm in all directions, including the out-of-plane direction, and the mean vector differences were in the range of 0.14–0.16 cm, indicating that DTS is a potentially highly reliable IGRT technique for HN treatment.

Furthermore, the Pearson correlation coefficients were calculated to compare the similarity of DTS positioning to the 2D radiograph and CBCT positioning. Interestingly, the correlations among DTS and CBCT methods were high (0.94–0.95) and the correlation between DTS methods and 2D methods were much lower (0.79–0.81). The correlations between 2D and CBCT methods were also consistently lower, at roughly 0.80. These results suggest that the DTS positioning results conform closely to the CBCT rather than the 2D method.

The daily measured rotational variation was comparable between the two 40° DTS methods and the CBCT method, with a mean difference of less than 0.4° in any of the three rotational axes (the 20° DTS methods were not studied). The Pearson correlation coefficients were 0.95 (40°DTS-sagittal to CBCT) and 0.96 (40° DTS-coronal to CBCT) over all three rotational angles. The existence of a small rotational error may not affect isocenter positioning. However, the resulting displacement at

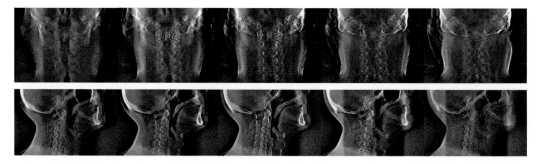

FIGURE 11.3 A set of DTS images reconstructed with a 44° scan angle, centered at gantry 0° for coronal-view DTS (a) and gantry 270° for sagittal-view DTS (b), respectively. (From Wu Q J, et al., *Int J Radiat Oncol Biol Phys*, 69: 598–606, 2007. With permission.)

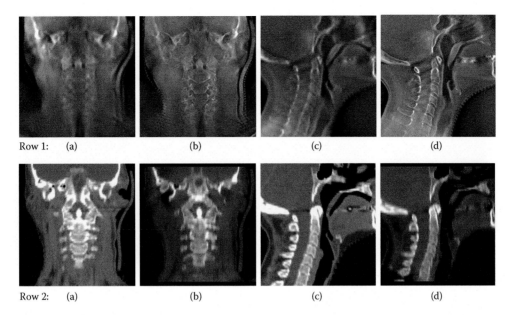

FIGURE 11.4 DTS (row 1) and CBCT (row 2) images of a head and neck cancer patient. Columns (a) and (c) are reference images, and columns (b) and (d) are their corresponding on-board images.

the far ends of a long treatment field may be problematic due to the projection of the error. Therefore, a complete correction of positioning error for H&N treatment with an elongated treatment volume should include rotational error correction. In such scenarios, 3D-based positioning techniques such as DTS or CBCT will have an advantage, as they directly provide six degrees of correction based on image content.

11.4 Image Guidance Using DTS for Prostate Cancer Treatment

A similar study to the head–neck site was performed for the prostate site, but the prostate study included the results of soft-tissue-based patient positioning (Yoo et al., 2009). A total of 92 image sessions from nine prostate cancer patients were analyzed. Figure 11.5 shows sample reference and corresponding on-board images used for localization in prostate cancer treatment. As shown, 2D radiography, represented in the form of digitally reconstructed radiographs (DRRs) computed from the planning CT image set as well as digital kV radiographs of the same projections, captures only bony anatomy information while both DTS and CBCT provide certain soft-tissue information along with bony anatomy. The coronal view DTS shows superior soft-tissue contrast compared to the sagittal view, as the increased lateral tissue thickness reduces the signal of the projection image in the sagittal direction. Tables 11.1B and C summarize the localization accuracy of different DTS methods for the prostate, compared to CBCT. When patient positioning was performed based on bony anatomy, the results from the DTS method were highly correlated to the results from the 3D CBCT method (accuracy ± 1 mm). The results of matching based on soft tissue (Table 11.1C) such as prostate showed a slightly lower

correlation than those based on bony anatomy (Table 11.1B) (accuracy ± 2 mm). In general, the sagittal-DTS method shows a larger variation from the CBCT method than the coronal-DTS method for matching of soft tissues.

When registering based on bony anatomy, the correlation of CBCT to DTS was higher (0.92–0.95) than the correlation between 2D and CBCT or DTS (0.81–0.83). When registering based on soft tissue, the correlation coefficients of CBCT to sagittal-DTS and to coronal-DTS were reduced to 0.84 and 0.92, respectively. Overall, the coronal-DTS and CBCT correlation was lowest in the vertical direction, as the vertical direction is the dimension of low resolution for coronal-DTS (i.e., the out-of-plane direction). Similarly, results in the lateral direction have the lowest correlation for comparison of sagittal-DTS with CBCT, as the lateral direction is the out-of-plane direction for the sagittal-DTS.

The results in Table 11.1 show that positioning verification using DTS has similar accuracy as CBCT when bony anatomy is used as the landmark. Coronal-DTS produces equivalent results to CBCT although sagittal-DTS alone is insufficient for soft-tissue-based positioning verification. These results suggest that DTS may provide comparable accuracy for soft-tissue-based target localization on a daily basis, with faster scanning time and less imaging dose.

11.5 Image Guidance Using DTS for Accelerated Partial Breast Treatment

Another interesting application of DTS imaging is for accelerated partial breast irradiation (APBI) treatments. In APBI treatments,

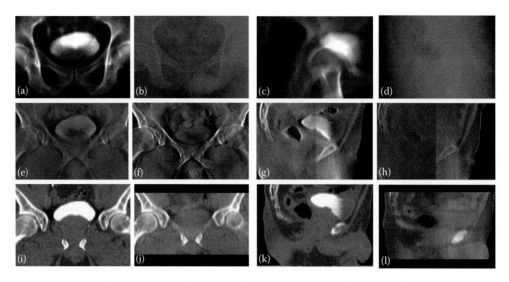

FIGURE 11.5 Reference images and on-board images of a prostate cancer patient. (a) AP DRR, (b) AP kV, (c) Lat DRR, (d) Lat kV, (e) Coronal RDTS, (f) Coronal DTS, (g) Sagittal RDTS, (h) Sagittal DTS, (i) Coronal planning CT, (j) Coronal CBCT, (k) Sagittal planning CT, and (l) Sagittal CBCT. All images were extracted at the isocenter plane. (From Yoo S, et al., *Int J Radiat Oncol Biol Phys,* 73: 296–305. 2009. With permission.)

TABLE 11.1. Patient positioning differences (DTS vs. CBCT) for the head and neck, and prostate

	A. Head and Neck (bony anatomy)			
	40° DTS-Sagittal	20° DTS-Sagittal	40° DTS-Coronal	20° DTS-Coronal
Vertical	0.7 (0.7)	0.8 (0.7)	0.7 (0.7)	0.7 (0.7)
Longitudinal	0.6 (0.6)	0.7 (0.7)	0.8 (0.7)	0.9 (0.7)
Lateral	0.7 (0.6)	0.9 (0.8)	0.8 (0.6)	0.8 (0.7)
Vector	1.4 (0.8)	1.6 (0.9)	1.5 (0.8)	1.6 (0.8)
	B. Prostate (bony anatomy)		C. Prostate (soft tissue)	
	40° DTS-Sagittal	40° DTS-Coronal	40° DTS-Sagittal	40° DTS-Coronal
Vertical	0.7 (0.8)	0.5 (0.7)	1.7 (1.7)	1.1 (1.2)
Longitudinal	0.4 (0.6)	0.4 (0.6)	1.0 (0.9)	0.7 (0.6)
Lateral	0.7 (0.6)	0.3 (0.6)	1.5 (1.4)	0.8 (0.7)
Vector	1.4 (0.8)	1.1 (0.8)	3.0 (1.7)	1.9 (1.1)

Source: From Wu Q J, et al., *Int J Radiat Oncol Biol Phys,* 69: 598–606, 2007; Yoo S et al., *Int J Radiat Oncol Biol Phys,* 73: 296–305, 2009. With permission.
Standard deviations shown in parentheses. All values are in mm.

the irradiated volume is relatively small compared to conventional tangential fields, and hence, there is particular interest in using 3D imaging techniques to guide patient positioning. Recent studies have reported that CBCT imaging can achieve 1–2 mm positioning accuracy for APBI setups (Fatunase et al., 2008; Purdie et al., 2007). However, the current CBCT techniques may not be optimal for APBI treatments in terms of radiation dose, acquisition time, and geometric clearance (Godfrey et al., 2006b; Zhang et al., 2009). Since the isocenter for breast patients is often placed several centimeters lateral to midline, near the chestwall, the couch often needs to be shifted medially (i.e.,

back to medial position) for CBCT data acquisition, to enable full gantry rotation of 360° without table or patient collisions. The contralateral breast and lung receive the same CBCT x-ray imaging dose (5–8 cGy) as the ipsilateral breast and lung (Kim et al., 2008). To protect healthy tissue and minimize secondary cancer occurrences, the dose to the contralateral breast and lung should be minimized if possible (Hall, 2006; Hall and Brenner, 2008; Fowble et al., 2001).

In DTS acquisition, contrary to CBCT acquisition, the patient can be left in the treatment position (no couch shift is necessary) because the gantry only has to rotate over a small angle. Furthermore, the contralateral breast and lung dose can be minimized because the scanning volume and angle can be selectively limited to the treatment site (Winey et al., 2009).

In a pilot study performed at our institution (Zhang et al., 2009), 10 patients receiving external-beam partial-breast irradiation were enrolled in an Institutional Review Board approved study to evaluate the utility of CBCT and DTS imaging in reducing patient set-up variations. To minimize statistical variation, the patient with only four CBCT scans was excluded from the study. For the other 9 evaluable patients, three had 10 CBCT scans, three had 9 scans, two had 8 scans, and two had 7 scans. Surgical clips were present at the excision bed in 6 of the 9 evaluable patients and were used for image registrations.

DTS scans were generated along coronal, sagittal, and oblique orientations. Due to the 15-cm detector shift applied in the half-fan CBCT scan mode, coronal DTS images were reconstructed using the projections between $180° + 22.5°$ (IEC convention) and $180° - 22.5°$ for right breast and the projections between $0° + 22.5°$ and $0° - 22.5°$ for the left breast. Sagittal DTS images were reconstructed using the projections between $270° + 22.5°$ and $270° - 22.5°$. Oblique DTS images were reconstructed using the projections between $225° + 22.5°$ and $225° - 22.5°$ for right breast and the projections between $315° + 22.5°$ and $315° - 22.5°$ for left breast.

Figures 11.6 and 11.7 show the coronal, sagittal, and oblique CBCT and DTS images for breast cancer patients with and without implanted surgical clips, respectively. As shown in both figures, it can be difficult to identify the tumor bed in one or both of the coronal and sagittal scans because bone and breast tissue contrast may strongly shade the tumor bed. However, the oblique scan orientation allows the breast tissue, bones, and lung to be well separated, and the soft–tissue contrast of the tumor bed appears sufficient for registration of the DTS images.

For patient positioning, the set of CBCT and DTS images for the first fraction were registered to each of the subsequent fraction sets of CBCT and DTS images in order to determine the translational shifts between fractions. In CBCT images, the registration was based on location of the soft tissue and surgical clips within the breast. In DTS images, the registration was based on the two clips closest to the treatment isocenter when surgical clips were available and based on the tumor bed itself when there were no surgical clips. Translational shifts of DTS images were compared to the translational shifts of the corresponding CBCT images to evaluate the registration accuracy.

Table 11.2 shows the positioning difference between the DTS and CBCT registrations for patients with (group A) and without (group B) surgical clips. DTS registrations based on the tumor bed had significantly lower accuracy than registrations based on surgical clips. For the oblique DTS, group B had comparatively larger root mean square (RMS) error values in the lateral and longitudinal directions than group A, and also for the vector sum. The RMS error along the vertical direction was not statistically different between the two groups. For group A, coronal DTS had smaller RMS error than sagittal and oblique DTS along the lateral direction and sagittal DTS had smaller RMS error than coronal and oblique DTS along the vertical direction. There was no significant difference in longitudinal RMS across the three DTS scan orientations.

Units are in millimeters. *P* value was calculated for the hypothesis that in-plane errors are smaller than out-of-plane errors.

Table 11.3 shows the positioning accuracy along both in-plane and out-of-plane directions for each DTS scan. For the six patients with surgical clips (group A), the off-plane accuracy was significantly lower than the in-plane accuracy for all three DTS scans. There was no significant difference between in-plane and off-plane accuracy for the three patients without surgical clips (group B).

In summary, in this pilot study for APBI patients, the positioning difference for DTS compared to CBCT localization was 1–2 mm. Oblique DTS scan orientations appear to be superior to coronal or sagittal scans for localization of tumor beds, and accuracy is

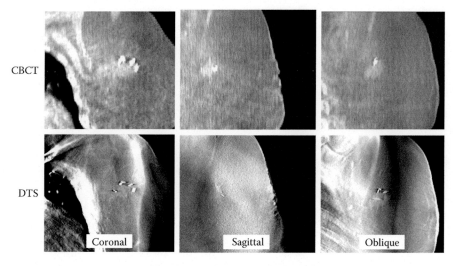

FIGURE 11.6 Three views of CBCT and DTS for a patient with surgical clips. While the surgical clips were visible in all three DTS scans, the tumor bed was clearly visible only in coronal and oblique scans. (From Zhang J, et al., *Int J Radiat Oncol Biol Phys,* 73: 952–7, 2009. With permission.)

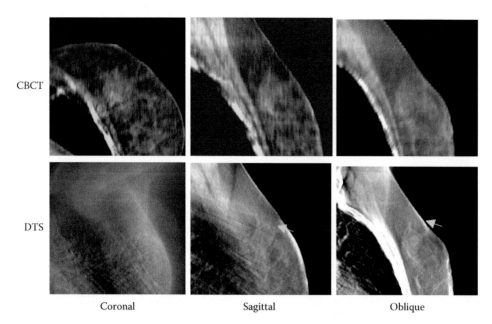

FIGURE 11.7 Three views of CBCT and DTS for a patient without surgical clips. The tumor bed (indicated by the arrows) is not visible in the coronal scan and is barely visible in the sagittal scan but is clearly visible in the oblique scan. (From Zhang J, et al., *Int J Radiat Oncol Biol Phys*, 73: 952–7, 2009. With permission.)

TABLE 11.2 Positioning difference between DTS and CBCT for three DTS scans, calculated as the RMS value

	Group A: 6 patients/52 fractions based on surgical clips			Group B: 3 patients/25 fractions based on tumor bed
	Coronal DTS	Sagittal DTS	Oblique DTS	Oblique DTS
Lateral	0.90	1.67	1.29	2.03
Vertical	1.31	1.28	1.35	1.24
Longitudinal	0.85	1.25	1.10	1.43
Vector	1.80	2.45	2.17	2.78

Source: From Zhang J, et al., *Int J Radiat Oncol Biol Phys*, 73: 952–7, 2009. With permission.
Unit: mm.

TABLE 11.3 In-plane and out-of-plane accuracy comparisons of the RMS values

	Group A: 6 patients/52 fractions based on surgical clips			Group B: 3 patients/25 fractions based on tumor bed
	Coronal DTS	Sagittal DTS	Oblique DTS	Oblique DTS
In-plane: longitudinal	0.85	1.28	1.10	1.43
In-plane: axial	0.90	1.25	0.96	1.75
Off-plane	1.31	1.67	1.60	1.62
p value	0.0001	0.01	0.0001	0.5

improved by the presence of surgical clips. Thus, for patients receiving (APBI), DTS localization offers comparable accuracy to CBCT localization for daily patient positioning while reducing mechanical constraints and imaging dose. These two factors are both clinically and biologically important for APBI treatments in which soft-tissue visibility and protection from x-ray imaging dose to the contralateral breast and lung are crucial.

11.6 Automatic Image Registration Using DTS

The three DTS image-guidance studies reported in the preceding sections were all based on manual, expert registration of reference RDTS and on-board DTS images, using visual recognition and correlation of complementary image features. This section discusses the feasibility of performing automatic registration of DTS images for IGRT patient positioning guidance.

Compared with manual registration, automatic registration is user independent, although expert-guidance for initial conditions may be important for certain techniques. A number of automatic image registration methods have been investigated in the literature (Maintz and Viergever, 1998). A wide spectrum of registration techniques have been developed for the registration of OBI images, such as 2D–2D registration of kV or MV portal images with DRRs (Asvestas et al., 2007; Dong and Boyer, 1995), 2D–3D registration of portal images with planning CT (Jans et al., 2006; Kim et al., 2005), and 3D–3D registrations of planning CTs with CBCTs (Paquin et al., 2009; Munbodh et al., 2006).

Automated registration algorithms for DTS image registration in radiation therapy are still under development. Unlike other image modalities, DTS images have high resolution in the reconstructed planes, but relatively low resolution along the plane-to-plane direction. This anisotropy of the resolution needs to be considered in developing the registration method for DTS (Godfrey et al., 2007). Automatic registration between RDTS and on-board DTS images is a critical step toward clinical implementation of DTS technology.

Figure 11.8 shows a prototype automatic DTS image registration scheme developed by our group, which incorporates the planning CT, multiple DRR and kV projection images, and RDTS and on-board DTS image sets. The DTS registration algorithm performs 6° rigid body alignment by maximizing the mutual information between the RDTS and on-board DTS volumes (Ren et al., 2008a). Both RDTS and on-board DTS images have very high in-plane resolution, but relatively low resolution along the out-of-plane direction due to the limited number of projections acquired. The continuous update and reprojection of the reference

DRR from the planning CT volume with each iteration ensures that the orientation of the low resolution axis in the RDTS matches that of the on-board DTS, providing optimal localization accuracy.

The registration robustness can be evaluated by calculating the capture range of the registration (Skerl et al., 2008). In this experiment, we considered a registration trial to be successful if its mean target registration error was less than 2 mm. The capture range was then defined as the range of the setup deviations for rotation [Rx, Ry, and Rz] and translation [Tx, Ty, and Tz], over which the registration trials were all successful. The larger the capture range, the more robust the registration. Table 11.4 displays the registration capture ranges for different scan angles (44° and 22°) and different region-of-interest (ROI) sizes for eight head-and-neck cancer patient cases (Section 11.3) (Ren et al., 2008a). The average capture ranges in single-axis simulations with a 44° scan angle and a large ROI covering the entire DTS volume were between −46° and +44° for rotations and between −58 and +64 mm for translations in the patient study. As shown, registration of a smaller ROI had smaller capture ranges than registration of the entire DTS volume. This is because less information is available for registration in the smaller ROI volume. Within the capture range of Table 11.4, the automatic registration technique also showed high accuracy of 1.4 mm, as shown in Table 11.5.

11.7 DTS for Respiratory Motion-Gated Treatment

For radiation treatment sites that are prone to respiratory motion (Balter et al., 1996; Berbeco et al., 2006; Blackall et al., 2006; Brandner et al., 2006; Rosu et al., 2003), such as liver and lung,

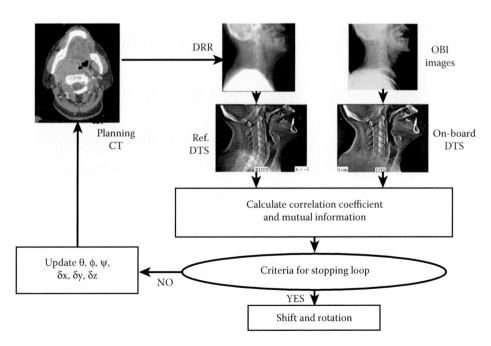

FIGURE 11.8   Automatic DTS registration system.

TABLE 11.4 The registration capture ranges for different scan angles (44° and 22°) and different ROI sizes in the head-and-neck cancer patient study

		Rx (°)	Ry (°)	Rz (°)	Tx (mm)	Ty (mm)	Tz (mm)
Entire volume registered	22° DTS	−20~20	−18~22	−36~38	−40~44	−44~58	−40~38
	44° DTS	−38~36	−34~36	−46~44	−50~58	−58~70	−64~60
ROI registered	22° DTS	−12~10	−8~8	−26~26	−26~18	−54~54	−38~52
	44° DTS	−20~32	−18~18	−18~20	−18~16	−52~56	−36~44

TABLE 11.5 The average, standard deviation, median, and 90th percentile of the mean target registration errors using a 44° DTS in the head-and-neck cancer patient study

	Average	STDEV	Median	90th percentile
Entire volume registered	1.4	0.4	1.4	1.8
ROI registered	1.4	0.3	1.4	1.7

Unit: mm.

reducing target motion has the advantage of eliminating the need for expanded internal target volumes (ITV) and reducing the normal tissue volumes exposed to high dose radiation. In order to minimize the motion, treatment using abdominal compression, under deep inspiration breath-hold (BH) or active breathing control (ABC), has been utilized (Balter et al., 2002; Dawson et al., 2001; Herfarth et al., 2000; Keall et al., 2006; Mageras and Yorke, 2004; Pattaranutaporn et al., 2001; Wong et al., 1999; Yokokawa and Shintani, 2002; Yoshitake et al., 2008).

Several studies investigated the reproducibility of organ position using ABC or BH for lung and liver cancer patients and have found a change in diaphragm position from day to day despite using ABC or BH in the same planned position (Dawson et al., 2001; Eccles et al., 2006). Therefore, quick daily imaging is preferred to verify the target position prior to treatment.

Due to its long scan duration (~1 min continuous scan), CBCT-based breath-hold localization has to be acquired over 3–4 breath holds. If used for BH treatment, the total time of acquiring a BH CBCT is about 3–4 min. DTS is a fast (< 10 s) alternative to CBCT for 3D imaging guidance in this scenario(Godfrey et al., 2006b). The BH DTS can be acquired over a single breath hold of less than 10 s versus several minutes for CBCT.

DTS-based IGRT for BH radiation treatment is currently being investigated at our institution. In this study, both treatment planning CT and on-board kV projection images for DTS reconstruction were acquired under breath hold. To be eligible for BH-gated treatment and imaging, patients were required to be able to hold their breath for at least 20 s. Each patient was instructed about the breath-hold technique and a brief session of practice was conducted prior to the treatment planning CT. The patients' BH levels were monitored by the RPM system (Guana, 2006; Kini et al., 2003). The motion of the abdomen surface, a surrogate of breathing motion, was tracked by the RPM infrared camera. A comfortable deep inspiration breath-hold level was set for each patient and the amplitude gating window was determined, as shown in Figure 11.9. This window established the upper and lower thresholds of the patient's breath-hold levels

and was saved as the reference for daily treatment throughout the treatment course. Then, BH treatment planning CT scans were acquired when the patient's BH levels were within these set thresholds. The scanning volumes were broken into segments of duration determined by the patient's length of a comfortable breath hold, as shown in Figure 11.9a. Each segment consisted of multiple axial slices of CT images. Between segments, the patient breathed freely until a stable breathing pattern was established. External marks, used for treatment position alignment with lasers, were also marked under BH.

Figure 11.9 shows the image data acquisition geometry and also illustrates how the BH segments are distributed during the image acquisition period for the different imaging modalities. The continuous CBCT scan takes about 1 min. When imaged under BH, the gantry rotation is typically broken into 3–4 segments to accommodate BH duration (~20 s), as shown in Figure 11.9b. Different segments cover different gantry projections and the composite of each BH image segment completes a full CBCT projection set. The total time for a complete CBCT scan including the breaks between BH sessions is about 3–5 min. Since DTS uses a small arc of gantry rotation, it can be acquired with only one BH segment. Two standard viewing angles, the coronal and the sagittal views, were reconstructed, as shown in Figure 11.9c. With breath hold used for acquisition of the planning CT and on-board kV projection images, DRR-kV projection image pairs, and complementary RDTS and DTS images can be computed and compared for treatment verification.

Figure 11.10 shows the BH RDTS-DTS images of a liver case. The dome of the liver, the tumor edges and the soft-tissue contrast between different organs are clearly visible. Based on these early results, DTS-based image guidance is expected to provide rapid and accurate target localization and verification for BH-gated radiation treatment.

11.8 Future DTS Research and Development

For patients who cannot endure breath-hold treatment, the 4D treatment planning protocol is used in our institution to properly account for respiration induced tumor motion and deformation. For this group of patients, a fast free-breathing CT is acquired, followed by a 4D-CT scan for treatment planning. The internal target volume (ITV) is formed by summing all the CTV from the 4D-CT images. Additional margin is added to the ITV to form the PTV for treatment planning. The verification of such 4D treatment is critical as patient breathing patterns

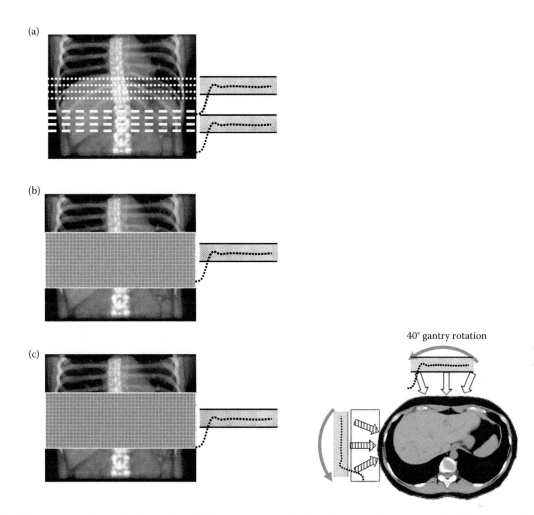

FIGURE 11.9 Distribution of the multiple breathhold (BH) segments over the imaging acquisition geometry. (a) CT geometry. Each BH segment covers a subset of CT slices and multiple BH segments are distributed in the superior to inferior direction. (b) CBCT geometry. Each BH segment covers a subset of projection images or gantry rotations. Multiple BH segments are distributed along the gantry rotation direction. (c) DTS geometry (coronal and sagittal). Single BH covers one imaging acquisition. Multiple BH segments are for different DTS views. (From Wu, Q J et al., *Int J Radiat Oncol Biol Phys,* 79(1): 289–296, 2011. With permission.)

can vary from fraction to fraction. CBCT has challenges for monitoring 4D target motion due to its data acquisition time cost and imaging dose per scan. 4D DTS, on the other hand, can be easily implemented by acquiring 4D projection images over 10–20° gantry angles with a total scan time of less than 1 min. These projections are then retrospectively sorted according to respiratory phase. Projections grouped by phase are then reconstructed into 4D DTS images. 4D DTS is currently under development by the authors and other groups (Maurer et al., 2008, 2009; Pang and Rowlands, 2005).

Another area of future study includes the combination of kV and MV image data to generate DTS reconstructions. The unique configuration of separate and orthogonal kV imaging and MV treatment beams and matching digital image receptors on modern radiation treatment machines allows for both kV and MV imaging. MV imaging with 6 MV x-rays provides complementary features to kV x-ray imaging at 100 kV, such as deeper penetration and reduced metal artifacts but yields less soft-tissue contrast. In the future, both kV and MV sources

with orthogonal orientations may be used for DTS imaging to improve the localization accuracy as well as image quality. Real-time tracking can provide high accuracy localization for a moving target and minimize the effect of motion. However, the kV and MV beams cross shooting the target interfere with each other with beam scattering, which affects the quality of images. We performed a clinical study investigating this effect (Luo et al., 2008). The kV and MV images were acquired for a gold implant marker that was used as a surrogate of the target and placed in an IMRT thorax phantom, a dynamic phantom, and a pelvis phantom to test the image quality in different situations. Contrast-to-noise ratio (CNR) was used to quantitatively describe the visibility of the target in the image. By comparing the ratio (R) of CNR with and without the MV beam on, the MV beam scatter was found to have dramatically reduced the target visibility in the kV images ($R = 0.47$). However, the kV scatter effect on the MV images was minor ($R = 0.93$). Considering a threshold of 1.0 CNR as a measure for the target visibility, a range of CNR from 1.3 to 4.2 was reached with appropriate tuning of

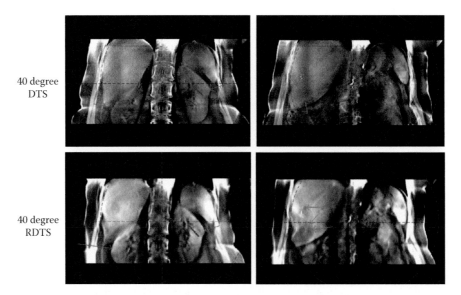

FIGURE 11.10 **(See color insert)** Breath-hold DTS and RDTS images for liver treatment. The pink arrows denote the kidney and lesion borders, and the red arrows point to the more detailed soft-tissue markings.

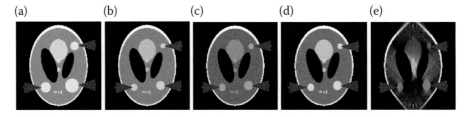

FIGURE 11.11 Reconstruction of the Shepp-Logan phantom using *a priori* CBCT imaging and filtered back projection (FBP) with 60 or 90° scan angles. Three tumors simulated are indicated by red arrows. (a) The prior CBCT image, (b) the new CBCT image, (c) the new CBCT image estimated from prior CBCT and 60° new projections, (d) the new CBCT image estimated from prior CBCT and 90° new projections, (e) FBP-based 90° DTS without *a priori* CBCT imaging. (From Ren L, et al., *Med Phys,* 35: 3110–5, 2008b. With permission.)

imaging parameters for different tumor sites, for simultaneous kV–MV imaging (Luo et al., 2008).

The current Feldkamp DTS reconstruction method does not provide full 3D volumetric information due to the limited angle of projection data acquired. This can impair the patient positioning accuracy using DTS images. Other novel methods are being developed to improve the estimation of the patient volumetric information from limited angle projection data (Badea et al., 1998; Kolitsi et al., 1993). One method is to use previous CBCT images as prior information to guide reconstruction of the new image volume as a deformation of the prior images. The deformation field can be solved by minimizing deformation energy and maintaining data fidelity (Ren et al., 2008b). Figure 11.11 shows early experimental results for the Shepp-Logan phantom test using the novel *a priori* method (Ren et al., 2008b). Three tumors of different sizes were simulated at initial sizes and different locations in the prior CBCT image (Figure 11.11a) and then simulated to experience tumor shrinkage in the new CBCT image (Figure 11.11b). As shown in Figure 11.11c and d, the shrinkage of tumors have been reconstructed accurately in the new CBCT images estimated

from the prior CBCT using new projections of 60° and 90°. The poorer fidelity, filtered back projection (FBP) DTS image reconstructed from 90° projections, without the use of the prior CBCT, is shown in Figure 11.11e for comparison.

11.9 Summary

CBCT technology will continue to improve. However, imaging limitations of CBCT technology for IGRT are driven by the mechanical limitations of mounting the CBCT on the gantry of a linear accelerator, increasing the possibility of equipment and patient collisions and reducing the sampling space, rather than the CBCT technology itself. Since DTS technology uses only a small subset of CBCT projections, DTS will always be faster and will have fewer clearance limitations than CBCT. There will always be an incremental benefit of DTS over CBCT in terms of imaging dose, acquisition time, and clearance. Thus, a tradeoff exists between the high image quality of CBCT and the high efficiency and clinical flexibility of DTS. Initial studies suggest that DTS-based image guidance may be appropriate for certain anatomic sites and treatment regimens, providing clinicians a means for avoiding some of the pitfalls of CBCT-based image guidance. Meanwhile, future DTS developments will likely continue to improve the potential for DTS-based image guidance.

Acknowledgments

Research in this manuscript has been supported by grants from NIH (5R21CA128368-02R21), Varian Medical Systems, and General Electric Medical Systems.

References

Asvestas P A, Delibasis K K, Mouravliansky N A, and Matsopoulos G K, 2007. ESTERR-PRO: a setup verification software system using electronic portal imaging. *Int J Biomed Imaging* **2007**: 61523.

Badea C, Kolitsi Z, and Pallikarakis N, 1998. A wavelet-based method for removal of out-of-plane structures in digital tomosynthesis. *Comput Med Imaging Graph* **22**: 309–15.

Badea C, Kolitsi Z, and Pallikarakis N, 2001. Image quality in extended arc filtered digital tomosynthesis. *Acta Radiol* **42**: 244–8.

Balter J M, Brock K K, Litzenberg D W, McShan D L, Lawrence T S, Ten Haken R, McGinn C J, Lam K L, and Dawson L A, 2002. Daily targeting of intrahepatic tumors for radiotherapy. *Int J Radiat Oncol Biol Phys* **52**: 266–71.

Balter J M, Ten Haken R K, Lawrence T S, Lam K L, and Robertson J M, 1996. Uncertainties in CT-based radiation therapy treatment planning associated with patient breathing. *Int J Radiat Oncol Biol Phys* **36**: 167–74.

Berbeco R I, Nishioka S, Shirato H, and Jiang S B, 2006. Residual motion of lung tumors in end-of-inhale respiratory gated radiotherapy based on external surrogates. *Med Phys* **33**: 4149–56.

Blackall J M, Ahmad S, Miquel M E, McClelland J R, Landau D B, and Hawkes D J, 2006. MRI-based measurements of respiratory motion variability and assessment of imaging strategies for radiotherapy planning. *Phys Med Biol* **51**: 4147–69.

Brandner E D, Wu A, Chen H, Heron D, Kalnicki S, Komanduri K, Gerszten K, Burton S, Ahmed I, and Shou Z, 2006. Abdominal organ motion measured using 4D CT. *Int J Radiat Oncol Biol Phys* **65**: 554–60.

Chang S, Frederick B, Liu X, Tracton G, Lawrence M, Lalush D, and Pizer S, 2009. Image-guided radiotherapy using Nanotube stationary Tomosynthesis technology. *Med Phys* **36**: 2478.

Dawson L A, Brock K K, Kazanjian S, Fitch D, McGinn C J, Lawrence T S, Ten Haken R K, and Balter J, 2001. The reproducibility of organ position using active breathing control (ABC) during liver radiotherapy. *Int J Radiat Oncol Biol Phys* **51**: 1410–21.

Dobbins J T, III and Godfrey D J, 2003. Digital x-ray tomosynthesis: current state of the art and clinical potential. *Phys Med Biol* **48**: R65–R106.

Dong L and Boyer A L, 1995. An image correlation procedure for digitally reconstructed radiographs and electronic portal images. *Int J Radiat Oncol Biol Phys* **33**: 1053–60.

Duryea J, Dobbins J T, III, and Lynch J A, 2003. Digital tomosynthesis of hand joints for arthritis assessment. *Med Phys* **30**: 325–33.

Eccles C, Brock K K, Bissonnette J P, Hawkins M, and Dawson L A, 2006. Reproducibility of liver position using active breathing coordinator for liver cancer radiotherapy. *Int J Radiat Oncol Biol Phys* **64**: 751–9

Fahrig R, Fox A J, Lownie S, and Holdsworth D W, 1997. Use of a C-arm system to generate true three-dimensional computed rotational angiograms: preliminary in vitro and in vivo results *AJNR Am J Neuroradiol* **18**: 1507–14.

Fatunase T, Wang Z, Yoo S, Hubbs J L, Prosnitz R G, Yin F F, and Marks L B, 2008. Assessment of the residual error in soft tissue setup in patients undergoing partial breast irradiation: results of a prospective study using cone-beam computed tomography. *Int J Radiat Oncol Biol Phys* **70**: 1025–34.

Feldkamp L A, Davis L C, and Kress J W, 1984. Practical cone-beam algorithm. *J Opt Soc Am A* **1**: 612–9.

Fowble B, Hanlon A, Freedman G, Nicolaou N, and Anderson P, 2001. Second cancers after conservative surgery and radiation for stages I-II breast cancer: identifying a subset of women at increased risk. *Int J Radiat Oncol Biol Phys* **51**: 679–90.

Fox T H, Elder E S, Crocker I R, Davis L W, Landry J C, and Johnstone P A, 2006. Clinical implementation and efficiency of kilovoltage image-guided radiation therapy. *J Am Coll Radiol* **3**: 38–44.

Godfrey D J, McAdams H P, and Dobbins J T, III, 2006a. Optimization of the matrix inversion tomosynthesis (MITS) impulse response and modulation transfer function characteristics for chest imaging. *Med Phys* **33**: 655–67.

Godfrey D J, Ren L, Yan H, Wu Q, Yoo S, Oldham M, and Yin F F, 2007. Evaluation of three types of reference image data for external beam radiotherapy target localization using digital tomosynthesis (DTS). *Med Phys* **34**: 3374–84.

Godfrey D J, Yin F F, Oldham M, Yoo S, and Willett C, 2006b. Digital tomosynthesis with an on-board kilovoltage imaging device. *Int J Radiat Oncol Biol Phys* **65**: 8–15.

Guana H, 2006. Time delay study of a CT simulator in respiratory gated CT scanning. *Med Phys* **33**: 815–9.

Hall E J, 2006. Intensity-modulated radiation therapy, protons, and the risk of second cancers. *Int J Radiat Oncol Biol Phys* **65**: 1–7.

Hall E J and Brenner D J, 2008. Cancer risks from diagnostic radiology. *Br J Radiol* **81**: 362–78.

Herfarth K K, Debus J, Lohr F, Bahner M L, Fritz P, Hoss A, Schlegel W, and Wannenmacher M F, 2000. Extracranial stereotactic radiation therapy: set-up accuracy of patients treated for liver metastases. *Int J Radiat Oncol Biol Phys* **46**: 329–35.

Jaffray D A, Drake D G, Moreau M, Martinez A A, and Wong J W, 1999. A radiographic and tomographic imaging system integrated into a medical linear accelerator for localization of bone and soft-tissue targets. *Int J Radiat Oncol Biol Phys* **45**: 773–89.

Jaffray D A, Siewerdsen J H, Wong J W, and Martinez A A, 2002. Flat-panel cone-beam computed tomography for image-guided radiation therapy. *Int J Radiat Oncol Biol Phys* **53**: 1337–49.

Jans H S, Syme A M, Rathee S, and Fallone B G, 2006. 3D interfractional patient position verification using 2D-3D registration of orthogonal images. *Med Phys* **33**: 1420–39.

Kak A C and Slaney M, 1999. *Principles of Computerized Tomographic Imaging.* SIAM (Society of Industrial and Applied Mathematics). Philadelphia.

Keall P J, Mageras G S, Balter J M, Emery R S, Forster K M, Jiang S B, Kapatoes J M, Low D A, Murphy M J, Murray B R, Ramsey C R, Van Herk M B, Vedam S S, Wong J W, and Yorke E, 2006. The management of respiratory motion in radiation oncology report of AAPM Task Group 76. *Med Phys* **33**: 3874–900.

Kim J, Yin F F, Zhao Y, and Kim J H, 2005. Effects of x-ray and CT image enhancements on the robustness and accuracy of a rigid 3D/2D image registration. *Med Phys* **32**: 866–73.

Kim S, Yoshizumi T T, Toncheva G, Yoo S, and Yin F F, 2008. Comparison of radiation doses between cone beam CT and multi detector CT: TLD measurements. *Radiat Prot Dosim* **132**: 339–45.

Kini V R, Vedam S S, Keall P J, Patil S, Chen C, and Mohan R, 2003. Patient training in respiratory-gated radiotherapy. *Med Dosim* **28**: 7–11.

Kolitsi Z, Panayiotakis G, and Pallikarakis N, 1993. A method for selective removal of out-of-plane structures in digital tomosynthesis. *Med Phys* **20**: 47–50.

Letourneau D, Wong J W, Oldham M, Gulam M, Watt L, Jaffray D A, Siewerdsen J H, and Martinez A A, 2005. Cone-beam-CT guided radiation therapy: technical implementation. *Radiother Oncol* **75**: 279–86.

Li H, Zhu X R, Zhang L, Dong L, Ahamad A, Chao K S, Morrison W H, Rosenthal D I, Schwartz D L, and Garden A S, 2006. Assessment of positioning accuracy of head and neck patients receiving IMRT using on-board imaging and cone beam CT. *Int J Radiat Oncol Biol Phys* **66**: S144.

Luo W, Yoo S, Wu Q J, Wang Z, and Yin F F, 2008. Analysis of image quality for real-time target tracking using simultaneous kV-MV imaging. *Med Phys* **35**: 5501–9.

Mageras G S and Yorke E, 2004. Deep inspiration breath hold and respiratory gating strategies for reducing organ motion in radiation treatment. *Semin Radiat Oncol* **14**: 65–75.

Maintz J B and Viergever M A, 1998. A survey of medical image registration. *Med Image Anal* **2**: 1–36.

Maltz J, Sprenger F, Fuerst J, Paidi A, Fadler F, and Bani-Hashemi A, 2009. Stationary-granty tomosynthesis system for on-line image guidance in radiation therapy based on a 52-source cold cathode x-ray tube. *Med Phys* **36**: 2762.

Maurer J, Godfrey D, Wang Z, and Yin F F, 2008. On-board four-dimensional digital tomosynthesis: first experimental results. *Med Phys* **35**: 3574–83.

Maurer J, Pan T, and Yin F F, 2009. Slow Gantry Rotation Acquisition Protocol for Four-Dimensional Digital Tomosynthesis. *Med Phys* **36**: 2725.

Messaris G, Kolitsi Z, Badea C, and Pallikarakis N, 1999. Three-dimensional localisation based on projectional and tomographic image correlation: an application for digital tomosynthesis. *Med Eng Phys* **21**: 101–9.

Munbodh R, Jaffray D A, Moseley D J, Chen Z, Knisely J P, Cathier P, and Duncan J S, 2006. Automated 2D-3D registration of a radiograph and a cone beam CT using line-segment enhancement. *Med Phys* **33**: 1398–411.

Niklason L T, Christian B T, Niklason L E, Kopans D B, Castleberry D E, Opsahl-Ong B H, Landberg C E, Slanetz P J, Giardino A A, Moore R, Albagli D, DeJule M C, Fitzgerald P F, Fobare D F, Giambattista B W, Kwasnick R F, Liu J, Lubowski S J, Possin G E, Richotte J F, Wei C Y, and Wirth R F, 1997. Digital tomosynthesis in breast imaging. *Radiology* **205**: 399–406.

Oldham M, Letourneau D, Watt L, Hugo G, Yan D, Lockman D, Kim L H, Chen P Y, Martinez A, and Wong J W, 2005. Cone-beam-CT guided radiation therapy: A model for on-line application. *Radiother Oncol* **75**: 271–8.

Pang G and Rowlands J A, 2005. Just-in-time tomography (JiTT): a new concept for image-guided radiation therapy. *Phys Med Biol* **50**: N323–30.

Paquin D, Levy D, and Xing L, 2009. Multiscale registration of planning CT and daily cone beam CT images for adaptive radiation therapy. *Med Phys* **36**: 4–11.

Pattaranutaporn P, Chansilpa Y, Ieumwananonthachai N, Kakanaporn C, Onnomdee K, Mungkung N, and Santisiri R, 2001. Three-dimensional conformal radiation therapy and periodic irradiation with the deep insipration breath-hold technique for hepatocellular carcinoma. *J Med Assoc Thai* **84**: 1692–700.

Pisani L, Lockman D, Jaffray D, Yan D, Martinez A, and Wong J, 2000. Setup error in radiotherapy: on-line correction using electronic kilovoltage and megavoltage radiographs. *Int J Radiat Oncol Biol Phys* **47**: 825–39.

Purdie T G, Bissonnette J P, Franks K, Bezjak A, Payne D, Sie F, Sharpe M B, and Jaffray D A, 2007. Cone-beam computed tomography for on-line image guidance of lung stereotactic radiotherapy: localization, verification, and intrafraction tumor position. *Int J Radiat Oncol Biol Phys* **68**: 243–52.

Ren L, Godfrey D J, Yan H, Wu Q J, and Yin F F, 2008a. Automatic registration between reference and on-board digital tomosynthesis images for positioning verification. *Med Phys* **35**: 664–72.

Ren L, Zhang J, Thongphiew D, Godfrey D J, Wu Q J, Zhou S M, and Yin F F, 2008b. A novel digital tomosynthesis (DTS) reconstruction method using a deformation field map. *Med Phys* **35**: 3110–5.

Rosu M, Dawson L A, Balter J M, McShan D L, Lawrence T S, and Ten Haken R K, 2003. Alterations in normal liver doses due to organ motion. *Int J Radiat Oncol Biol Phys* **57**: 1472–9.

Sharpe M B, Moseley D J, Haycocks T, Siewerdsen J H, and Jaffray D A, 2003. An integrated volumetric imaging and guidance system for targeting of soft-tissue structures in radiotherapy. *Int J Radiat Oncol Biol Phys* **57**: S183.

Siddon R L, 1985. Prism representation: a 3D ray-tracing algorithm for radiotherapy applications. *Phys Med Biol* **30**: 817–24.

Skerl D, Likar B, and Pernus F, 2008. A protocol for evaluation of similarity measures for non-rigid registration. *Med Image Anal* **12**: 42–54.

Sorcini B and Tilikidis A, 2006. Clinical application of image-guided radiotherapy, IGRT (on the Varian OBI platform). *Cancer Radiother* **10**: 252–7.

Suit H, Goldberg S, Niemierko A, Ancukiewicz M, Hall E, Goitein M, Wong W, and Paganetti H, 2007. Secondary carcinogenesis in patients treated with radiation: a review of data on radiation-induced cancers in human, non-human primate, canine and rodent subjects. *Radiat Res* **167**: 12–42.

Wang Z, Wu Q J, Marks L B, Larrier N, and Yin F F, 2007. Cone-beam CT localization of internal target volumes for stereotactic body radiotherapy of lung lesions. *Int J Radiat Oncol Biol Phys* **69**: 1618–24.

Winey B, Zygmanski P, and Lyatskaya Y, 2009. Evaluation of radiation dose delivered by cone beam CT and tomosynthesis employed for setup of external breast irradiation. *Med Phys* **36**: 164–73.

Wong J W, Sharpe M B, Jaffray D A, Kini V R, Robertson J M, Stromberg J S, and Martinez A A, 1999. The use of active breathing control (ABC) to reduce margin for breathing motion. *Int J Radiat Oncol Biol Phys* **44**: 911–9.

Wu Q J, Godfrey D J, Wang Z, Zhang J, Zhou S, Yoo S, Brizel D M, and Yin F F, 2007. On-board patient positioning for head-and-neck IMRT: comparing digital tomosynthesis to kilovoltage radiography and cone-beam computed tomography. *Int J Radiat Oncol Biol Phys* **69**: 598–606.

Yin F F, Wang Z, Yoo S, Jackie Q, Kirkpatrick J, Larrier N, Meyer J, Willett C G, and Marks L B, 2008. Integration of cone-beam CT in stereotactic body radiation therapy. *Technol Cancer Res Treat* **7**: 133–40.

Yokokawa T and Shintani H, 2002. Development of picture and voice gated intermittent irradiation system connected without linear accelerator for voluntary breath-hold synchronized with respiration. *Nippon Igaku Hoshasen Gakkai Zasshi* **62**: 290–1.

Yoo S, Wu Q J, Godfrey D, Yan H, Ren L, Das S, Lee W R, and Yin F F, 2009. Clinical evaluation of positioning verification using digital tomosynthesis and bony anatomy and soft tissues for prostate image-guided radiotherapy. *Int J Radiat Oncol Biol Phys* **73**: 296–305.

Yoshitake T, Nakamura K, Shioyama Y, Nomoto S, Ohga S, Toba T, Shiinoki T, Anai S, Terashima H, Kishimoto J, and Honda H, 2008. Breath-hold monitoring and visual feedback for radiotherapy using a charge-coupled device camera and a head-mounted display: system development and feasibility. *Radiat Med* **26**: 50–5.

Zhang J, Wu Q J, Godfrey D J, Fatunase T, Marks L B, and Yin F F, 2009. Comparing digital tomosynthesis to cone-beam CT for position verification in patients undergoing partial breast irradiation. *Int J Radiat Oncol Biol Phys* **73**: 952–7.

12

Image Registration and Segmentation in Radiation Therapy

Michael B. Sharpe
University of Toronto

Michael Velec
University Health Network

Kristy K. Brock
University of Toronto

12.1 Introduction

The treatment of cancer patients with radiation therapy requires a variety of medical imaging studies to support treatment planning, to guide delivery, and to assess response in follow-up exams. Treatment planning and delivery demand precise delineation of targets and healthy tissues where organ function should be preserved. An ever-broadening selection of imaging modalities is used to localize anatomy and to characterize physiological processes. Informing treatment planning and guidance procedures with disparate information requires clear objectives, as well as accurate and consistent methods for building an appropriate patient model.

Computed tomography (CT) has become the standard for establishing a primary model of the patient for treatment planning. CT imaging provides a geometrically accurate and robust *static* representation of the patient's anatomy and estimates the distribution of tissue density, which is an important radiological property for computing dose distributions [1–4]. Classifying tissues by density alone is not always sufficient and other imaging modalities provide complimentary information to enhance the delineation of soft tissues. In some cases, tissue characterization includes assessments of organ movement or the distribution of physiological and metabolic activity within an organ. For example, respiratory-correlated CT imaging, or "4DCT," has also emerged as an innovative means of characterizing organ movement related to breathing and estimating its contribution for determining planning target

volume (PTV) margins [5–8]. Other imaging modalities, such as contrast-enhanced CT, magnetic resonance imaging (MR), and positron-emission tomography (PET), are used increasingly to augment the collective understanding of the disease and surrounding vasculature, organ motion, and normal organ function [9–17]. MRI and PET offer a wealth of options (higher field strength, pulse sequences, novel agents) to aid in the discrimination of tumors and normal tissues for radiation therapy.

While the wide variety of imaging modalities available to support treatment planning provide increasingly detailed anatomical and physiological information, integrating the required information into one model of the patient can be challenging because the imaging studies frequently take place at various locations on different imaging devices, and with variable imaging parameters. The rendering of a self-consistent patient model requires a recapitulation of the patient position for each imaging modality, and the creation of a temporal sample, or "snapshot," of the patient's anatomy at the time of imaging. Variations in body position and natural physiological processes tend to introduce systematic and random geometric variation, resulting in radiation treatment risks of compromised target coverage or unnecessary irradiation of normal tissues [18].

When a variety of three-dimensional (3D) imaging modalities are used, and when similar exams are repeated at different points in time, image registration is required to establish a correspondence between imaging studies and to support geometric targeting in image-guided radiation treatment (IGRT) [19–21]. Image registration must resolve geometric discrepancies that exist between multimodality image sets while preserving the salient information that is required for patient care. There is a growing role for image registration and segmentation of anatomical structures in modern radiotherapy and a range of technologies are available to potentially fulfill these requirements.

This chapter offers a review of the role of registration and related technologies in radiotherapy processes. Common and emerging technologies are summarized, examples of their limitations are illustrated, and current quality assurance (QA) practices pertaining to image registration are reviewed. Additional detailed information on algorithms and implementations is included in the bibliography that accompanies this chapter.

12.2 Image Registration Concepts

Image *registration* establishes the geometric correspondence between images. It is used to compute the alignment, or transformation, that positions images in the same frame of reference. Image *fusion* uses visualization techniques to display the complimentary data simultaneously in each image set, both within and across modalities. These procedures are illustrated in Figures 12.1 and 12.2, using the numerals and minute graduations of a clock. In Figure 12.1, a rotation and translation aligns the numerals with the graduations. Their alignment is subsequently visualized in Figure 12.2, via fusion overlay (left) or "split-screen" view (right). In clinical practice, these two functions are closely linked and referred to almost interchangeably. These concepts, and the underlying mathematics and principles, have been described and reviewed widely [19,22,23].

As mentioned previously, a treatment planning CT, obtained with set criteria for patient positioning and imaging parameters, serves as the primary patient model and frame of reference. Other imaging modalities (e.g., MRI, PET) enhance the accuracy and precision of organ delineation for treatment planning and delivery. When images of an individual patient are acquired with different modalities, they usually have different coordinate systems and record anatomical discrepancies related to body position, organ filling, and weight change at different points in time. Image registration is the process of establishing a correspondence of the information available in each image within a common coordinate system to facilitate their comparison.

To perform image registration, a transformation model is required. For example, a rigid body transform is a model that employs linear translations and rotations to register image coordinates (Figures 12.1 and 12.2). Rigid registrations can be manipulated manually with appropriate tools to achieve a visual match or automatically optimized with the aid of a metric, which objectively describes the degree of similarity between images as they are aligned using the registration model (discussed in the next section). Image registration can be viewed as a four-step process that involves: (1) identifying common information to guide the registration; (2) using this information to formulate an objective correspondence; (3) creating a means of alignment where no common information exists; and (4), computing and applying a transformation map. These four steps are explored in more detail below.

12.2.1 Common Information

Image registration is guided by information that is common to both image sets. For example, it is sometimes possible to identify the tumor boundary on volumetric images used for guidance [24–27]. However, it is important to emphasize that image registration is motivated by the need for additional information that is not common to both image sets. Other common anatomical features can serve as a surrogate for guiding the image registration, as summarized in Figure 12.3. The visible anatomy, or surrogate, identified to guide the registration process has an impact on the accuracy and precision of actual information of interest.

Surrogates for image registration can be as straightforward as surface markers (i.e., tattoos) placed on the patient's skin and aligned to room laser coordinates. Choosing a surrogate in close proximity to the organ or disease of interest can improve the registration. The skeleton or the diaphragm are useful surrogates for wide range of imaging modalities [28–32], and the implantation of radiographically visible markers can create a highly effective surrogate for indicating the position of a treatment volume [14,33–36]. However, both approaches can be confounded by deformation of the target volume [37], and implanting markers for guidance may be associated with a small risk of infection or tumor seeding along the needle track [38–40].

Image registration using the tumor-bearing organ or adjacent organs can also be performed. However, the accuracy of its surrogacy depends on the amount of deformation that the organ and tumor undergo, as well as any differences in coupling between the organ motion and the tumor motion. The degree of uncertainty between the surrogate and the target for treatment should be included in the PTV margins in the treatment design. These uncertainties can be determined from comparative and repeat image studies where the tumor and the surrogate are visible.

12.2.2 Establishing Correspondence

Once an appropriate localization surrogate is identified, a method of establishing correspondence must be determined. This can be as simple as identifying points such as seed locations, or a more advanced application based on the intensity information in some portion of the image. The correspondence of surrogates is expressed as a similarity measure, or registration metric. A wide range of formulations and methods exist for deriving a registration metric and are reviewed elsewhere [22,23]. Common registration metrics are based on the distance between corresponding anatomical points, line-segments, or delineated surfaces, or by comparison of the grayscale intensities of image elements. An appropriate registration metric accounts for the clinical objectives in feature alignment in 2D and 3D images, and reflects the capabilities of the underlying transformation model [41–48]. Three common methods for calculating correspondence

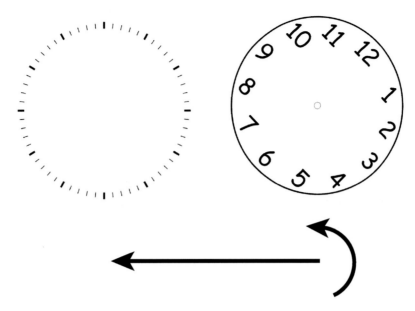

FIGURE 12.1 Registration of the numerals and minute graduations of a clock. A rotation and translation aligns the numerals with the graduations.

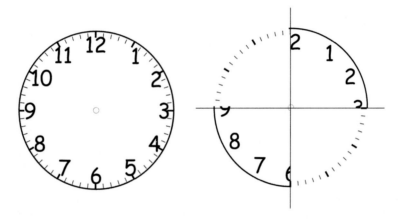

FIGURE 12.2 Visualization of the clock registration via a fusion overlay (left) or "split-screen" view (right).

of surrogates are described below: alignment by points, alignment by surfaces, and alignment by intensity pattern.

12.2.2.1 Point Alignment

The alignment of volumetric images using points requires the identification of at least three pairs of non-coplanar points. This approach is used commonly with the application of implanted gold seed markers in the prostate, which can be seen on megavoltage (MV) and kilovoltage (kV) portal images and kV cone beam CT (CBCT) images [49]. A reference CT or set of digitally reconstructed radiographs (DRRs) for orthogonal or beams-eye-views (BEVs) are obtained from planning that include visible seed locations. The reference CT and/or DRRs are compared with CBCT volumetric images and/or MV or kV portal radiographs obtained during treatment. In the absence of tissue deformation or seed migration resulting in different marker locations from when implanted, the position of the markers on the reference and secondary images can be matched exactly

using a rigid registration model that includes translation and rotation. In general, exact rigidity is not the case for soft tissue anatomy, and the residual error of all the seeds must be minimized. A registration metric for the rigid registration of three markers, α, β, and γ, can be expressed as the least-squares distance between corresponding vector positions in images 1 and 2:

$$F(\alpha, \beta, \gamma) = \min \sum \left[(\vec{\alpha}_1 - \vec{\alpha}_2)^2 + (\vec{\beta}_1 - \vec{\beta}_2)^2 + (\vec{\gamma}_1 - \vec{\gamma}_2)^2 \right] \quad (12.1)$$

Marker implants have been shown widely to be a very effective method of registering the prostate prior to treatment. Importantly, clinical use requires the evaluation of registration residual error. A study performed at Princess Margaret Hospital, where repeat MR images were obtained of the prostate and implanted marker seeds, indicated the potential for substantial deformation to exist following registration of the prostate using

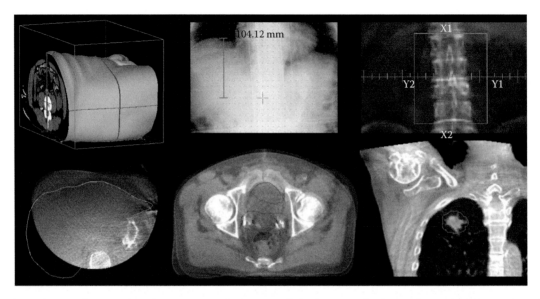

FIGURE 12.3 (See color insert) Examples of surrogates in radiotherapy include: the external body and alignment of skin marks with room lasers (top-left); registration based on neighboring organs may include the diaphragm (top-center) or bony-anatomy (top-right); tumor bearing organ alignment such as the liver (bottom-left); registration based on implanted markers in or near the tumor (bottom-center); direct alignment of the tumor itself (bottom-right).

two metrics for residual error, one translation-based, and one based on combined translation and rotation [37]. In 10% of the patients, more than 50% of the prostate surface was misaligned by more than 3 mm after alignment of the seeds, with the worst case exhibiting 1.3 cm of deformation following translation and 1.1 cm of deformation following translation and rotation. Figure 12.4 shows the worst case of the 29 patients examined: the mesh represents the prostate surface position at the first MR image and the colorwash display represents the prostate surface at the second MR image. The colorwash intensities indicate the vector magnitude differences in prostate surface positions the first and second MR images.

12.2.2.2 Surface Alignment

The delineation of anatomical regions of interest is an integral part of radiotherapy treatment planning and can be a convenient basis for a registration surrogate. Target, target-bearing organ, and adjacent or other structure surfaces can be delineated manually or automatically using intensity-gradient thresholds, or by more advanced image processing methods for surface detection [50–53]. Once delineated and identified in a pair of images, these surfaces can be used for registration. Surface alignment is similar to point-based alignment, where the aim is to minimize the distance between the collections of points defining the two surfaces. This method is commonly referred to as chamfer matching [43,54,55].

In the IGRT setting, alignment of the liver prior to treatment is an important example to illustrate the value of surface registration for neighboring organs and the tumor-bearing organ. Simple 2D registration for liver position has been performed using the spine (bony vertebral bodies) to determine the left–right and anterior–posterior position and the dome of the diaphragm for the superior-inferior position. Kirilova et

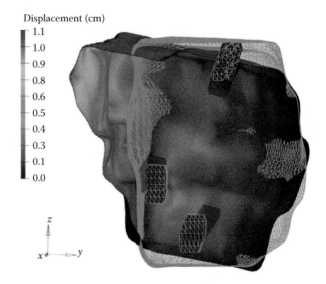

FIGURE 12.4 (See color insert) Sagittal slice showing the interior surface of a repeated MR (displacement colorwash) and initial MR mesh (pink). Residual error due prostate deformation over 1 cm was observed even after rigid registration based on translations and rotations of the implanted seeds.

al. have shown using fluoroscopy and cine MR that there can be substantial differences of over 2 cm in the superior–inferior motion of the tumor compared to its position defined by the diaphragm [56]. It is important to understand these uncertainties when calculating a PTV margin as well as when performing registration when images are obtained at breath hold.

In contrast, with volumetric imaging (CT, MR, CBCT), registration of the surface of the organ can be performed to increase the precision of registration by improving the relationship between the surrogate, the tumor-bearing organ, and the tumor, i.e., the tumor-bearing organ will provide a closer surrogate for the tumor position than neighboring organs, such as bone. Surface registration can be performed manually, by registering the contours from the planning scan onto the images from the pretreatment images, or by identification of the entire organ surface, either through manual contouring or autosegmentation.

Again, referring to the liver registration example, the planning CT liver contour (a stack of 2D contours) can then be registered to the liver contoured on the kV CBCT to enable a registration matching of the entire organ volume. Even with good alignment (surface metrics), it is important to note that this surface registration remains only a surrogate for tumor registration. The organ may deform, prohibiting a rigid registration, even with rotation, to perfectly align these contours [57]. The online (immediately prior to treatment) registration of 13 patients treated under a liver cancer protocol with rigid registration to fit the contours from the CT scan onto the kV CBCT images obtained prior to treatment were subsequently analyzed with deformable registration. Results showed that four of these patients (31%) exhibited residual, regional deformation of the liver, with more than 5% of the liver volume deformed by more than 5 mm. This deformation, without detection, could potentially impact the positioning of the tumor in the radiation treatment field [58]. Therefore, it is critical to know what part of the anatomy offers greatest accuracy for alignment, and the degree of this uncertainty must be reflected in PTV margins, even with online image guidance every day.

In lung cancer therapy, surface image registration benefits from the contrast between the lung and the tumor, often allowing the tumor to be visualized on pretreatment volumetric images. In this case, alignment of the tumor itself to the planning scan volumes at the time of treatment can be performed. In addition, some tumors encompass the entire organ, such as the prostate [26,59,60]. Registration fidelity is therefore dependent on the tumor itself, and residual errors, due to deformation and changes in anatomy over the course of treatment, can be visualized after registration. It is important to note that the anatomy outside of that surrogate surface may also be getting a significant dose (i.e., critical normal tissue), regardless of which surrogate controls the registration. The impact of the registration on this nearby anatomy must be considered, as well.

12.2.3 Intensity-Based Alignment

The information inherent in the image, that is, the intensity of each voxel, can be used to drive the registration using automated registration methods. Alignment by intensity is performed by identifying a metric that describes the similarity of the voxel intensities between the two images, a transformation is then applied to the secondary image, and the similarity metric is recalculated. This process is repeated several times through an iterative optimization algorithm to find the optimal transformation that leads to the best similarity between the images. The similarity metric can be calculated using several different techniques and three of the most common, the sum of the squared difference, cross correlation, and mutual information methods, are now described.

12.2.3.1 Sum of the Squared Difference

The sum of the squared difference (SSD) between two gray-scale images is minimized by transforming the secondary image, B, with respect to the primary image, A:

$$\text{SSD}(\vec{A}, \vec{B}) = \sum (\vec{A} - \vec{B})^2 \tag{12.2}$$

The difference is calculated iteratively for each voxel in the images as the secondary image is transformed. This metric is beneficial as it is simple to implement and computation is very efficient; however, application is limited to images that are of the same modality and have a direct gray-scale correspondence (i.e., 2 CT images) [61,62].

12.2.3.2 Cross-Correlation Coefficient

Cross correlation is one of the commonly adopted registration metrics available in commercial treatment planning systems. Local normalization can be used to account for local intensity variations between images. Normalized cross correlation (NCC) is similar to SSD, in that it compares the two images, A and B, on a voxel-by-voxel basis in an iterative fashion:

$$\text{NCC}(\vec{A}, \vec{B}) = \frac{\sum (\vec{A} - |\vec{A}|)(\vec{B} - |\vec{B}|)}{\sqrt{\sum (\vec{A} - |\vec{A}|)^2} \sqrt{\sum (\vec{B} - |\vec{B}|)^2}}, \tag{12.3}$$

for a comparison of images A and B, where $|A|$ and $|B|$ are the global or local mean value of the voxels in images A and B, respectively. Essentially, this method evaluates the difference between two images as a function of the variation of intensities in that image. For example, if image A has a white region of interest (ROI) on a black background and image B shows the same ROI as a light gray ROI on a dark gray background, NCC would recognize that the ROIs correspond in the two images by examining the relationship between the ROI and the background in each image. Cross correlation is more intensive computationally, compared to SSD, but it is less sensitive to local noise and small differences between corresponding images [63–69].

12.2.3.3 Mutual Information

Mutual information (MI) image registration is based on information theory. The registration metric examines the correspondence of the entropy, or information, contained in the two images [70–73]. Equation 4 shows a common expression for mutual information, where the joint entropy, or combined information content in a pair of images is equal to the entropy of image A, $H(\vec{A})$, plus the entropy of image B, $H(\vec{B})$, minus the joint entropy contained in images A and B, $H(\vec{A}, \vec{B})$:

$$\text{MI}(\vec{A}, \vec{B}) = H(\vec{A}) + H(\vec{B}) - H(\vec{A}, \vec{B}) \tag{12.4}$$

If the two images are completely independent of each other, $H(A, B)$ is 0. MI can be used for same modality images, when there is a difference in image contrast, or for images obtained from different modalities. This method is more complex than either SSD or NCC, can be extremely robust, offers great flexibility on its application, and is often the algorithm and metric of choice for images of different modalities [71–77].

12.2.3 Computing Correspondence

In clinical practice, the accuracy and precision of image registration depends the transformation model and registration metric used to drive it. The majority of commercially available registration algorithms use rigid body transformations, computing the correspondence achievable with linear transformations and rotations.

It is useful to perform rigid registration of the gross alignment of images acquired in different reference frames and often in anatomical locations with a limited range of organ movement, such as the brain. In general, most anatomical sites will benefit from more advanced transformation models to address deforming anatomy. In the thorax, for example, complex motions can be observed with diaphragm contraction, as the lungs inflate, the ribs flex, and the spine remains stationary, at least within a single imaging study. Repeat scans of the head and neck show linear motion of the skull, but differential variations position of the vertebra of the neck. Longer term studies over time can reveal substantial anatomical changes related to weight loss and treatment response, which cannot be accounted for by rotation and translation alone. In each of these cases, deformation is occurring and must be accounted for by a more sophisticated interpolation method. A few common methods are briefly described later in the chapter. But first, some general strategies for the application of rigid body transforms can improve the utility of registration for specific tasks. These "focal registration" strategies include the use of limiting boundaries or other volumetric structures to exclude peripheral information that would otherwise confound a rigid registration metric.

When an automated registration is performed using an intensity-based method, the registration will examine the intensity throughout the entire image. If substantial deformation occurs between the two images, optimization of a "global" metric may not produce the best a clinical result. For example, if a patient with head and neck cancer is imaged with two modalities and the neck flexure differs between scans, their alignment would, in general, require a deformable registration model. However, clinically relevant information can still be obtained from the rigid registration of the two images. If the registration is done manually, the user focuses the registration on the region that is deemed most important. It is possible to translate this technique into an automated approach by limiting the region of the image that is used for the registration. By limiting the region, the algorithm only calculates, and therefore optimizes, the correspondence in the selected area. The region can be identified using a "clip box" or a cube-based region of interest or a free-form region of interest that is tailored to specific anatomy (i.e., organ delineation).

An example is shown in Figure 12.5 for a head and neck case using a commercially available radiation therapy guidance software package (Synergy XVI R3.5 General Release software, Elekta Limited, Crawley, UK). In this example, a clip box is incorporated to perform localized image guidance at the time of treatment. The algorithm sets a threshold for the bones and then performs a surface match on the segmented bone [43]. The reference image is a planning CT image, and the secondary image is a kV CBCT image. In the upper row of Figure 12.5, the clip box is placed on the neck, resulting in good registration of the neck but poor registration of the skull, due to deformation resulting from neck flexion between the primary (green) and secondary (purple) images. In the middle row, the clip box is placed around the sphenoid bone, resulting in good registration of the skull and poor registration of the neck, and in the bottom row of the figure, the clip box encompasses the C6-C7 vertebrae. Each of these scenarios yields a different rigid registration result. Clearly, the registration must be tailored to match the clinical application.

The clip box concept has been extended to use more general anatomical ROIs to limit the registration region. This approach allows a more tailored control of the registration but can require more user intervention, i.e., contouring the ROI. For treatment planning purposes, contoured ROIs are often already available, so registration can take advantage of this more tailored "clip box" (Figure 12.6).

The example shown in Figure 12.6 is an inhale and exhale breath-hold image of the abdomen for a liver cancer patient. The primary image, on the left, is at exhale breath hold. The liver has been contoured, indicated by the yellow outline. The image in the middle is at inhale breath hold. The spine and ribs have not moved substantially between the two image sets and will cause problems for a rigid registration algorithm; however, if the liver contour is used to limit the registration, the results, shown on the right, are very good for the liver, which is the clinically important ROI in this case. This registration was performed using mutual information in a commercially available treatment planning system (Pinnacle³, Philips Medical Systems, Madison, WI).

It is important to establish the priority of organ contours in treatment planning and guidance procedures. It is also critical to understand the relative risks and benefits of registrations, when tradeoffs are being made, for their clinical consequences. It is possible a more detail examination of alignment discrepancies could require manipulation of the patient's positioning or the creation of a new treatment plan that adapts to new anatomy. For example, if a clip box is used to focus the registration on a lung tumor, to overcome registration errors due to deformation, but the results of the registration places the spinal cord into the high dose region, caution should be taken before treatment of the patient.

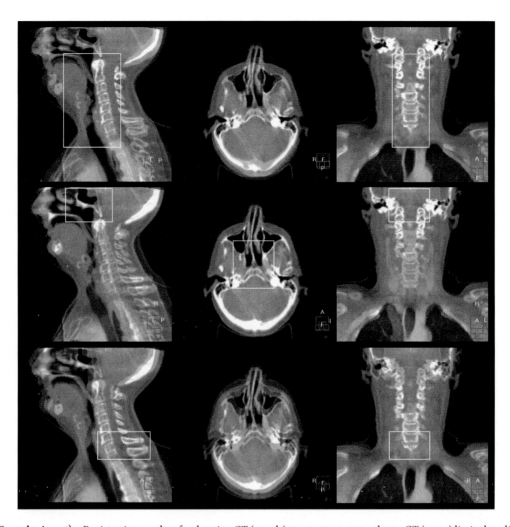

FIGURE 12.5 (See color insert) Registration results of a planning CT (purple) to a treatment cone-beam CT (green) limited to clipboxes. Clipbox around the entire cervical neck (top) resulted in translations (mm) of 0.2 left–right (LR), 4.5 superior–inferior (SI) 3.4 anterior posterior (AP), and rotations (°) of 6.0 pitch, −0.4 roll, and −0.3 yaw. Clipbox centered over the sphenoid bone (middle) resulted in −0.6 LR, 2.7 SI, −7.3 AP, and −0.9 pitch, −0.8 roll, and 0.4 yaw. Clipbox around the C6-C7 vertebrae (bottom) resulted in 1.4 LR, 3.3 SI, 5.8 AP, and 1.3 pitch, 0.9 roll, and −0.7 yaw.

12.2.3.1 Deformable Registration

As illustrated above, the human body is clearly able to move and deform with physiological motion, patient positioning, and treatment response. Deformable registration models have been the subject of ongoing research activities, specifically in radiation therapy over the last decade. Recently, a multi-institution study was performed to compare the results of several deformable registration algorithms using the same clinical data [78]. Although beyond the scope of this chapter to describe each deformable registration algorithm in detail, three of the often used algorithms are summarized: fluid and optical flow techniques, spline-based methods, and biomechanical models.

In a fluid flow approach, the deformations in the images are modeled as the movement of a viscous fluid. The algorithm optimizes a similarity metric, as described above (i.e., SSD, NCC, or MI), while constraining the interpolation by the laws of continuum mechanics. This method is currently being investigated by several groups for 4D CT registration [79–81],

intracavitary brachytherapy [82], and brain anatomy [83,84]. The approach can be fully automatic, invertible, and has shown accuracy of less than 4 mm in the lung. Two potential limitations include accommodating non-continuous motion, such as the stationary spine next to the moving lung, and accommodating a lack of intensity correspondence, such as an image with a full rectum being registered to an image with an empty rectum. For multimodality registration, this algorithm must be implemented with MI.

Optical flow uses the differences between the images and the gradient of the image as two forces to drive the registration and therefore has an inherent similarity metric, which is similar to SSD. This approach is often referred to as the "Demon's approach," which was first implemented by Thirion [85]. Additional forces, such as an active force, based on the gradient in the moving image, can be added to improve the outcome of the registration [68,86]. This algorithm has been investigated in the head and neck and prostate radiotherapy [68]. As with the

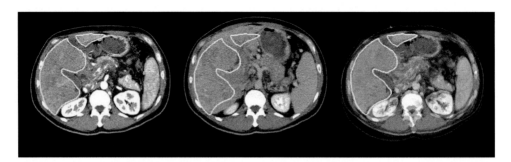

FIGURE 12.6 (See color insert) Exhale breath-hold CT (left) and inhale breath-hold CT (middle) is acquired in the same position with the exhale liver contour overlaid. Results (right) of mutual information-based registration limited to the liver, between exhale CT (gray scale) and inhale CT (thermal scale).

fluid flow algorithms, accommodating noncontinuous motion and lack of intensity correspondence may be a limitation in some instances. Research is ongoing to solve these potential problems.

A spline-based approach deforms the image using control points that are placed in specific locations (thin-plate spline) or on a regular grid (B-spline). The control points guide the deformation of the image as a similarity metric is optimized. In a thin-plate spline approach, each control point effects the deformation of the entire image. The extent depends on the distance to the control point, making this approach best for single organ registration. In contrast, the control points in B-spline only affect a local area of the registration, allowing for multiorgan registration to be performed because a local registration can be preferentially weighted for each organ of interest. Spline approaches have been used in a variety of anatomical sites, including liver [72,87–90], lung [62,91–93], and prostate [94–96]. The algorithm can be fully automated and efficient, and an accuracy of 1.0–3.5 mm has been shown. Potential limitations are the same as the fluid and optical flow methods, accommodating noncontinuous motion and lack of intensity correspondence. The fluid flow, optical flow, and spline methods share the benefit that contouring or organ segmentation is typically not required.

A biomechanical approach deforms the image according to the material properties of the tissue, that is, if the material is hard or soft. The approach is typically implemented using a finite element model of the anatomy in the image, which represents each ROI as a series of connected nodes, forming tetrahedrons that approximate the ROI surface. Tetrahedron geometric relationships are solved using finite element analysis. Boundary conditions are required that describe tissue motion and deformation, and the model may incorporate relevant biomechanical parameters such as the tissue stiffness and compressibility. Empirical tissue motion can be determined using a similarity metric, often by deforming the contoured ROI on one image to the contoured ROI on a secondary image, subject to constraints imposed by the biomechanical tissue properties. This approach has been used for several anatomical sites, including the thorax [97–99], abdomen [97,100,101], and pelvis [102–104]. Accuracy of 1.2–2.5 mm has been shown. Potential limitations include the dependence of contours on the registration and the uncertainty in defining the biomechanical properties of the anatomy being modeled.

12.2.4 Image Registration Procedures

Image registration tasks are performed by clinical practitioners, including radiation oncologists, radiation therapists, and medical physicists. Users must possess sufficient skills to allow them to exercise expert judgment when completing the task. Image registration can be performed manually, by adjusting the registration between two images and viewing the fusion of the images to assess accuracy, automatically, using one of several algorithms, or using a combination of manual and automated registration, where the user may initialize the registration, run the automated algorithm, and then make any needed small adjustments. It should be noted that a combination of manual and automated registration should only be performed in the case of rigid registration. Manual adjusting of deformable registration can lead to additional uncertainties that cannot be viewed using simple fusion tools. In practice, the user should always have the final approval of the registration results. Because the vast majority of commercially available systems rely on rigid registration at this time, expert approval is especially true in situations involving significant soft tissue deformation, for example, in the abdomen and pelvis. The user must find a best compromise to register deforming anatomy in multiple imaging modalities.

12.3 Applications in Image-Guided Radiation Therapy

Image registration and fusion integrate complimentary imaging modalities in radiation treatment planning and in target localization for IGRT. Image registration also has a role in evaluating dosimetric changes that may be occurring during the treatment course (due to anatomical changes in target or normal tissues), and for monitoring tumor and normal tissue responses to evaluate the efficacy of treatment. Thus, image registration is required for the planning image and any follow-up images.

The problem of anatomical variation is increased further over the course of treatment as radiotherapy often extends over an interval lasting several weeks. The patient is required to be in the same position as the model created for treatment planning and limited deviations between the intended position and the actual position are anticipated and accommodated with the definition of the PTV [105]. However, the PTV increases the irradiated volume to ensure target coverage at the cost of exposing more of the surrounding normal tissue. Larger than expected deviations from the planned patient position and progressive response to treatment are clearly significant concerns.

To address these potential errors, image-guided radiation therapy (IGRT) aids in the frequent, often daily, use of imaging to assess and control the accuracy and precision of treatment delivery [20]. Guidance is supported by a variety of technologies, as covered in other chapters herein, including radiographic portal imagers [42,64,106–108], ultrasound systems [109–114], in-room CT scanners [115–118], and other forms of tomographic imaging [25,27,119–123]. Serial imaging with each fraction offers an opportunity to actively localize treatment to improve accuracy and precision using a variety of online and offline corrections strategies, all of which include the important process of image registration to enable treatment decisions to be made [124–128].

The process of planning and delivering radiation therapy are considered distinct events delineated in time, although it is possible to imagine a much closer integration of these activities in the future. Image registration in planning establishes correspondence between imaging modalities for patient modeling. With each return visit for treatment the planned setup is reproduced and registration of planning and treatment images is performed, as depicted in Figure 12.7.

12.3.1 Treatment Planning

Modern treatment planning is founded on volumetric CT images, and augmented by additional modalities such as MR and PET. Ideally, these supplemental exams are temporally and geometrically concordant with the initial planning CT. In practice, however, these modalities are scheduled for different appointments and at different geographic locations throughout a hospital. Variations occur with body position, organ filling, and other changes that can lead to geometric uncertainties following image registration. Importantly, the planning CT is considered the *primary* model of the patient state over the course of therapy, and rigid body registration models should be evaluated carefully to verify there is acceptable consistency between imaging modalities.

Differences seen in the secondary modalities are minimized during registration to build a self-consistent static model. If the secondary images were acquired to aid in the delineation of the disease, for example, the visible tumor or tumor-bearing organ would be the focus for aligning with the primary image, as shown in Figure 12.8.

It is important to note that image registration can be performed at the time of image acquisition with some modalities. For example, respiration-correlated CT or "4D-CT" is designed to assess volumetric organ movement due to breathing over short time interval [79]. These types of images are formatted to reconstruct different breathing phases that are organized into a series of related imaging studies. Anatomy in the images that is not subject to breathing motion in the 4DCT images tends

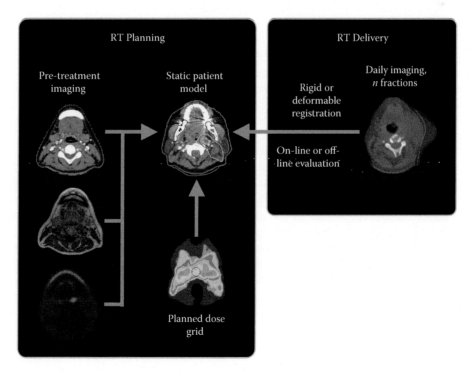

FIGURE 12.7 Simulation and image-guided treatment process: each arrow indicates the inclusion of an image into the planning and delivery, thus requiring image registration.

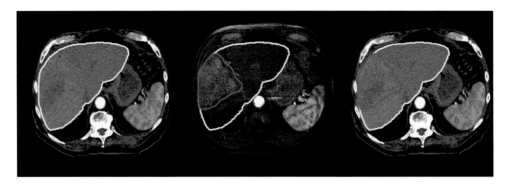

FIGURE 12.8 (See color insert) Registration of the liver (yellow) between noncontrast CT (left) and MR (middle) allows the segmented MR tumor (red) to be mapped onto the planning CT (right).

to be registered inherently when acquired in the same scanning session as the primary CT exam. Similarly, the PET and CT images acquired with hybrid PET-CT systems are inherently registered [129–131].

12.3.2 Treatment Delivery

Image registration must also support accurate and precise guidance of treatment delivery by relating the images obtained just prior to treatment delivery with the models created for treatment planning. With each patient visit over a course of fractionated radiation therapy, the patient is aligned nominally to the machine isocenter. Images are acquired and registered to the planning CT, and the target location is refined to fall within a defined tolerance interval by adjusting the patient set up (6 degrees of freedom: 3 translations and 3 rotations). This process has evolved over time but became formalized with image matching of MV portal radiographs with a DRR generated from the planning CT, where positional corrections are implemented by simple couch translations, or manipulation of the patient's position on the couch [42,63,64,106–108,132,133].

The widespread adoption of CBCT and other tomography technologies has made it possible to guide treatment routinely using images of soft-tissue [25,134–136]. The registration of treatment images with the planning CT aids the evaluation of target location relative to the machine isocenter and the position of normal tissues that lie adjacent and peripheral to the target. This process increases the accuracy and precision of daily treatment, assuring that objectives for target coverage and normal tissue sparing are translated properly from the planning context to the delivery of each treatment fraction.

Guiding treatment differs from the treatment planning context because images are not expected to be perfectly concordant over time. Instead of a static geometry, the images from each treatment session represent a temporal sample of the changing patient geometry. Relative to the initial plan, each treatment image incorporates residual setup variations, small shifts in the relative position of organs and targets, and other anatomical changes. Residual setup errors and deformation are undesirable but are anticipated and managed using appropriately designed PTV margins. The availability of soft-tissue imaging for IGRT

has spawned an area of active research and development to understand and mitigate the clinical consequences of residual uncertainties.

12.3.3 Adaptive Treatment Planning

Current applications of IGRT increase targeting accuracy and minimize setup uncertainties, predominantly through *on line* evaluation using rigid registration. Soft-tissue images can also provide record of residual variations and anatomical changes over the treatment course. Experience gained with MV portal imaging has led to strategies that include *offline* components for determining statistical trends in systematic and random errors [125,137]. Statistics generated with offline strategies support the assessment and adjustment of PTV margins to exploit the precision inherent to an individual patient's treatment course [138,139].

Routine IGRT leads naturally to the need to formally "serialize" information. That is, to arrange images in chronological order with registration to establish a relationship to the initial plan. The transformation model then supports computation and mapping of dose distributions representing individual treatments in the planning reference image, as illustrated in Figure 12.9. Deformable registration and anatomical structure mapping will provide a better estimate of anatomical changes (Δ) during and subsequent to therapy, as well as accumulation of the actual dose delivered (Σ) [103,140,141]. Formal dose accumulation may improve the prediction of response, compared to nominal planned distributions. When this process is managed actively during a course of therapy, adaptation to accumulating anatomical changes will be possible. Deformable registrations of both anatomy and dose are critically important steps of the adaptive radiation treatment process.

12.3.4 Treatment Response

Innovations in image registration support an emerging approach to patient care in which images are used to establish a link between treatment planning, control of delivery, treatment adaptation, and patient assessment for follow-up exams. These innovations will establish a more quantitative relationship between

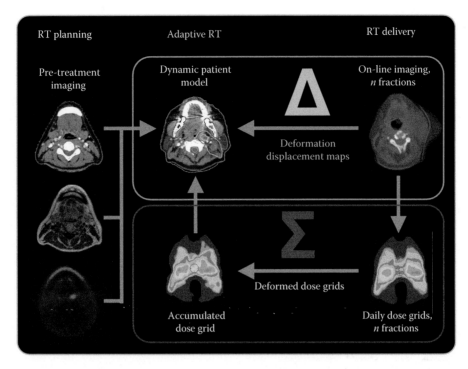

FIGURE 12.9 Schema for adaptive radiotherapy to using deformable registration of treatment imaging to account for anatomic changes (Δ), and allowing the change in accumulated dose (Σ) to be calculated.

images acquired for diagnosis, therapy, and follow-up. The correlation of "all" of a patient's images over time, using robust registration techniques, will provide a high-fidelity patient model for treatment planning, enable a more accurate estimation of the actual dose delivered, and thus provide improved clinical assessment of radiation therapy via patient follow-up exams for both assessment of tumor response and normal tissue toxicity.

12.4 Quality Assurance

Models and algorithms have limitations in image registration, and it is important to understand the principles and uncertainties inherent in their application. In addition, studies have shown that variations in the software implementation of the same algorithm can lead to variations in algorithm performance. Therefore, one cannot assume that the accuracy of two algorithms is equivalent, even if the underlying technique (i.e., Demon's algorithm) is the nominally the same [78,142].

Image registration in planning and delivery requires verification of the results. Presently, rigid registration is predominant in commercial software offered for treatment planning and target localization applications, although deformable registration is beginning to be offered. Several groups have recommended guidelines for QA of image registration in radiosurgery and general planning, and many of these recommendations are appropriate for image registration used for IGRT [143–148]. The International Atomic Energy Agency (IAEA), for example, recommends the appropriate use of software matched to the anatomical site and the number of imaging modalities employed [148]. They recommend assessment of: the technical principles in use, any bias to a particular imaging modality, constraints imposed on image acquisition, support for 2D and/or 3D registration, the degree and behavior of automation, the type of model (i.e., rigid or deformable), and dependence on image acquisition parameters or reliance on segmented structures.

The IAEA and American Association of Physicists in Medicine (AAPM) also recommend combined objective and visual queues for evaluating registrations [143,148]. Recently, the AAPM formed Task Group 132 to review techniques for image registration, to identify issues related to their clinical implementation, to determine the best methods to assess accuracy, and to outline issues related to acceptance and QA. A key recommendation of the task group will be the need to perform process oriented "end-to-end" testing of image registration tasks, spanning network-connected systems for image acquisition, planning, and delivery. This comprehensive testing could be achieved, for example, using a geometric or anthropomorphic phantom that allows assessment of the accuracy and consistency of geometry, numerical gray-scale intensities, image registration and tissue parameters, demographic information, etc.

There is a demand for objective metrics of registration quality within radiotherapy and image-guided surgery [149–151]. Phantom testing can determine if algorithms reproduce known displacements or changes in orientation under varying conditions [144,146,147]. Phantoms also help to confirm basic performance metrics like geometric scale calibration and orientation, as well as the limits of linearity, accuracy, and precision. However, phantom studies, whether with static or dynamic phantoms, do not completely capture factors that challenge and degrade registration algorithm performance, such as variations in slice thickness, resolution, distortion, noise, tissue deformation, and patient movement. In practice, process QA is required to monitor and manage these factors, and to achieve consistent practice. However, phantoms in standardized form do offer a "best-case" scenario for users to understand the behavior and limitations of the algorithms' registration metrics and transformation models.

Setup variation and deformation in individual patients are the most limiting factors in image registration. It is a difficult to generate systematic evidence and make specific recommendations in this area, although a standardized, multi-modality phantom may be of assistance. Fortunately, the cross-comparison of many common imaging modalities inherently includes redundant structures, which help in the visual validation of each patient-specific procedure [97,152,153]. As illustrated in Figure 12.10, this type of qualitative assessment of accuracy can be achieved through image overlay, side-by-side comparison, split-screens, checker-board displays, and a variety of other visualization techniques [19,21]. More quantitative validation can be computed by identifying naturally occurring or implanted fiducials in the body, such as vascular calcifications [154], the bronchial bifurcations in the lung, or via implanted gold seeds in the prostate. The accuracy of identifying these landmarks or marks will limit the confidence of the accuracy assessment, but studies have demonstrated good reproducibility for naturally occurring fiducials in the liver and lung [92,97,100] as well as for implanted seeds in the prostate [14,33,35,36]. The predicted displacement between the fiducials from the registration can be compared to the actual displacement of the fiducials between the two images. Repeat registrations can also be performed to quantify the variability in registration results. Quantitative accuracy assessment is important when a new algorithm is purchased or developed; however, it is not feasible to perform quantitative validation for each patient during routine clinical use.

In the absence of quantitative accuracy, qualitative accuracy can be performed by visual assessment of the results of the registration. Image overlay is a visual method of assessing the differences. Examples of image overlay have been demonstrated throughout the chapter. Figure 12.5 employs a color overlay, where one image is green, the other is purple, and where they agree the image turns gray. This display is a very effective way of visualizing differences, as areas that lack correspondence stand out. Figure 12.10 shows another color overlay, where one image is gray-scale and the other is a thermal scale, where the variation in intensity is displayed as a range of red and orange. This display allows visualization of both images. In addition, both images may be shown in gray-scale and a checkerboard or sliding window can be used to see the correspondence between both images. Figure 12.10 also shows an example of a checkerboard, dividing the image into four quadrants, with the diagonal quadrants displaying the same image regions of

misregistrations can be seen clearly. The position of the quadrant can move interactively, allowing the user to see the registration at different regions of the image. The number of divisions can also be increased, allowing more comparisons of fine features to be examined. It should be noted, however, that in the absence of detailed anatomy, visual, qualitative QA can give the user a false sense of accuracy assessment, especially when using deformable registration.

Modern IGRT routinely involves frequent/daily imaging to direct radiation therapy procedures, with the implication that the role of image registration has expanded greatly. Traditionally, QA of registration tools occurs within the planning context and depends on a limited number of "upstream" imaging devices [143,148]. In general, image registration has been limited to the treatment planning context and has been a "one time" event involving only few staff and a limited need for physicians to delegate decision making. Subsequent treatment delivery involved guidance by radiographs and has relied on separate guidelines for QA and clinical practice [155]. However, imaging data now accompanies planning data when it is transferred to treatment management systems and individual linear accelerators, where it serves as a reference image. Each delivery system, in turn, is capable of generating new datasets that are fed back into planning systems to support vector-based dose accumulation and assessment of anatomical changes, as illustrated in Figures 12.3, 12.6, and 12.9. It is likely that images will be stored on externally administered data storage. In order to complete and evaluate routine volumetric image registration tasks, a stable infrastructure must be maintained. Thus, QA programs for equipment and software in the IGRT era must assure operability and stability spanning across multiple imaging platforms, and QA practices must reflect the integration of planning and delivery across information management systems and network infrastructure. Software, knowledge, and decision making are disseminated throughout, and potentially beyond, the radiation therapy department. Consequently, a strong emphasis on standard guidelines for consistent practice and communication of expected results is required to support a working culture that is process driven, vigilant to exceptions, and able to reduce the burden of patient-specific QA.

12.5 Discussion

Image registration allows the radiotherapy process to be contemplated as a closed-loop intervention with the potential to improve the accuracy of each step of the process by connecting tasks, as shown in Figure 12.11. The process begins with multimodality imaging for accurate target and normal tissue definition [12,13,41,69,156]. Deformable registration is expected to reduce the uncertainty in the correspondence of these multiple sources of information and thus will improve target delineation. Accurate motion assessment is another important imaging application, and it is related to accurate target delineation

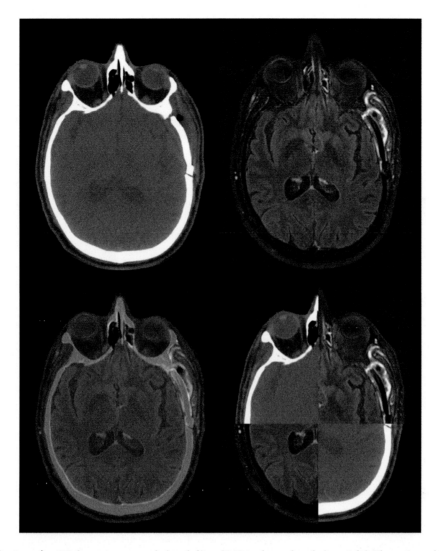

FIGURE 12.10 (See color insert) CT shown in gray-scale (top-left) and MR in thermal-scale (top-right). The registered images can be displayed in color overlay, (bottom-left), or checkerboard (bottom-right).

[27,79,157–161]. When multiple examples of geometry of the patient are obtained, such as 4DCT scans, a more accurate deformation map between breathing phases can be generated. In treatment delivery, accurate tumor guidance for online image registration may be improved using deformable registration [27,57,122,162,163]. Finally, in accurate response follow up, the response assessment of the tumor and changes in the normal tissue can be improved using deformable registration to compare the pre-treatment images with those obtained following the completion of treatment [100,164–167]. Thus, the impact of image registration is pervasive throughout the state-of-the-art image-guided radiotherapy process.

The routine use of IGRT leads to the requirement to "serialize" and register each image set to the treatment planning context. The potential to assess anatomical change quantitatively and to perform accurate dose accumulation are some of the anticipated benefits of an integrated approach to IGRT. Radiation therapy supports a strong culture of QA using prescriptive tests for

equipment, and logical intervals and tolerances for acceptance, commissioning, and periodic routine QA [168]. With regard to the specific QA aspects for image registration, these principles are maintained in recent literature. However, there are no uniform consensus recommendations for a comprehensive and prescriptive QA program for image registration used in the radiation treatment process.

It is feasible to confirm the quantitative performance of imaging devices, registration software, and networked storage and retrieval using phantom studies, but there is a strong need to rely on visual checks to assure consistent and unified practice in individual patient cases. The provision of a robustly tested infrastructure within documented and well-exercised clinical processes will increase confidence in patient-specific situations. To minimize the possibility of human or algorithm error, clinical image acquisition and registration processes should be maintained in an integrated fashion where possible, to assure it is logical, sequential, and reproducible [169].

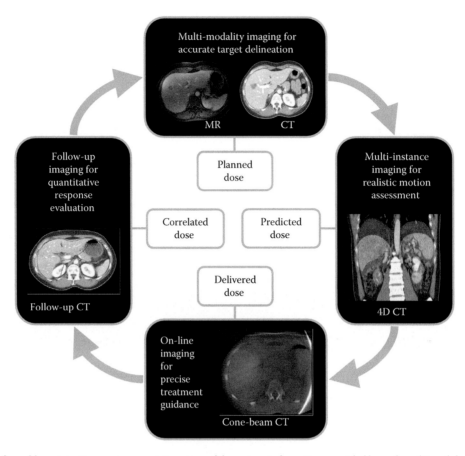

FIGURE 12.11 Deformable registration can improve integration of the unique information provided by each multimodal, multi-instance image, for the purposes of diagnosis and target delineation, treatment planning, online target localization, and follow-up response assessment. This process can also be used accumulate dose throughout treatment, providing improved correlation with outcomes. The example shown is of stereotactic-body radiotherapy of the liver.

12.6 Summary

Advances in image registration allow multimodality imaging and volumetric imaging at the time of treatment to be fully integrated into the radiotherapy process. The increasing use of multimodality imaging for treatment planning and the growing use of volumetric imaging for image guidance has demanded automated registration algorithms that are efficient and accurate. The four components of registration are (1) determining common surrogates, (2) calculating the correspondence between surrogates, (3) interpolating between surrogates, and (4) evaluating and displaying results. Several surrogates can be used depending on the application, including points, surfaces, and image intensities. Calculating the correspondence depends on the surrogate and can be as simple as minimizing the difference, for points and surfaces, or complex, such as mutual information for comparing image intensities. The appropriate surrogate and correspondence must be selected for each clinical problem and the limitations of the surrogates must be understood and included in the PTV margins for the treatment delivery. Currently, most commercially available systems interpolate the image space

between the surrogates using a linear translation, accounting for rotation and translation only. This limitation applies mainly for soft tissue, which deforms due to physiological motion, flexibility in patient positioning, and anatomical changes over the course of treatment. Deformable registration algorithms, which allow for more complex interpolations, are currently being developed. Local improvements in linear registration can be achieved in the presence of deformation by optimizing the registration to focus on the ROI that is most important. The use of clip boxes or ROI delineations can restrict the algorithm to the ROI of importance; however, caution should be used to ensure that the misregistrations outside of the ROI would not significantly violate planning or treatment constraints.

Quality assurance of image registration results is very important. Quantitative approaches are possible but are less efficient and should be performed offline to evaluate a new registration algorithm or application to a new anatomical site. Qualitative evaluation, such as looking at image overlays, is very efficient and should be used to ensure that each registration is acceptable prior to proceeding with the treatment or planning process.

Image registration can complete integration of the radiotherapy process. As registration becomes fully integrated into the radiotherapy process, improvements may be possible in target delineation, motion assessment, image guidance, and response assessment. Research is actively pursuing deformable registration algorithms, which will further improve the registration process and reduce the need for user intervention for optimization of linear registration in the presence of deformation.

Acknowledgments

The authors are grateful for the contributions of the faculty, students, and staff of Princess Margaret Hospital, especially Laura Dawson, Douglas Moseley, Tim Craig, and David Jaffray.

References

1. Sontag, MR, Battista, JJ, Bronskill, MJ, Cunningham, JR. Implications of computed tomography for inhomogeneity corrections in photon beam dose calculations. *Radiol.* 1977;124:143–149.
2. Sherouse, GW, Novins, K, Chaney, EL. Computation of digitally reconstructed radiographs for use in radiotherapy treatment design. *Int. J. Radiat. Oncol. Biol. Phys.* 1990;18:651–658.
3. Sherouse, GW, Chaney, EL. The portable virtual simulator. *Int. J. Radiat. Oncol. Biol. Phys.* 1991;21:475–482.
4. Thomas, SJ. Relative electron density calibration of CT scanners for radiotherapy treatment planning. *Br. J. Radiol.* 1999;72:781–786.
5. Shirato, H, Shimizu, S, Kitamura, K, et al. Four-dimensional treatment planning and fluoroscopic real-time tumor tracking radiotherapy for moving tumor. *Int. J. Radiat. Oncol. Biol. Phys.* 2000;48:435–442.
6. Vedam, SS, Keall, PJ, Kini, VR, Mostafavi, H, Shukla, HP, Mohan, R. Acquiring a four-dimensional computed tomography dataset using an external respiratory signal. *Phys. Med. Biol.* 2003;48:45–62.
7. Keall, P. 4-dimensional computed tomography imaging and treatment planning. *Semin. Radiat. Oncol.* 2004;14:81–90.
8. Mageras, GS, Pevsner, A, Yorke, ED, et al. Measurement of lung tumor motion using respiration-correlated CT. *Int. J. Radiat. Oncol. Biol. Phys.* 2004;60:933–941.
9. Khoo, VS, Dearnaley, DP, Finnigan, DJ, Padhani, A, Tanner, SF, Leach, MO. Magnetic resonance imaging (MRI): considerations and applications in radiotherapy treatment planning. *Radiother. Oncol.* 1997;42:1–15.
10. Ling, CC, Humm, J, Larson, S, et al. Towards multidimensional radiotherapy (MD-CRT): biological imaging and biological conformality. *Int. J. Radiat. Oncol. Biol. Phys.* 2000;47:551–560.
11. Schad, LR. Improved target volume characterization in stereotactic treatment planning of brain lesions by using high-resolution BOLD MR-venography. *MMR Biomed.* 2001;14:478–483.
12. Krempien, RC, Daeuber, S, Hensley, FW, Wannenmacher, M, Harms, W. Image fusion of CT and MRI data enables improved target volume definition in 3D-brachytherapy treatment planning. *Brachytherapy* 2003;2:164–171.
13. Krempien, RC, Schubert, K, Zierhut, D, et al. Open low-field magnetic resonance imaging in radiation therapy treatment planning. *Int. J. Radiat. Oncol. Biol. Phys.* 2002;53:1350–1360.
14. Parker, CC, Damyanovich, A, Haycocks, T, Haider, M, Bayley, A, Catton, CN. Magnetic resonance imaging in the radiation treatment planning of localized prostate cancer using intra-prostatic fiducial markers for computed tomography co-registration. *Radiother. Oncol.* 2003;66:217–224.
15. Yap, JT, Carney, JP, Hall, NC, Townsend, DW. Image-guided cancer therapy using PET/CT. *Cancer J.* 2004;10:221–233.
16. Black, QC, Grills, IS, Kestin, LL, et al. Defining a radiotherapy target with positron emission tomography. *Int. J. Radiat. Oncol. Biol. Phys.* 2004;60:1272–1282.
17. Ghilezan, MJ, Jaffray, DA, Siewerdsen, JH, et al. Prostate gland motion assessed with cine-magnetic resonance imaging (cine-MRI). *Int. J. Radiat. Oncol. Biol. Phys.* 2005;62:406–417.
18. Mageras, GS. Introduction: management of target localization uncertainties in external-beam therapy. *Semin. Radiat. Oncol.* 2005;15:133–135.
19. Kessler, ML. Image registration and data fusion in radiation therapy. *Br. J. Radiol.* 2006;79 (Spec No 1):S99–S108.
20. Dawson, LA, Sharpe, MB. Image-guided radiotherapy: rationale, benefits, and limitations. *Lancet Oncol.* 2006;7:848–858.
21. Brock, KK. Image registration in intensity-modulated radiation therapy, image-guided radiation therapy and stereotactic body radiation therapy. Basel, Switzerland: Karger. 2007.
22. Modersitzki, J. *Numerical methods for image registration.* Oxford: Oxford University Press. 2004.
23. Leondes, CT. *Biomechanical systems technology.* Singapore: World Scientific. 2007.
24. Welsh, JS, Bradley, K, Manon, R, et al. Megavoltage CT imaging for adaptive helical tomotherapy of lung cancer. *Int. J. Radiat. Oncol. Biol. Phys.* 2003;57:S429.
25. Letourneau, D, Wong, JW, Oldham, M, et al. Cone-beam-CT guided radiation therapy: technical implementation. *Radiother. Oncol.* 2005;75:279–286.
26. Letourneau, D, Martinez, AA, Lockman, D, et al. Assessment of residual error for online cone-beam CT-guided treatment of prostate cancer patients. *Int. J. Radiat. Oncol. Biol. Phys.* 2005;62:1239–1246.
27. Sonke, JJ, Zijp, L, Remeijer, P, Van Herk, M. Respiratory correlated cone beam CT. *Med. Phys.* 2005;32:1176–1186.
28. Wong, JW, Sharpe, MB, Jaffray, DA, et al. The use of active breathing control (ABC) to reduce margin for breathing motion. *Int. J. Radiat. Oncol. Biol. Phys.* 1999;44:911–919.

29. Dawson, LA, Eccles, C, Bissonnette, JP, Brock, KK. Accuracy of daily image guidance for hypofractionated liver radiotherapy with active breathing control. *Int. J. Radiat. Oncol. Biol. Phys.* 2005;62:1247–1252.

30. Eccles, C, Brock, KK, Bissonnette, JP, Hawkins, M, Dawson, LA. Reproducibility of liver position using active breathing coordinator for liver cancer radiotherapy. *Int. J. Radiat. Oncol. Biol. Phys.* 2006;64:751–759.

31. Dawson, LA, Brock, KK, Kazanjian, S, et al. The reproducibility of organ position using active breathing control (ABC) during liver radiotherapy. *Int. J. Radiat. Oncol. Biol. Phys.* 2001;51:1410–1421.

32. Stromberg, JS, Sharpe, MB, Kim, LH, et al. Active breathing control (ABC) for Hodgkin's disease: reduction in normal tissue irradiation with deep inspiration and implications for treatment. Int. *J. Radiat. Oncol. Biol. Phys.* 2000;48:797–806.

33. Dehnad, H, Nederveen, AJ, van der Heide, UA, van Moorselaar, RJ, Hofman, P, Lagendijk, JJ. Clinical feasibility study for the use of implanted gold seeds in the prostate as reliable positioning markers during megavoltage irradiation. *Radiother. Oncol.* 2003;67:295–302.

34. Balter, JM, Sandler, HM, Lam, K, Bree, RL, Lichter, AS, Ten Haken, RK. Measurement of prostate movement over the course of routine radiotherapy using implanted markers. *Int. J. Radiat. Oncol. Biol. Phys.* 1995;31:113–118.

35. Balter, JM, Lam, KL, Sandler, HM, Littles, JF, Bree, RL, Ten Haken, RK. Automated localization of the prostate at the time of treatment using implanted radiopaque markers: technical feasibility. *Int. J. Radiat. Oncol. Biol. Phys.* 1995;33:1281–1286.

36. Litzenberg, D, Dawson, LA, Sandler, H, et al. Daily prostate targeting using implanted radiopaque markers. *Int. J. Radiat. Oncol. Biol. Phys.* 2002;52:699–703.

37. Nichol, AM, Brock, KK, Lockwood, GA, et al. A magnetic resonance imaging study of prostate deformation relative to implanted gold fiducial markers. *Int. J. Radiat. Oncol. Biol. Phys.* 2007;67:48–56.

38. Haddad, FS, Somsin, AA. Seeding and perineal implantation of prostatic cancer in the track of the biopsy needle: three case reports and a review of the literature. *J. Surg. Oncol.* 1987;35:184–191.

39. Rodgers, MS, Collinson, R, Desai, S, Stubbs, RS, McCall, JL. Risk of dissemination with biopsy of colorectal liver metastases. *Dis. Colon Rectum.* 2003;46:454–458.

40. Clayman, G, Cohen, JI, Adams, GL. Neoplastic seeding of squamous cell carcinoma of the oropharynx. *Head Neck.* 1993;15:245–248.

41. Kessler, ML, Pitluck, S, Petti, P, Castro, JR. Integration of multimodality imaging data for radiotherapy treatment planning. *Int. J. Radiat. Oncol. Biol. Phys.* 1991;21:1653–1667.

42. Balter, JM, Pelizzari, CA, Chen, GT. Correlation of projection radiographs in radiation therapy using open curve segments and points. *Med. Phys.* 1992;19:329–334.

43. Van Herk, M, Kooy, HM. Automatic three-dimensional correlation of CT-CT, CT-MRI, and CT- SPECT using chamfer matching. *Med. Phys.* 1994;21:1163–1178.

44. Kooy, HM, Van Herk, M, Barnes, PD, et al. Image fusion for stereotactic radiotherapy and radiosurgery treatment planning. *Int. J. Radiat. Oncol. Biol. Phys.* 1994;28:1229–1234.

45. Gilhuijs, KG, Touw, A, Vanherk, M, et al. Optimization of automatic portal image analysis. *Med. Phys.* 1995;22:1089–1099.

46. Gilhuijs, KG, van de Ven, PJ, Van Herk, M. Automatic three-dimensional inspection of patient setup in radiation therapy using portal images, simulator images, and computed tomography data. *Med. Phys.* 1996;23:389–399.

47. Gilhuijs, KG, Drukker, K, Touw, A, van de Ven, PJ, Van Herk, M. Interactive three dimensional inspection of patient setup in radiation therapy using digital portal images and computed tomography data. *Int. J. Radiat. Oncol. Biol. Phys.* 1996;34:873–885.

48. Ploeger, LS, Betgen, A, Gilhuijs, KG, Van Herk, M. Feasibility of geometrical verification of patient set-up using body contours and computed tomography data. *Radiother. Oncol.* 2003;66:225–233.

49. Moseley, DJ, White, EA, Wiltshire, KL, et al. Comparison of localization performance with implanted fiducial markers and cone-beam computed tomography for on-line image-guided radiotherapy of the prostate. *Int. J. Radiat. Oncol. Biol. Phys.* 2007; 67:942–953.

50. Pekar, V, McNutt, TR, Kaus, MR. Automated model-based organ delineation for radiotherapy planning in prostatic region. *Int. J. Radiat. Oncol. Biol. Phys.* 2004;60:973–980.

51. Chaney, EL, Pizer, SM. Defining Anatomical Structures from Medical Images. *Semin. Radiat. Oncol.* 1992;2:215–225.

52. Pizer, SM, Fritsch, DS, Yushkevich, PA, Johnson, VE, Chaney, EL. Segmentation, registration, and measurement of shape variation via image object shape. *Trans. Med. Imaging* 1999; 18:851–865.

53. Pizer, SM, Fletcher, PT, Joshi, S, et al. A method and software for segmentation of anatomic object ensembles by deformable m-reps. *Med. Phys.* 2005;32:1335–1345.

54. Van Herk, M, Gilhuijs, KG, de Munck, J, Touw, A. Effect of image artifacts, organ motion, and poor segmentation on the reliability and accuracy of three-dimensional chamfer matching. *Comput. Aided Surg.* 1997;2:346–355.

55. Cai, J, Chu, JC, Recine, D, et al. CT and PET lung image registration and fusion in radiotherapy treatment planning using the chamfer-matching method. *Int. J. Radiat. Oncol. Biol. Phys.* 1999;43:883–891.

56. Kirilova, A, Lockwood, G, Choi, P, et al. Three-dimensional motion of liver tumors using cine-magnetic resonance imaging. *Int. J. Radiat. Oncol. Biol. Phys.* 2008;71:1189–1195.

57. Hawkins, MA, Brock, KK, Eccles, C, Moseley, D, Jaffray, D, Dawson, LA. Assessment of residual error in liver position using kV cone-beam computed tomography for liver cancer high-precision radiation therapy. *Int. J. Radiat. Oncol. Biol. Phys.* 2006;66:610–619.

58. Brock, KK, Hawkins, M, Eccles, C, et al. Improving image-guided target localization through deformable registration. *Acta. Oncol.* 2008;47:1279–1285.

59. Smitsmans, MH, Wolthaus, JW, Artignan, X, et al. Automatic localization of the prostate for on-line or off-line image-guided radiotherapy. *Int. J. Radiat. Oncol. Biol. Phys.* 2004;60:623–635.

60. Schaly, B, Bauman, GS, Song, W, Battista, JJ, Van Dyk, J. Dosimetric impact of image-guided 3D conformal radiation therapy of prostate cancer. *Phys. Med. Biol.* 2005;50:3083–3101.

61. Keall, PJ, Joshi, S, Vedam, SS, Siebers, JV, Kini, VR, Mohan, R. Four-dimensional radiotherapy planning for DMLC-based respiratory motion tracking. *Med. Phys.* 2005;32:942–951.

62. Rietzel, E, Chen, GT, Choi, NC, Willet, CG. Four-dimensional image-based treatment planning: Target volume segmentation and dose calculation in the presence of respiratory motion. *Int. J. Radiat. Oncol. Biol. Phys.* 2005;61:1535–1550.

63. Moseley, J, Munro, P. A semiautomatic method for registration of portal images. *Med. Phys.* 1994;21:551–558.

64. Dong, L, Boyer, AL. An image correlation procedure for digitally reconstructed radiographs and electronic portal images. *Int. J. Radiat. Oncol. Biol. Phys.* 1995;33:1053–1060.

65. Dong, L, Boyer, AL. A portal image alignment and patient setup verification procedure using moments and correlation techniques. *Phys. Med. Biol.* 1996;41:697–723.

66. McParland, BJ, Kumaradas, JC, Portal, I, et al. Digital portal image registration by sequential anatomical matchpoint and image correlations for real-time continuous field alignment verification. *Med. Phys.* 1995;22:1063–1075.

67. Fitchard, EE, Aldridge, JS, Reckwerdt, PJ, Mackie, TR. Registration of synthetic tomographic projection data sets using cross-correlation. *Phys. Med. Biol.* 1998;43:1645–1657.

68. Wang, H, Dong, L, Lii, MF, et al. Implementation and validation of a three-dimensional deformable registration algorithm for targeted prostate cancer radiotherapy. *Int. J. Radiat. Oncol. Biol. Phys.* 2005;61:725–735.

69. Schad, LR, Boesecke, R, Schlegel, W, et al. Three dimensional image correlation of CT, MR, and PET studies in radiotherapy treatment planning of brain tumors. *J. Comput. Assist. Tomogr.* 1987;11:948–954.

70. Maes, F, Collignon, A, Vandermeulen, D, Marchal, G, Suetens, P. Multimodality image registration by maximization of mutual information. *IEEE Trans. Med. Imaging* 1997;16:187–198.

71. Wells, WM, III, Viola, P, Atsumi, H, Nakajima, S, Kikinis, R. Multi-modal volume registration by maximization of mutual information. *Med. Image Anal.* 1996;1:35–51.

72. Meyer, CR, Boes, JL, Kim, B, et al. Demonstration of accuracy and clinical versatility of mutual information for automatic multimodality image fusion using affine and thin-plate spline warped geometric deformations. *Med. Image Anal.* 1997;1:195–206.

73. Maes, F, Vandermeulen, D, Suetens, P. Comparative evaluation of multiresolution optimization strategies for multimodality image registration by maximization of mutual information. *Med. Image Anal.* 1999;3:373–386.

74. Plattard, D, Soret, M, Troccaz, J, et al. Patient set-up using portal images: 2D/2D image registration using mutual information. *Comput. Aided Surg.* 2000;5:246–262.

75. Kim, J, Fessler, JA, Lam, KL, Balter, JM, Ten Haken, RK. A feasibility study of mutual information based setup error estimation for radiotherapy. *Med. Phys.* 2001;28:2507–2517.

76. Chen, HM, Varshney, PK. Mutual information-based CT-MR brain image registration using generalized partial volume joint histogram estimation. *IEEE Trans. Med. Imaging* 2003;22:1111–1119.

77. D'Agostino, E, Maes, F, Vandermeulen, D, Suetens, P. A viscous fluid model for multimodal non-rigid image registration using mutual information. *Med. Image Anal.* 2003;7:565–575.

78. Brock, KK. Results of a Multi-Institution Deformable Registration Accuracy Study (MIDRAS). *Int. J. Radiat. Oncol. Biol. Phys.* 76:583–596.

79. Keall, PJ, Starkschall, G, Shukla, H, et al. Acquiring 4D thoracic CT scans using a multislice helical method. *Phys. Med. Biol.* 2004;49:2053–2067.

80. Keall, P. 4-dimensional computed tomography imaging and treatment planning. *Semin. Radiat. Oncol.* 2004;14:81–90.

81. Keall, PJ, Siebers, JV, Joshi, S, Mohan, R. Monte Carlo as a four-dimensional radiotherapy treatment-planning tool to account for respiratory motion. *Phys. Med. Biol.* 2004;49:3639–3648.

82. Christensen, GE, Carlson, B, Chao, KS, et al. Image-based dose planning of intracavitary brachytherapy: registration of serial-imaging studies using deformable anatomic templates. *Int. J. Radiat. Oncol. Biol. Phys.* 2001;51:227–243.

83. Christensen, GE, Joshi, SC, Miller, MI. Volumetric transformation of brain anatomy. *IEEE Trans. Med. Imaging* 1997;16:864–877.

84. Haller, JW, Banerjee, A, Christensen, GE, et al. Three-dimensional hippocampal MR morphometry with high-dimensional transformation of a neuroanatomic atlas. *Radiology* 1997;202:504–510.

85. Thirion, JP. Image matching as a diffusion process: an analogy with Maxwell's demons. *Med. Image Anal.* 1998;2:243–260.

86. Wang, H, Dong, L, O'Daniel, J, et al. Validation of an accelerated 'demons' algorithm for deformable image registration in radiation therapy. *Phys. Med. Biol.* 2005;50:2887–2905.

87. Brock, KK, McShan, DL, Ten Haken, RK, Hollister, SJ, Dawson, LA, Balter, JM. Inclusion of organ deformation in dose calculations. *Med. Phys.* 2003;30:290–295.

88. Brock, KM, Balter, JM, Dawson, LA, Kessler, ML, Meyer, CR. Automated generation of a four-dimensional model of the liver using warping and mutual information. *Med. Phys.* 2003;30:1128–1133.

89. Park, H, Bland, PH, Brock, KK, Meyer, CR. Adaptive registration using local information measures. *Med. Image Anal.* 2004;8:465–473.

90. Rohlfing, T, Maurer, CR, Jr., O'Dell, WG, Zhong, J. Modeling liver motion and deformation during the respiratory cycle using intensity-based nonrigid registration of gated MR images. *Med. Phys.* 2004;31:427–432.

91. Rosu, M, Chetty, IJ, Balter, JM, Kessler, ML, McShan, DL, Ten Haken, RK. Dose reconstruction in deforming lung anatomy: dose grid size effects and clinical implications. *Med. Phys.* 2005;32:2487–2495.

92. Coselmon, MM, Balter, JM, McShan, DL, Kessler, ML. Mutual information based CT registration of the lung at exhale and inhale breathing states using thin-plate splines. *Med. Phys.* 2004;31:2942–2948.

93. Paganetti, H, Jiang, H, Adams, JA, Chen, GT, Rietzel, E. Monte Carlo simulations with time-dependent geometries to investigate effects of organ motion with high temporal resolution. *Int. J. Radiat. Oncol. Biol. Phys.* 2004;60:942–950.

94. Schaly, B, Bauman, GS, Battista, JJ, Van Dyk, J. Validation of contour-driven thin-plate splines for tracking fraction-to-fraction changes in anatomy and radiation therapy dose mapping. *Phys. Med. Biol.* 2005;50:459–475.

95. Venugopal, N, McCurdy, B, Hnatov, A, Dubey, A. A feasibility study to investigate the use of thin-plate splines to account for prostate deformation. *Phys. Med. Biol.* 2005;50:2871–2885.

96. Schaly, B, Kempe, JA, Bauman, GS, Battista, JJ, Van Dyk, J. Tracking the dose distribution in radiation therapy by accounting for variable anatomy. *Phys. Med. Biol.* 2004;49:791–805.

97. Brock, KK, Sharpe, MB, Dawson, LA, Kim, SM, Jaffray, DA. Accuracy of finite element model-based multi-organ deformable image registration. *Med. Phys.* 2005;32:1647–1659.

98. Schnabel, JA, Tanner, C, Castellano-Smith, AD, et al. Validation of nonrigid image registration using finite-element methods: application to breast MR images. *IEEE Trans. Med. Imaging* 2003;22:238–247.

99. Zhang, T, Orton, NP, Mackie, TR, Paliwal, BR. Technical note: A novel boundary condition using contact elements for finite element based deformable image registration. Med. Phys. 2004;31:2412–2415.

100. Brock, KK, Dawson, LA, Sharpe, MB, Moseley, DJ, Jaffray, DA. Feasibility of a novel deformable image registration technique to facilitate classification, targeting, and monitoring of tumor and normal tissue. *Int. J. Radiat. Oncol. Biol. Phys.* 2006;64:1245–1254.

101. Brock, KK, Hollister, SJ, Dawson, LA, Balter, JM. Technical note: creating a four-dimensional model of the liver using finite element analysis. *Med. Phys.* 2002;29:1403–1405.

102. Liang, J, Yan, D. Reducing uncertainties in volumetric image based deformable organ registration. *Med. Phys.* 2003;30:2116–2122.

103. Yan, D, Jaffray, DA, Wong, JW. A model to accumulate fractionated dose in a deforming organ. *Int. J. Radiat. Oncol. Biol. Phys.* 1999;44:665–675.

104. Bharatha, A, Hirose, M, Hata, N, et al. Evaluation of three-dimensional finite element-based deformable registration of pre- and intraoperative prostate imaging. *Med. Phys.* 2001;28:2551–2560.

105. ICRU. *Prescribing, recording, and reporting photon beam therapy.* Washington, DC: International Commission on Radiation Units and Measurements. 1993.

106. Van Herk, M, Meertens, H. A matrix ionisation chamber imaging device for on-line patient setup verification during radiotherapy. *Radiother. Oncol.* 1988;11:369–378.

107. Munro, P, Rawlinson, JA, Fenster, A. A digital fluoroscopic imaging device for radiotherapy localization. *Int. J. Radiat. Oncol. Biol. Phys.* 1990;18:641–649.

108. Michalski, JM, Graham, MV, Bosch, WR, et al. Prospective clinical evaluation of an electronic portal imaging device. *Int. J. Radiat. Oncol. Biol. Phys.* 1996;34:943–951.

109. Mohan, DS, Kupelian, PA, Willoughby, TR. Short-course intensity-modulated radiotherapy for localized prostate cancer with daily transabdominal ultrasound localization of the prostate gland. *Int. J. Radiat. Oncol. Biol. Phys* 2000;46:575–580.

110. Huang, E, Dong, L, Chandra, A, et al. Intrafraction prostate motion during IMRT for prostate cancer. *Int. J. Radiat. Oncol. Biol. Phys.* 2002;53:261–268.

111. Morr, J, Dipetrillo, T, Tsai, JS, Engler, M, Wazer, DE. Implementation and utility of a daily ultrasound-based localization system with intensity-modulated radiotherapy for prostate cancer. *Int. J. Radiat. Oncol. Biol. Phys.* 2002;53:1124–1129.

112. Serago, CF, Chungbin, SJ, Buskirk, SJ, Ezzell, GA, Collie, AC, Vora, SA. Initial experience with ultrasound localization for positioning prostate cancer patients for external beam radiotherapy. *Int. J. Radiat. Oncol. Biol. Phys.* 2002;53:1130–1138.

113. Langen, KM, Pouliot, J, Anezinos, C, et al. Evaluation of ultrasound-based prostate localization for image-guided radiotherapy. *Int. J. Radiat. Oncol. Biol. Phys.* 2003;57:635–644.

114. Artignan, X, Smitsmans, MH, Lebesque, JV, Jaffray, DA, van Her, M, Bartelink, H. Online ultrasound image guidance for radiotherapy of prostate cancer: impact of image acquisition on prostate displacement. *Int. J. Radiat. Oncol. Biol. Phys.* 2004;59:595–601.

115. Cheng, CW, Wong, J, Grimm, L, Chow, M, Uematsu, M, Fung, A. Commissioning and clinical implementation of a sliding gantry CT scanner installed in an existing treatment room and early clinical experience for precise tumor localization. *Am. J. Clin. Oncol.* 2003;26:e28–e36.

116. Paskalev, K, Ma, C, Jacob, R, Price, R. Clinical evaluation of a CT gantry on rails as a daily target localization tool. *Int. J. Radiat. Oncol. Biol. Phys.* 2003;57:S266.

117. Shiu, AS, Chang, EL, Ye, JS, et al. Near simultaneous computed tomography image-guided stereotactic spinal radiotherapy: an emerging paradigm for achieving true stereotaxy. *Int. J. Radiat. Oncol. Biol. Phys.* 2003; 57:605–613.

118. Wong, JR, Grimm, L, Uematsu, M, et al. Image-guided radiotherapy for prostate cancer by CT-linear accelerator combination: prostate movements and dosimetric considerations. *Int. J. Radiat. Oncol. Biol. Phys.* 2005;61:561–569.

119. Mackie, TR, Holmes, T, Swerdloff, S, et al. Tomotherapy: a new concept for the delivery of dynamic conformal radiotherapy. *Med. Phys.* 1993;20:1709–1719.

120. Welsh, JS, Bradley, K, Ruchala, KJ, et al. Megavoltage computed tomography imaging: a potential tool to guide and improve the delivery of thoracic radiation therapy. *Clin. Lung Cancer.* 2004;5:303–306.

121. Jaffray, DA, Siewerdsen, JH, Wong, JW, Martinez, AA. Flat-panel cone-beam computed tomography for image-guided radiation therapy. *Int. J. Radiat. Oncol. Biol. Phys.* 2002;53:1337–1349.

122. Ford, EC, Chang, J, Mueller, K, et al. Cone-beam CT with megavoltage beams and an amorphous silicon electronic portal imaging device: potential for verification of radiotherapy of lung cancer. *Med. Phys.* 2002;29:2913–2924.

123. Pouliot, J, Bani-Hashemi, A, Chen, J, et al. Low-dose megavoltage cone-beam CT for radiation therapy. *Int. J. Radiat. Oncol. Biol. Phys.* 2005;61:552–560.

124. Bel, A, Van Herk, M, Bartelink, H, Lebesque, JV. A verification procedure to improve patient set-up accuracy using portal images. *Radiother. Oncol.* 1993;29:253–260.

125. Van Herk, M. Errors and margins in radiotherapy. *Semin. Radiat. Oncol.* 2004;14:52–64.

126. Birkner, M, Yan, D, Alber, M, Liang, J, Nusslin, F. Adapting inverse planning to patient and organ geometrical variation: algorithm and implementation. *Med. Phys.* 2003;30:2822–2831.

127. Yan, D, Lockman, D, Brabbins, D, Tyburski, L, Martinez, A. An off-line strategy for constructing a patient-specific planning target volume in adaptive treatment process for prostate cancer. *Int. J. Radiat. Oncol. Biol. Phys.* 2000; 48:289–302.

128. Yan, D, Vicini, FA, Wong, JW, Martinez, AA. Adaptive radiation therapy. *Phys. Med. Biol.* 1997;42:123–132.

129. Kluetz, PG, Meltzer, CC, Villemagne, VL, et al. Combined PET/CT Imaging in Oncology. Impact on Patient Management. *Clin. Positron Imaging.* 2000;3:223–230.

130. Townsend, DW, Cherry, SR. Combining anatomy and function: the path to true image fusion. *Eur. Radiol.* 2001;11:1968–1974.

131. Beyer, T, Townsend, DW, Blodgett, TM. Dual-modality PET/CT tomography for clinical oncology. *Quat. J. Nucl. Med.* 2002;46:24–34.

132. Gilhuijs, KG, el Gayed, AA, Van Herk, M, Vijlbrief, RE. An algorithm for automatic analysis of portal images: clinical evaluation for prostate treatments. *Radiother. Oncol.* 1993;29:261–268.

133. Van Herk, M, Bel, A, Gilhuijs, KG, Vijlbrief, RE. A comprehensive system for the analysis of portal images. *Radiat. Oncol.* 1993;29:221–229.

134. Purdie, TG, Bissonnette, JP, Franks, K, et al. Cone-beam computed tomography for on-line image guidance of lung stereotactic radiotherapy: localization, verification, and intrafraction tumor position. *Int. J. Radiat. Oncol. Biol. Phys.* 2007;68:243–252.

135. Sharpe, MB, Moseley, DJ, Purdie, TG, Islam, M, Siewerdsen, JH, Jaffray, DA. The stability of mechanical calibration for a kV cone beam computed tomography system integrated with linear accelerator. *Med. Phys.* 2006;33:136–144.

136. Jaffray, DA. Emergent technologies for 3-dimensional image-guided radiation delivery. *Semin. Radiat. Oncol.* 2005;15:208–216.

137. Yan, D, Lockman, D, Martinez, A, et al. Computed tomography guided management of interfractional patient variation. *Semin. Radiat. Oncol.* 2005;15:168–179.

138. Lujan, AE, Ten Haken, RK, Larsen, EW, Balter, JM. Quantization of setup uncertainties in 3-D dose calculations. *Med. Phys.* 1999;26:2397–2402.

139. Craig, T, Battista, J, Moiseenko, V, Van Dyk, J. Considerations for the implementation of target volume protocols in radiation therapy. *Int. J. Radiat. Oncol. Biol. Phys.* 2001;49:241–250.

140. Schaly, B, Kempe, JA, Bauman, GS, Battista, JJ, Van Dyk, J. Tracking the dose distribution in radiation therapy by accounting for variable anatomy. *Phys. Med. Biol.* 2004;49:791–805.

141. Mohan, R, Zhang, X, Wang, H, et al. Use of deformed intensity distributions for on-line modification of image-guided IMRT to account for interfractional anatomic changes. *Int. J. Radiat. Oncol. Biol. Phys.* 2005; 61:1258–1266.

142. Kashani, R, Hub, M, Kessler, ML, Balter, JM. Technical note: a physical phantom for assessment of accuracy of deformable alignment algorithms *Med. Phys.* 2007;34:2785–2788.

143. Fraass, B, Doppke, K, Hunt, M, et al. American Association of Physicists in Medicine Radiation Therapy Committee Task Group 53: quality assurance for clinical radiotherapy treatment planning. *Med. Phys.* 1998;25:1773–1829.

144. Mutic, S, Dempsey, JF, Bosch, WR, et al. Multimodality image registration quality assurance for conformal three-dimensional treatment planning. *Int. J. Radiat. Oncol. Biol. Phys.* 2001;51:255–260.

145. Yu, C, Apuzzo, ML, Zee, CS, Petrovich, Z. A phantom study of the geometric accuracy of computed tomographic and magnetic resonance imaging stereotactic localization with the Leksell stereotactic system. *Neurosurgery* 2001;48:1092–1098.

146. Moore, CS, Liney, GP, Beavis, AW. Quality assurance of registration of CT and MRI data sets for treatment planning of radiotherapy for head and neck cancers. *J. Appl. Clin. Med. Phys.* 2004; 5:25–35.

147. Lavely, WC, Scarfone, C, Cevikalp, H, et al. Phantom validation of coregistration of PET and CT for image-guided radiotherapy. *Med. Phys.* 2004;31:1083–1092.

148. *Commissioning and quality assurance of computerized planning systems for radiation treatment of cancer*. Vienna: International Atomic Energy Agency. 2004.

149. Rucklidge, W. *Efficient visual recognition using the Hausdorff distance*. Berlin ; New York: Springer. 1996.

150. Jannin, P, Grova, C, Maurer, C. Model for defining and reporting reference-based validation protocols in medical image processing. *Int. J. Comp. Assisted Radiol. Surg.* 2006;1:63–73.

151. Crum, WR, Camara, O, Hill, DL. Generalized overlap measures for evaluation and validation in medical image analysis. *IEEE Trans. Med. Imaging* 2006;25:1451–1461.

152. Hosten, N, Wust, P, Beier, J, Lemke, AJ, Felix, R. MRI-assisted specification/localization of target volumes. Aspects of quality control. *Strahlenther Onkol* 1998;174 (Suppl 2):13–18.

153. Castillo, R, Castillo, E, Guerra, R, et al. A framework for evaluation of deformable image registration spatial accuracy using large landmark point sets. *Phys. Med. Biol.* 2009;54:1849–1870.

154. Zeng, GG, McGowan, TS, Larsen, TM, et al. Calcifications are potential surrogates for prostate localization in image-guided radiotherapy. *Int. J. Radiat. Oncol. Biol. Phys.* 2008;72:963–966.

155. Herman, MG, Balter, JM, Jaffray, DA, et al. Clinical use of electronic portal imaging: report of AAPM Radiation Therapy Committee Task Group 58. *Med. Phys.* 2001;28:712–737.

156. Sailer, SL, Rosenman, JG, Soltys, M, Cullip, TJ, Chen, J. Improving treatment planning accuracy through multimodality imaging. *Int. J. Radiat. Oncol. Biol. Phys.* 1996;35:117–124.

157. Ford, EC, Mageras, GS, Yorke, E, Ling, CC. Respiration-correlated spiral CT: a method of measuring respiratory-induced anatomic motion for radiation treatment planning. *Med. Phys.* 2003;30:88–97.

158. Rietzel, E, Rosenthal, SJ, Gierga, DP, Willet, CG, Chen, GT. Moving targets: detection and tracking of internal organ motion for treatment planning and patient set-up. *Radiother. Oncol.* 2004;73 (Suppl 2):S68–S72.

159. Sonke, JJ, Brand, B, Van Herk, M. Focal spot motion of linear accelerators and its effect on portal image analysis. *Med. Phys.* 2003;30:1067–1075.

160. Erdi, YE, Nehmeh, SA, Pan, T, et al. The CT motion quantitation of lung lesions and its impact on PET-measured SUVs. *J. Nucl. Med.* 2004;45:1287–1292.

161. Pevsner, A, Davis, B, Joshi, S, et al. Evaluation of an automated deformable image matching method for quantifying lung motion in respiration-correlated CT images. *Med. Phys.* 2006;33:369–376.

162. Jaffray, DA, Drake, DG, Moreau, M, Martinez, AA, Wong, JW. A radiographic and tomographic imaging system integrated into a medical linear accelerator for localization of bone and soft-tissue targets. *Int. J. Radiat. Oncol. Biol. Phys.* 1999;45:773–789.

163. Letourneau, D, Watt, L, Gulam, M, Oldham, M, Wong, J. Implementation of an on-board kilovoltage cone-beam CT imaging system for clinical applications. *Int. J. Radiat. Oncol. Biol. Phys.* 2003;57:S185.

164. Park, JO, Lee, SI, Song, SY, et al. Measuring response in solid tumors: comparison of RECIST and WHO response criteria. *Jpn. J. Clin. Oncol.* 2003;33:533–537.

165. McHugh, K, Kao, S. Response evaluation criteria in solid tumours (RECIST): problems and need for modifications in paediatric oncology? *Br. J. Radiol.* 2003;76:433–436.

166. Prasad, SR, Saini, S, Sumner, JE, Hahn, PF, Sahani, D, Boland, GW. Radiological measurement of breast cancer metastases to lung and liver: comparison between WHO (bidimensional) and RECIST (unidimensional) guidelines. *J. Comput. Assist. Tomogr.* 2003;27:380–384.

167. Kimura, M, Tominaga, T. Outstanding problems with response evaluation criteria in solid tumors (RECIST) in breast cancer. *Breast Cancer* 2002;9:153–159.

168. Kutcher, GJ, Coia, L, Gillin, M, et al. Comprehensive QA for radiation oncology: report of AAPM Radiation Therapy Committee Task Group 40. *Med. Phys.* 1994; 21:581–618.

169. Sharpe, M, Brock, KK. Quality assurance of serial 3D image registration, fusion, and segmentation. *Int. J. Radiat. Oncol. Biol. Phys.* 2008;71:S33–S37.

Index